SPECIAL PROBLEMS IN HEMODIALYSIS PATIENTS

Edited by **Maria Goretti Penido**

Special Problems in Hemodialysis Patients
Edited by Maria Goretti Penido

Published by InTech
Janeza Trdine 9, 51000 Rijeka, Croatia

Publishing Process Manager Masa Vidovic

Technical Editor Teodora Smiljanic

Cover Designer InTech Design Team

Additional hard copies can be obtained from orders@intechopen.com

Special Problems in Hemodialysis Patients, Edited by Maria Goretti Penido
p. cm.
ISBN 978-953-307-396-5

For EU product safety concerns:
IN TECH d.o.o., Prolaz Marije Krucifikse Kozulić 3, 51000 Rijeka, Croatia,
info@intechopen.com or visit our website at intechopen.com.

Meet the editor

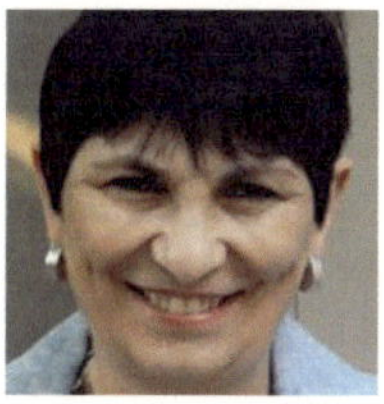

Dr. Maria Goretti Moreira Guimarães Penido, MD, PhD is Associate Professor of Pediatrics and Pediatric Nephrology at the Federal University of Minas Gerais, School of Medicine, Department of Pediatrics and Pediatric Nephrology Unit. She graduated medicine in 1980 at the Federal University of Minas Gerais, and obtained her Master Degree in Pediatric Nephrology in 1995 at the same institution, as well as a PhD in Pediatric Nephrology in 2000. She was a Postdoctoral Fellow in the Bone and Mineral Disorders Clinic and Research Laboratory, Section of Pediatric Nephrology, The Children's Mercy Hospitals and Clinics, University of Missouri, Kansas City School of Medicine, US. She is member of the Unity of Pediatric Nephrology, Clinics Hospital, School of Medicine, Federal University of Minas Gerais, Belo Horizonte, Brazil.

Contents

Preface

This book provides an overview of special cases in hemodialysis patients. Authors have contributed their most interesting findings in dealing with patients suffering of other diseases simultaneously, such as diabetes, cardiovascular disease and other health problems.

Each chapter has been thoroughly revised and updated so the readers are acquainted with the latest data and observations in these complex cases, where several aspects are to be considered. The book is comprehensive and not limited to a partial discussion of hemodialysis. To accomplish this we are pleased to have been able to summarize state of the art knowledge in each chapter of the book.

This book provides practical and accessible information. It is quite comprehensive as it covers various special circumstances in hemodialysis patients and their treatment. We wish to thank each author for taking considerable time and effort to ensure their chapter provides state of the art information. We hope that readers achieve the same level of acquisition of new knowledge as we have attained by editing this book.

Dr. Maria Goretti Penido
Department of Pediatrics
School of Medicine
Federal University of Minas Gerais
Minas Gerais
Brasil

1

Gastroesophageal Reflux Disease in Chronic Renal Failure Patients

Yoshiaki Kawaguchi and Tetsuya Mine
Tokai University School of Medicine
Japan

1. Introduction

Gastroesophageal reflux disease (GERD) is one of acid-related gastrointestinal disorders, because GERD develops when excessively acidic gastric contents reflux into the esophagus. The condition is believed mainly to be due to an increase in the number of transient LES relaxations. Other major mechanisms include decreased clearance of esophageal contents and reflux owing to impaired peristalsis, decreased gastric emptying with resultant reflux into the esophagus, and increased gastric acid production with a resultant increase in the potency of the reflux. Chronic renal failure (CRF) is associated with an increased incidence of acid-related gastrointestinal disorders (1-3). Therefore we can predict high morbidity of GERD in CRF patients, but the association between GERD and CRF remains unclear.

In our study (4) by questionnaire for the diagnosis of reflux disease (QUEST) produced by Carlsson et al. (5), the prevalence of GERD was 24.2% in the 418 stable hemodialysis (HD) patients who did not undergo endoscopic examination. Compared to the reported prevalence of GERD in 6010 Japanese adults (16.3%) (6), the prevalence of GERD in CRF patients who underwent HD (24.2%) was increased.

In the gastroendoscopic findings of the 156 CRF patients who underwent endoscopic examination, the prevalence of GERD was 34.0%. Especially, in symptomatic cases, the prevalence of GERD was 44.0% (7).

Although we are now aware of the increasing prevalence of symptomatic GERD in HD patients, little is known about the gastroendoscopic findings and the prevalence of endoscopical GERD in CRF patients. In this chapter, I would like to explain about GERD in CRF patients.

2. Epidemiology

The overall proportion of reflux esophagitis in 6010 Japanese adults was 16.3% in prospective evaluation by gastroendoscopy (6). Several studies using endoscopic examination suggested that the overall prevalence of reflux esophagitis in Western countries was around 10%-20% (8, 9). These data indicated that reflux esophagitis is a common disease in Japan.

2.1 Evaluation by QUEST

We examined 418 stable CRF patients (257 men [62%] and 161 women [38%], mean age: 64.9 ± 10.2 [± standard deviation, SD] [range: 23-91] years) who underwent HD in the HD clinics and did not necessarily undergo gastroendoscopy (Table 1) (4). Instead of gastroendoscopy, QUEST, a structured questionnaire for the assessment of symptomatic GERD, was used to diagnose GERD in this study. We diagnosed GERD in those with a score of four points or more. In these 418 stable HD patients, the prevalence of GERD was 101 patients (24.2%) (Table 1) (4). Compared to the reported prevalence of GERD in Japan (16.3%) (6), the prevalence of GERD in CRF patients (24.2%), especially who underwent HD, is increased. This increased prevalence of GERD in HD patients was in accordance with the results (36%) of the autopsy study of 78 HD patients (10).

We also examined the risk factor for GERD in HD patients by using a questionnaire added to QUEST (4). The questionnaire included questions about age, sex, BMI (height and weight), presence of upper gastrointestinal symptoms, etiology of renal disease, past history, alcohol consumption and smoking habits. And we checked medications, laboratory data (BUN, Cr, K, Ca, P, TP, Hb, Ht), blood pressure (BP) and cardiothoracic ratio (CTR). As for these clinical findings, we compared the GERD group with the non-GERD group. Mean age was 62.2 ± 11.4 (± SD) years (range: 35-85) in GERD group and 65.8 ± 12.2 (± SD) years (range: 23-91) in non-GERD group. GERD group consisted of 64 males (63%) and 37 females (37%), on the other hand non-GERD group consisted of 193 males (61%) and 124 females (39%). Mean BMI was 20.8 ± 5.6 (± SD) (range: 14.7-28.2) in GERD group and 20.7 ± 6.2 (± SD) (range: 14.1-30) in non-GERD group. 79 patients (18.9%) were smoker, 51% of those were GERD group. 91 patients (22.1%) were alcohol drinker, 54% of those were GERD group. Diabetic nephropathy was seen in total 120 patients (29.2%) who consisted of 28 GERD patients (27%) and 92 non-GERD patients(29%). Mean CTR was 51.2 ± 10.1 (± SD) (range: 40.5-61.8) in GERD group and 51.9 ± 10.6 (± SD) (range: 39.5-77.6) in non-GERD group. Mean systolic BP was 158.5 ± 16.2 (± SD) (range: 120-210) in GERD group and 155.7 ± 15.8 (± SD) (range: 90-230) in non-GERD group. Mean diastolic BP was 78.6 ± 12.1 (± SD) (range: 55-110) in GERD group and 78.6 ± 12.5 (± SD) (range: 45-110) in non-GERD group. There were no statistically significant differences in age, sex, BMI, alcohol consumption, smoking, etiology of CRF, CTR, BP, laboratory data and medications between the GERD group and non-GERD group (Table 2, Fig. 1, 2).

The risk factor for this increased GERD in CRF patients was not clear. Evaluation of the prevalence of reflux esophagitis of HD patients needs further exploration by endoscopy.

2.2 Evaluation by endoscopic examination

In an endoscopic surveillance study in adults, no difference was seen in the incidence of esophagitis between patients with CRF and healthy controls (11). On the other hand, in an uncontrolled study using 24 hour pH-metry, Ruley et al found that 73% (16 of 22) of children with CRF had significant GERD.

We examined 156 CRF patients (97 men [62%] and 59 women [38%], mean age: 64.2 ± 12.3 [± SD] [range: 29-89] years) whose creatinine level was more than 2 mg/dl and who underwent endoscopy examination (7). This group involved 42 patients (27%) with some upper GI symptoms, 55 patients (35%) with DM and 87 patients (56%) with HT (Table 3). To investigate renal function, we classified the patients into three categories based on the creatinine level and as follows: 2< Cr. < 5 (44 patients [28%]), Cr. 5< and patients on pre-dialysis (53 patients [34%]), Cr. 5< and patients on hemodialysis (59 patients [38%]) (Table 3). As we could not examine glomerular filtration rate (GFR) of all patients, we used serum creatinine level as renal function. These clinical findings were compared with the gastroendoscopic findings retrospectively. The prevalence of GERD was highest (53 patients

	Patients (n = 418)
Mean age (years)	64.9 ± 10.2 (range: 23-91)
Sex	
Male	257 (61.5%)
Female	161 (38.5%)
BMI	20.7 ± 5.9 (range: 14.1-30.0)
Smoker	79 (18.9%)
Alcohol Drinker	91 (22.1%)
QUEST score (more than 4)	101 (24.2%)
Etiology of Renal Disease	
Chronic Glomerulonephritis	121 (29.4%)
Diabetic Nephropathy	120 (29.2%)
Nephrosclerosis	75 (18.2%)
Polycystic Kidney	24 (5.8%)
Others	71 (17.3%)

Data are given as the mean ± standard deviation (SD) or as the number of patients (n)

Table 1. Clinical characteristics of 418 Stable HD Patients.

	GERD Group (n = 101)	Non-GERD Group (n=317)	
Mean age (years)	62.2 ± 11.4 (range: 35-85)	65.8 ± 12.2 (range: 23-91)	**NS**
Sex			
Male	64 (63%)	193 (61%)	**NS**
Female	37 (37%)	124 (39%)	**NS**
Mean Body Mass Index	20.8 ± 5.6 (range: 14.7-28.2)	20.7 ± 6.2 (range: 14.1-30.0)	**NS**
Smoker	40 (51%)	39 (49%)	**NS**
Alcohol Drinker	49 (54%)	42 (46%)	**NS**
Prevalence of Diabetes mellitus	27 (27%)	92 (29%)	**NS**
Mean Cardiothoracic Ratio (%)	51.2 ± 10.1 (range: 40.5-61.8)	51.9 ± 10.6 (range: 39.5-77.6)	**NS**
Mean Blood Pressure			
Systolic (mmHg)	158.5 ± 16.2 (range: 120-210)	155.7 ± 15.8 (range: 90-230)	**NS**
Diastolic (mmHg)	78.6 ± 12.1 (range: 55-110)	78.6 ± 12.5 (range: 45-110)	**NS**

Data are given as the mean ± standard deviation (SD) or as the number of patients (n)
NS, not significant

Table 2. Comparison between GERD Group and Non-GERD Group in 418 Stable CRF Patients.

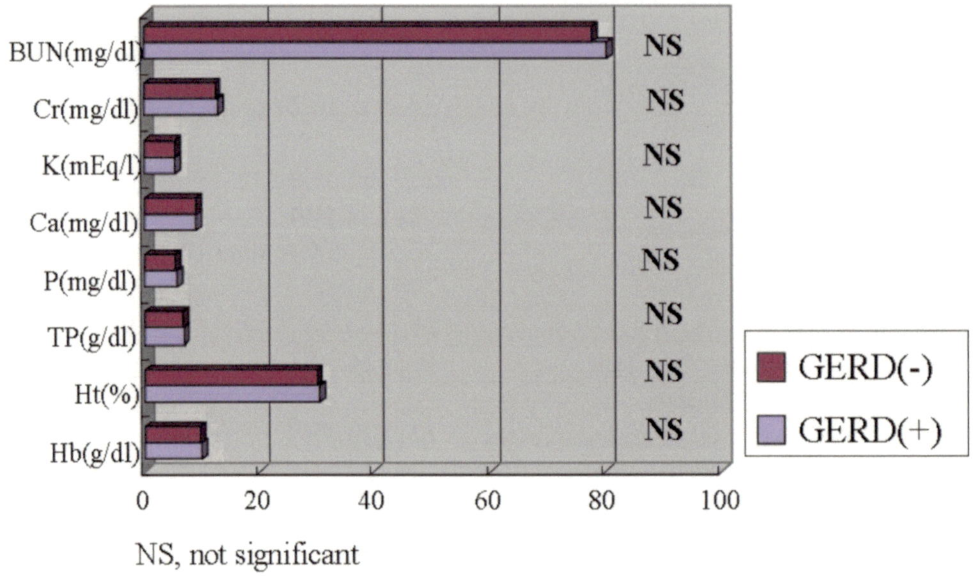

Fig. 1. Comparison of laboratory data between GERD group and non-GERD group.

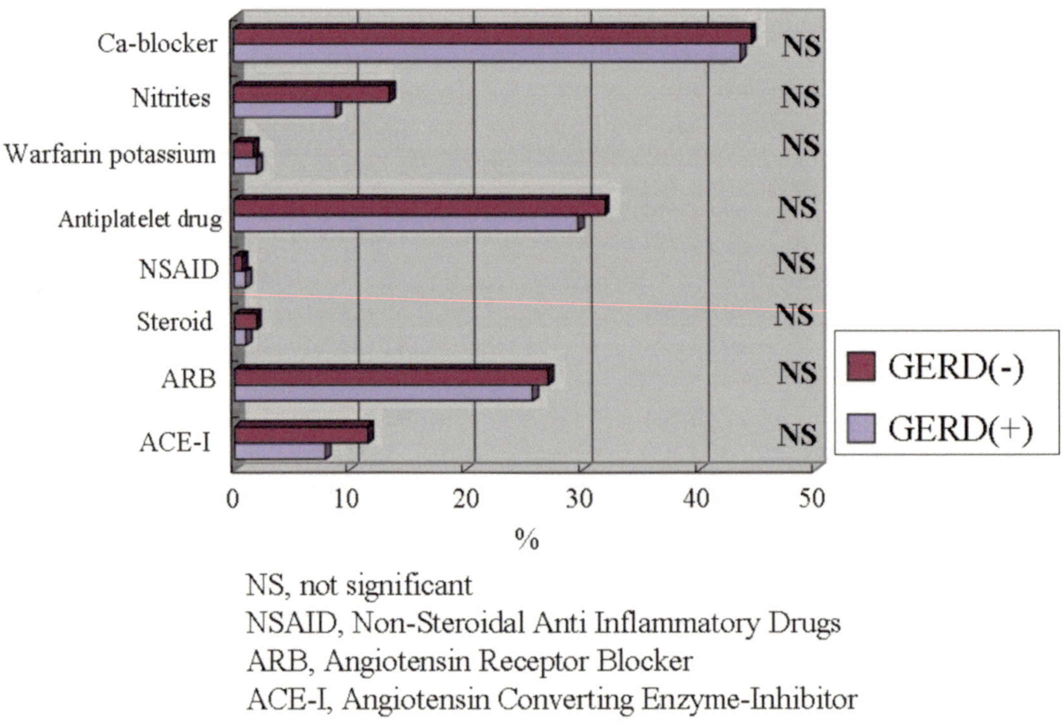

Fig. 2. Comparison of medications between GERD group and non-GERD group.

[34.0%]) in the gastroendoscopic findings of the 156 CRF patients who underwent endoscopic examination (Fig.3). Gastric ulcer and ulcer scar, erosion, hemorrhagic change (hematin), angiodysplasia and gastric antral vascular ectasia (GAVE) were seen in 39 patients (25%), 42 patients (27%), 41 patients (26%), 8 patients (5%) and 5 patients (3%), respectively (Fig.3). In the evaluation of 42 patients (27%) with some upper GI symptoms, 22 patients (52%) underwent hemodialysis, and the prevalence of GERD was highest (18 patients [44.0%]) in the gastroendoscopic findings. And in relationships between renal function and gastrointestinal symptoms, as renal function became worse, symptomatic cases tended to increase. There were statistically significant differences between the patients on hemodialysis and pre-dialysis (Fig.4). In relationships between renal function and gastroendoscopic findings, in the patients on hemodialysis the frequency of GERD and erosion increased, especially the prevalence of GERD was highest (50.0%). There were statistically significant differences between the patients on hemodialysis and pre-dialysis (Fig.5). The severity of GERD tended to be mild. In the patients with GERD, 77% was grade M or A of modified Los Angels grading system. Esophageal herniation was seen in 19 patients (32%) (Fig.6).

Although mechanisms exist that potentially lead to an increase of GERD in CRF, their existence would be insufficient to suggest that the incidence of GERD is increased in CRF patients without further study.

	Patients (n = 156)
Mean age (years)	64.2 ± 12.3 (range: 29-89)
Sex	
Male	97
Female	59
Cases with Upper GI Symptoms	42
Renal function	
2 < Cr. < 5	44
Cr. 5 <, without hemodialysis	53
Cr. 5 <, with hemodialysis	59
Complications	
Diabetes Mellitus	55
Hypertension	87

Data are given as the mean ± standard deviation (SD) or as the number of patients (n)

Table 3. Clinical characteristics of 156 CRF patients.

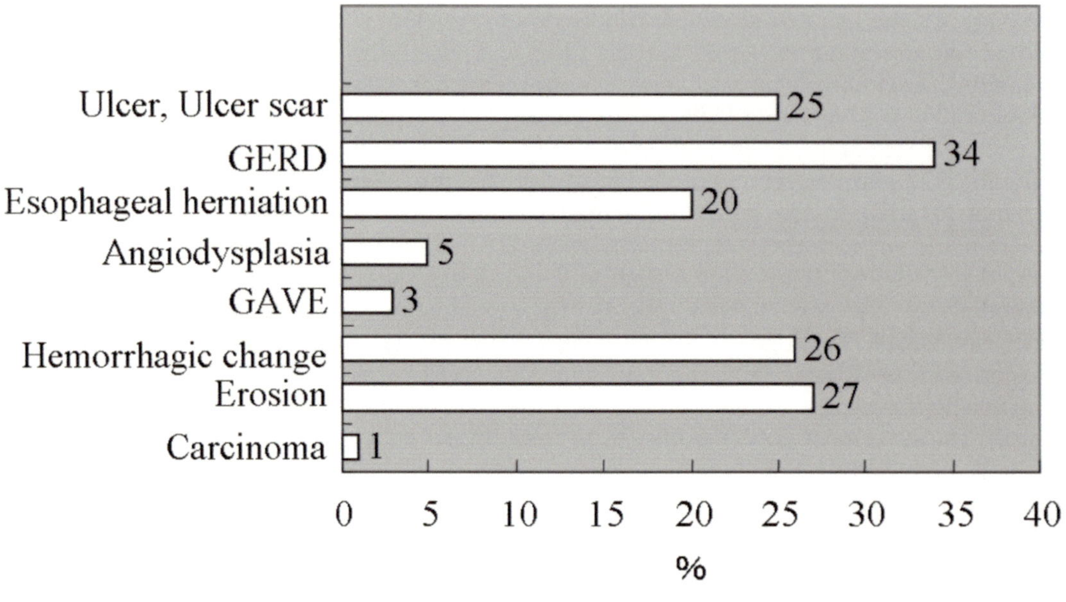

Fig. 3. Gastroendoscopic findings of 156 CRF patients who underwent endoscopic examination.

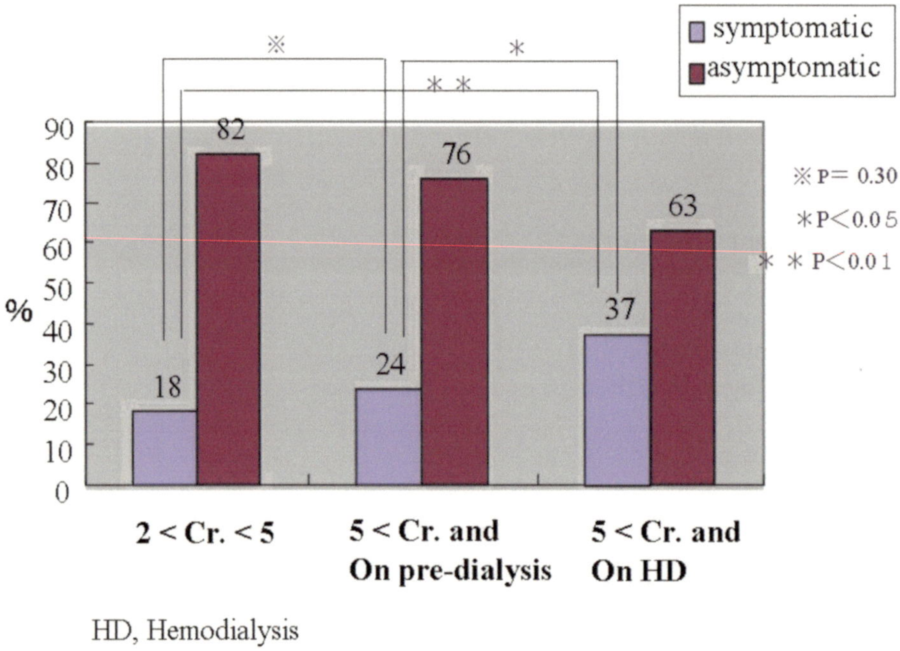

Fig. 4. Relationships between renal function and gastrointestinal symptoms.

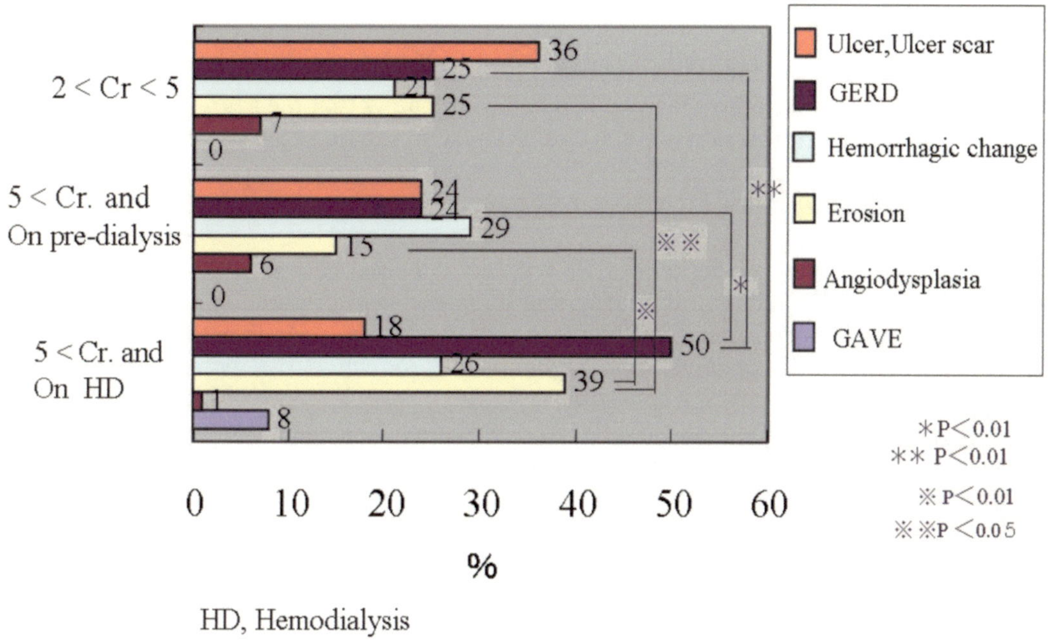

Fig. 5. Relationships between renal function and gastroendoscopic findings.

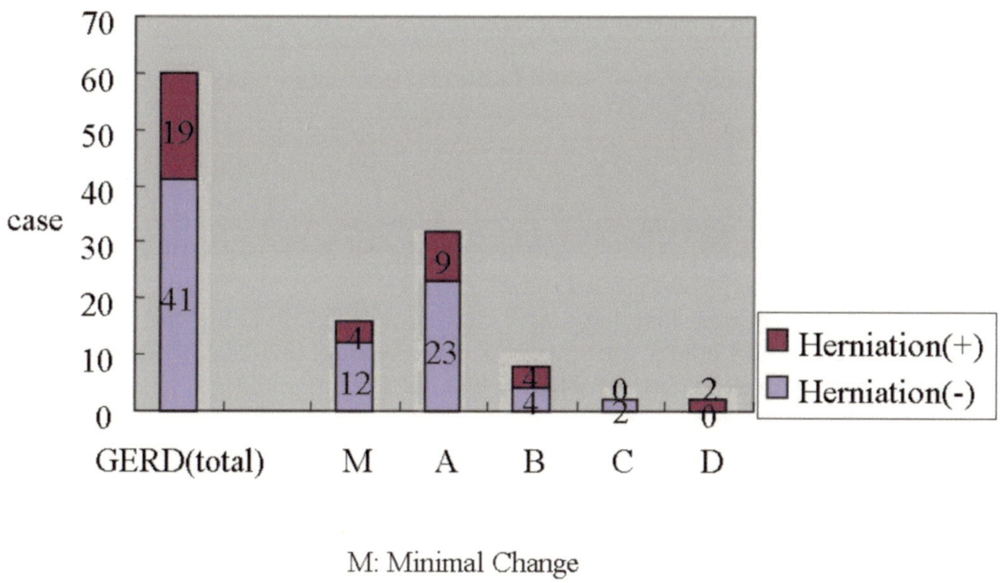

Fig. 6. Relationships between severity of GERD and esophageal herniation.

3. Pathophysiology

The pathophysiology of GERD is multifactorial and depends on interaction between aggressive factors and defensive factors. It is believed mainly that the aggressive factor is an increased gastric acid production and the defensive factor is a decreased gastric emptying.

3.1 Aggressive factors

3.1.1 Hypergastrinemia

We have to consider the association of CRF with an increased gastric acid production as an aggressive factor. Although we cannot say that increased acid production occurs in all CRF patients, some patients certainly have increase acid production. Hypergastrinemia is in fact present (12, 13) in CRF patients, and higher acid production can occur secondary to hypergastrinemia, which can be a consequence of decreased clearance of gastrin owing to a reduced glomerular filtration rate (GFR). And Straathof *et al.* reported that postprandial plasma concentrations of gastrin decrease lower esophageal sphincter pressure and increase the transient lower esophageal sphincter relaxations associated with reflux (14). In our study, the prevalence of GERD tended to increase as renal function become worse, although we could not examine serum gastrin level (7). But hypergastrinemia may also be in part to due increased secretion, because the density of G cells is increased in CRF patients (15, 16) possibly owing to a hyperthyroid state. Elevated serum gastrin causes an increase in acid production by the parietal cells. However, when measured in CRF patients, large variations in the mean gastric acid production actually occur from achlorhydria to hyperchlorhydria (17). Indeed, achlorhydria has been suggested as the stimulus for hypergastrinemia, because a feedback mechanism exists between the G cells and the low-acid state that stimulates the secretion of gastrin.

Serum gastrin may be an important factor as both an aggressive and a defensive factor.

3.1.2 Helicobacter pylori infection

On the other hand several studies have shown that rates of *Helicobacter pylori* (*H. pylori*) infection in CRF are lower than expected (17-20). Shousha *et al.* found that the prevalence of antral *H. pylori* was significantly less in patients with renal disease (24%) than in a control group (42%) (19). These lower rates of *H. pylori*, which lead to hyperacidity state in stomach, may potentially be a mechanism by which CRF can be associated with GERD. *H. pylori* infection also may be an important factor for GERD.

Some researchers reported that long-term dialysis reduced the prevalence of *H. pylori* infection (21–23), while others found no such correlation (24, 25). Nakajima et al. (22) reported that in Japanese patients on HD the mean duration of HD was significantly longer in *H. pylori*-negative patients than in *H. pylori*-positive patients. More recently, Sugimoto et al. (23) have shown that the prevalence of *H. pylori* infection serially decreased within 4 years in identical patients on HD, particularly among patients on HD for less than 4 years. Moriyama et al. (26) reported that such an inverse association between *H. pylori* and HD was again confirmed, and such a trend was obvious in patients on HD for more than 8 years.

It is widely accepted that reflux esophagitis is associated with *H. pylori* infection in the general population (27, 28). However, only two studies have investigated the correlation between *H. pylori* infection and reflux esophagitis in patients with CRF (29, 30). In a case-control study by Cekin et al. (30), *H. pylori* infection was found to be protective against reflux esophagitis in patients on HD; in contrast, in another study of patients prior to renal transplantation, reflux esophagitis was found irrespective *H. pylori* infection (29). These results suggest that long-term HD is an independent risk factor of reflux esophagitis.

3.2 Defensive factors

Then we also have to consider the association of CRF with a decreased gastric emptying as a defensive factor. Nausea and vomiting are often encountered in CRF and can be caused by delayed gastric emptying. The association of CRF with delayed gastric emptying seems to depend on the type of patient. A patient on peritoneal dialysis would be expected to have delayed gastric emptying simply due to the physical impairment caused by the peritoneal fluid. A lot of CRF patients have DM and HT as complications. We can also predict decreased gastric emptying by DM neuropathy and LES relaxations by Ca-antagonists and nitrites. CRF patients in our study also involved 55 patients (35%) with DM and 87 patients (56%) with HT, although we could not show the association of GERD with DM or HT (4). Results in other CRF patients, such as patients with uremia but not on dialysis, or patients on HD, have yielded conflicting results. Three studies demonstrated delayed gastric emptying in uremic predialysis patients (31-33). The researchers have also documented delayed gastric emptying in hemodialysis patients particularly patients who are hypoalbuminemic (32, 33). In our study, as for total protein, the differences between GERD group and Non-GERD group were not statistically significant (Fig. 1) (4). The situation is meddled by other studies that have not demonstrated decreased gastric emptying in hemodialysis patients (33-36).

The reasons for the discrepancy between the various results are likely multifactorial. One of the confounding factors is whether the patient is pre-dialysis, on peritoneal dialysis, or on hemodialysis. Ko et al demonstrated that uremic patients undergoing dialysis had gastric rhythm disturbance that deteriorated after HD (37). Dumitrascu et al demonstrated that patients with CRF had delayed gastric emptying if parasympathetic and sympathetic neuropathy were both present (38). DM is at increased risk of autonomic neuropathy, and they certainly constitute a large proportion of patients with CRF. In our study diabetic nephropathy was 29.2% of 418 stable HD patients (Table 1) and the differences between GERD group and Non-GERD group were not statistically significant (Fig. 1) (4). As the other risk factor of GERD, we examined age, sex, BMI, alcohol, smoking, etiology of renal disease, laboratory data (BUN, Cr., K, Ca, P, TP, Ht, Hb) and some medications, but the differences between GERD group and Non-GERD group were not statistically significant (Fig. 1, 2) (4).

4. Conclusions

CRF, especially HD patients, seem to be associated with an increased incidence of GERD, though the pathophysiology of GERD is multifactorial and complicated. We should keep GERD in mind, when we see CRF patients.

We used QUEST or endoscopy for the diagnosis of GERD. Though endoscopy is highly useful for the diagnosis of reflux esophagitis, endoscopic examination has not been used to evaluate the prevalence of reflux esophagitis in a large population of HD patients. Because many HD patients have the other diseases, we cannot undergo endoscopy easily. QUEST is thought to be accurate since upper GI symptoms in HD are correlated well with GERD (39). And we think that GERD diagnosed by QUEST is nearly equal to symptomatic GERD. But we need to pay attention that symptomatic GERD is not always equal to endoscopic GERD.

5. References

Ala-Kaila K, Vaajalahti P, Karvonen AL. Gastric *Helicobacter* and upper gastrointestinal symptoms in chronic renal failure. *Ann Med* 1991; 23:403-6.

Ala-Kaila K. Upper gastrointestinal findings in chronic renal failure. *Scand J Gastroenterol* 1987; 22:372-6.

Ayhan HC, Sedat B, Murat G, Banu B, Gurden G, Ebru D, *et al*. Gastroesophageal reflux disease in chronic renal failure patients with upper GI symptoms: multivariate analysis of pathogenic factors. *Am J Gastroenterol* 2002; 97:1352-6.

Berstad A, Weberg R, Froyshov LI. Relationship of hiatus hernia to reflux oesophagitis. *Scand J Gastroenterol* 1986; 21: 55-58.

Brown-Cartwright D, Smith HJ, Feldman M. Gastric emptying of an indigestible solid in patients with end-stage renal disease on continuous ambulatory peritoneal dialysis. *Gastroenterology* 1998; 95:49-51.

Carlei F, Caruso U, Lezoche E. Hyperplasia of antral G cells in uraemic patients. *Digestion* 1984; 29:26-30.

Carlsson R, Dent J, Bolling-Sternevald E, Johnsson F, Junghard O, Lauristen K, *et al*. The usefulness of a structured questionnaire in the assessment of symptomatic gastroesophageal reflux disease. *Scand J Gastroenterol* 1998; 33:1023-9.

Cekin AH, Boyacioglu S, Gursoy M, Bilezikci B, Gur G, Akin ED, et al. Gastroesophageal reflux disease in chronic renal failure patients with upper GI symptoms: multivariate analysis of pathogenic factors. Am J Gastroenterol. 2002;97: 1352–6.

Crivelli O, Pera A, Lombardo L. Antral G and D cell counts in chronic renal failure. *Scand J Gastroenterol* 1979; 14:327-31.

Dumitrascu DL, Barnert J, Kirschner T. Antral emptying of semisolid meal measured by real-time ultrasonography in chronic renal failure. *Dig Dis Sci* 1995; 40: 636-44.

Furukawa N, Iwakiri R, Koyama T *et al*. Proportion of reflux esophagitis in 6010 Japanese adults: prospective evaluation by endoscopy. *J Gastroenterol* 1999; 34: 441-4.

Hallgren R, Karlsson FA, Lundqvist G. Serum levels of immunoreactive gastrin: influence of kidney function. *Gut* 1978; 19:207-13.

Huang JJ, Huang CJ, Ruaan MK, Chen KW, Yen TS, Sheu BS. Diagnostic efficacy of (13) C-urea breath test for *Helicobacter pylori* infection in hemodialysis patients. Am J Kidney Dis. 2000;36:124–9.

Kang JY. The gastrointestinal tract in uremia. *Dig Dis Sci* 1993; 38(2): 257-68.

Kao CH, Hsu YH, Wang SJ. Delayed gastric emptying in patients with chronic renal failure. *Nucl Med Commun* 1996; 17:164-7.

Kawaguchi Y, Mine T, Kawana I, Yasuzaki H, Kokuho T, Toya Y, Ohnishi T, Umemura S. Gastroesophageal Reflux Disease in Hemodialysis Patients. Tokai J Exp Clin Med. 2009; 34: 48-52.

Kawaguchi Y, Mine T, Kawana I, Yasuzaki H, Kokuho T, Toya Y, Ohnishi T, Umemura S. Gastroesophageal Reflux Disease in Chronic Renal Failure Patients: evaluation by endoscopic examination. Tokai J Exp Clin Med. 2009; 34:

Ko CW, Chang CS, Wu MJ. Gastric dysrhythmia in uremic patients on maintenance hemodialysis. *Scand J Gastroenterol* 1998; 33: 1047-51.

Koike T, Ohara S, Sekine H, Iijima K, Kato K, Shimosegawa T, et al. *Helicobacter pylori* infection inhibits reflux esophagitis by inducing atrophic gastritis. Am J Gastroenterol. 1999;94:3468–72.

Korman MG, Laver MC, Hansky J. Hypergastrinaemia in chronic renal failure. *Br Med J* 1972; 1(794): 209-10.

Labenz J, Blum AL, Bayerdorffer E, Meining A, Stolte M, Borsch G. Curing *Helicobacter pylori* infection in patients with duodenal ulcer may provoke reflux esophagitis. Gastroenterology. 1997;112:1442–7.

Margolis DM, Saylor JL, Geisse G *et al*. Upper gastrointestinal disease in chronic renal failure. A prospective study. *Arch Intern Med* 1978; 138(8): 1214-17.

McNamee PT, Moore GW, McGeown MG *et al*. Gastric emptying in chronic renal failure. *Br Med J (Clin Res Ed)* 1985; 291:310-11.

Milito G, Taccone-Gallucci M, Brancaleone C *et al*. Assessment of the upper gastrointestinal tract in hemodialysis patients awaiting renal transplantation. *Am J Gastroenterol* 1983; 78:328-31.

Milito G, Taccone-Gallucci M, Brancaleone C, *et al*. The gastrointestinal tract in uremic patients on long-term hemodialysis. *Kidney Int* 1985; 17(suppl):157-60.

Moriyama T, Matsymoto T, Hirakawa K, Ikeda H, Tsuruya K, et al. *Helicobacter pylori* status and esophagogastroduodenal mucosal lesions in patients with end-stage renal failure on maintenance hemodialysis. J Gastroenterol. 2010;45:515-522.

Munoz de Bustillo E, Sanchez Tomero JA, Sanz JC, Moreno JA, Jimenez I, Lopez-Brea M, et al. Eradication and follow-up of *Helicobacter pylori* infection in hemodialysis patients. Nephron. 1998;79:55–60.

N.D. Vaziri, B Dure-Smith, R Miller, M.K.Mirahmadi. Pathology of gastrointestinal tract in chronic hemodialysis patients: an autopsy study of 78 cases. *Am J Gastroenterol* 1985; 80:608-11.

Nakajima F, Sakaguchi M, Amemoto K, Oka H, Kubo M, Shibahara N, et al. Prevalence of *Helicobacter pylori* antibodies in long-term dialysis patients. Nephrology. 2004;9:73–6.

Offerhause GJA, Kreuning J, Valentijn RM *et al*. Campylobacter pylori. Prevalence and significance in patients with chronic renal failure. *Clin Nephrol* 1989; 32:239-41.

Ollyo JB, Monnier P, Fontolliet CF. The natural history, proportion and incidence of reflux oesophagitis. *Gullet* 1993; 3: (Suppl) 3-10.

Özgur O, Boyacioglu S, Ozdogan M, Gur G, Telatar H, Haberal M. *Helicobacter pylori* infection in haemodialysis patients and real transplant recipients. Nephrol Dial Transplant. 1997;12:289–91.

Ravelli AM, Lederman SE, Bisset WM *et al*. Foregut motor function in chronic renal failure. *Arch Dis Child* 1992; 67:1343-7.

Shousha S, Arnaout AH, Abbas SH *et al*. Antral *Helicobacter pylori* in patients with chronic renal failure. *J Clin Pathol* 1990; 4(5): 397-9.

Soffer EE, Geva B, Helman C *et al*. Gastric emptying in chonic renal failure patients on hemodialysis. *J Clin Gastroenterol* 1987; 9(6): 651-3.

Sotoudehmanesh R, Ali Asgari A, Ansari R, Nouraie M. Endoscopic findings in end-stage renal disease. Endoscopy. 2003; 35:502–5.

Straathof JWA, Lamers CBHW, Masclee AAM. Effect of gastrin-17 on lower esophageal sphincter characteristics in man. *Dig Dis Sci* 1997; 42:2547-51.

Sugimoto M, Sakai K, Kita M, Imanishi J, Yamaoka Y. Prevalence of *Helicobacter pylori* infection in long-term hemodialysis patients. Kidney Int. 2009;75:96–103.

Wright RA, Clemente R, Wathen R. Gastric emptying in patients with chronic renal failure receiving hemodialysis. *Arch Intern Med* 1984; 144:495-6.

2

Hepatitis B Virus (HBV) Variants in Hemodialysis Patients

Selma A. Gomes, Francisco C. Mello and Natalia M. Araujo
Laboratório de Virologia Molecular, Instituto Oswaldo Cruz, FIOCRUZ, Rio de Janeiro, RJ Brazil

1. Introduction

In this chapter we discuss the global epidemiology of hepatitis B virus (HBV) in the general population and compare the data with those from populations at higher risk for hepatitis B infection, as hemodialysis patients. We discuss disease burden, HBV genotype distribution, and patterns of HBV transmission in the general population and among hemodialysis patients. We focus on the importance of detecting occult HBV infection in hemodialysis. Finally, we compare HBV variants detected in the general population with those detected by nosocomial transmission in hemodialysis units.

2. History of hepatitis B virus

HBV is an etiologic agent of acute and chronic liver disease in humans. About one-third of people infected with HBV have a completely "silent" disease. When symptoms are present, they may be mild or severe. The most common early symptoms are mild fever, headache, muscle aches, fatigue, loss of appetite, nausea, vomiting and diarrhea. Later symptoms may include dark coffee-colored, rather than dark yellow, urine, clay-colored stools, abdominal pain, and yellowing of the skin and whites of the eyes (jaundice). Several reports of the occurrence of epidemic jaundice are found from the period before the Christian era, and were initially described by Hippocrates (400 BC). However, only in the late nineteenth century, after smallpox vaccination (vaccine prepared from human lymph) of 1,289 shipyard workers in Bremen, Germany, of which 15% became jaundiced, it became clear the association of this illness with an agent of parenteral transmission (Lurman, 1885).
During the first half of the twentieth century, outbreaks of hepatitis of "long incubation period" (30-180 days) were observed in many countries and have been associated with blood transfusions, use of injectable drugs, unsterilized needles and syringes, and vaccine administration, for example, an outbreak of hepatitis/jaundice occurred in militaries who were vaccinated against yellow fever during the Second World War (Krugman, 1989).
The 1940s was the period in which distinguished the presence of more than one viral agent for the epidemic of jaundice. In 1947, MacCallum appointed the terms "hepatitis A virus" (HAV) and "hepatitis B virus" (HBV), referring to the presumed etiologic agents of hepatitis of short incubation period (18 to 37 days) and long incubation period (30 to 180 days), respectively. This terminology was adopted by the committee of viral hepatitis of the World Health Organization, staying until nowadays (Hollinger, 1991).

In 1965, Blumberg and colleagues published what would become one of the most important revelations about viral hepatitis. With the aim of studying polymorphic hereditary characteristics, Blumberg and his team examined thousands of serum samples from different geographic areas of the world. During the course of the investigation, the team found that a serum sample from an Australian aborigine contained an antigen that reacted specifically with an antibody present in the serum of a hemophiliac patient in the United States. Subsequent studies revealed that this "Australia antigen" was relatively rare in the population of North America and Western Europe, but prevalent in some African and Asian regions and among patients with leukemia, Down syndrome and acute hepatitis (Bayer et al., 1968; Blumberg et al., 1967). In 1968, the correlation of the Australia antigen (now called the surface antigen of hepatitis B or HBsAg) with HBV, could be established (Okochi&Murakami, 1968; Prince, 1968). Subsequently, the purification of HBV was performed from serum of carriers of Australia antigen and the complete particle or virion was detected by electron microscopy (Dane et al., 1970).

3. HBV routes of transmission

HBV is present in high titers in blood and exudates of acutely and chronically infected persons. More moderate viral titers are found in semen, urine, saliva, and nasopharyngeal fluid (Alter et al., 1977; Davison et al., 1987). HBV is present in the blood of individuals positive for hepatitis B e antigen (HBeAg, a marker of high infectivity) at a concentration of approximately 10^8 to 10^9 viral particles per milliliter (mL) of blood (Dane et al., 1970). By comparison, human immunodeficiency virus (HIV) is present in blood at much lower concentrations: 10^3 to 10^4 viral particles/mL for a person with AIDS and 10 to 100/mL for a person with asymptomatic HIV infection (Ho et al., 1989). The risk of HBV transmission after percutaneous exposure to HBeAg-positive blood is approximately 100-fold higher than the risk of HIV transmission after percutaneous exposure to HIV infected blood (CDC, 2011). In addition, HBV is an extremely resistant virus, capable of withstanding extreme temperature and humidity. HBV retains infectivity when stored at 30°C to 32°C for at least 6 months and when frozen at -15°C for 15 years. HBV present in blood can resist drying on a surface for at least a week (Hollinger&Liang, 2001). These characteristics explain why HBV is so highly transmissible by a variety of percutaneous procedures, with an annual global estimation of 8–16 million new HBV infections due to the use of unsafe injections (Simonsen et al., 1999).

HBV transmission occurs mainly by percutaneous or mucosal exposure to infected blood. It also occurs through perinatal exposure, sexual intercourse, exposure to blood products (needles shared by intravenous drug users, by skin lesions) and through organ transplantation. In areas of high incidence of HBV infection, dissemination occurs mainly in children, either at birth (perinatal) or during the first years of life by horizontal transmission among family members (Margolis et al., 1991). Perinatal transmission from mother to child may occur during birth by newborn exposure to blood or amniotic fluid. In areas of low prevalence, the infection occurs primarily in adults. Individuals at high risk for HBV infection are injecting drug users (Alter, 1993; Oliveira et al., 1999), homosexual or heterosexual individuals with multiple sexual partners (Piot et al., 1990), health professionals (Beltrami et al., 2000) and polytransfused patients. Patients undergoing hemodialysis are at high risk of acquiring HBV (Canero-Velasco et al., 1998; Covic et al., 1999; Vladutiu et al., 2000).

4. Clinical features

It is believed that the HBV itself does not exert a direct cytopathic effect on hepatocytes (Alberti et al., 1983). Hepatitis B infection can, however, vary from an acute self-limited to a severe form of fulminant hepatitis. The course of HBV infection can be extremely variable. It may be unapparent or patients may develop symptoms. Asymptomatic cases can be identified by detecting biochemical or virus specific serological alterations. Symptoms range from mild to severe. It is estimated that about 90-95% of infected adults will recover from the infection, and less than 1% of individuals may develop a fulminant hepatitis. However, children up to 5 years old, have over 90% of chance of becoming chronic carriers due to the immature immune system. Patients with acute hepatitis may recover completely or progress to chronic hepatitis. Acute hepatitis can be divided into four clinical phases (a) incubation period that usually ranges from 30 to 180 days; (b) pre-icteric phase, ranging from several days to more than a week. This phase is typically characterized by mild fever, fatigability, anorexia, nausea and vomiting. At this stage, patients may refer diffuse abdominal pain, intolerance to various foods, taste disturbances, abdominal discomfort. The occurrence of arthritis, arthralgia and myalgia are described as well as the observation rubelliform rashes (McIntyre, 1990). Physical examination may reveal a mild hepatomegaly; (c) icteric phase that is characterized by the appearance of dark, golden-brown urine, followed by pale stools and discoloration of the mucous membranes, conjunctivae, and skin. This icteric phase begins within 10 days of the initial symptoms in over 85% of the HBV cases and; (d) convalescent period. In this stage, with the evolution of the disease, painful hepatomegaly and splenomegaly, and any gastrointestinal symptoms and those related to jaundice, if present, will gradually diminish. This recovery period lasts on average 20 to 30 days.

5. HBV open reading frames

HBV represents the prototype of *Hepadnaviridae* family (genus *Orthohepadnavirus*) where a group of singular few viruses with genomes composed by a partial double stranded DNA replicating via reverse transcriptase were clustered. HBV is one of the smallest genomes of human viruses, with about 3.2 Kb. The HBV genome is fully coding with four open reading frames designated pre-S/S, pre-C/C, P and X. All the virus genes are overlapped at least to one other open reading frame, and due to this characteristic, HBV may produce about 50% more proteins than expected for the size of its genome (Ganem&Varmus, 1987). The genomic pre-S/S region encodes the viral surface proteins (HBsAg) that is abundant in serum of infected individual. The pre-C/C region is responsible for the synthesis of the proteins that form HBV capsid, named core antigen (HBcAg). This region also synthesizes the e antigen (HBeAg) that is secreted from HBV particles and is found free in the serum of infected individuals. HBeAg is an important marker of active replication. The open reading frame for the polymerase (P gene) encodes the viral polymerase with activity of reverse transcriptase, and RNAseH. This protein is the target of anti-HBV drugs (see Topic 9). A small gene named X synthesizes a regulatory protein, called protein X (HBxAg). Almost all HBV proteins and antibodies against these products are important markers for HBV serological detection.

6. HBV serological and molecular markers of infection

From a clinical point of view, viral hepatitis has very similar symptoms. The etiological diagnosis to identify the causative agent of infection can be performed by serological techniques, immuno-histochemical and molecular research. Biochemical tests of liver function, such as determination of transaminases (alanine aminotransferase - ALT and aspartate aminotransferase - AST) and bilirubin are also performed for diagnostic purposes, because their serum levels increase during episodes of hepatocellular injury or necrosis due to viral infection (Sjogren, 1994). The symptoms start with the elevation of aminotransferases, and patients become positive to anti-HBc IgM. Anti-HBc IgM together with HBsAg, is the key to diagnosing acute infection, since the IgG fraction of this antibody serves only as evidence of immune memory. Despite being a long-lasting antibody, anti-HBc does not confer immunity to the individual, it does not have neutralizing capacity (Sjogren, 1994). The early disease markers of virus replication (HBeAg and HBV-DNA) are found in high titers. As the infection sets in, the host immune response modulates the infection and progressively decreases viral replication. Individuals who present satisfactory immune response can resolve viral replication, usually within the first 3 months of illness, giving rise to anti-HBe antibody, which is associated with a poor replication of HBV. The absence of the seroconversion HBeAg/anti-HBe within the first 3 months of acute illness is a sign of poor prognosis, indicating failure of the immune system and tendency to chronicity of the process. Upon the termination of viral replication, HBsAg gradually disappears and, after a few weeks, anti-HBs emerges, thus, conferring immunity to the patient. Chronic hepatitis is determined by the persistence of HBsAg in serum for more than six months after the onset of infection. In chronic patients, markers of viral replication and clinical manifestations are dependent on the virus-host interactions (Sjogren, 1994).

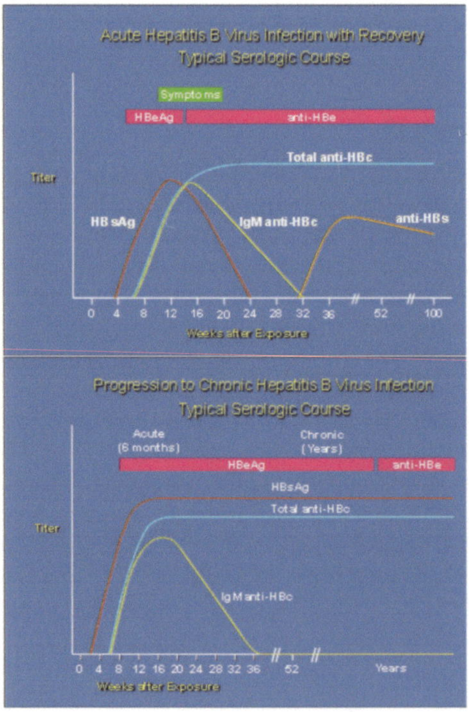

Fig. 1. Typical serologic course of acute and chronic HBV infections. Available in <http://www.cdc.gov/ncidod/diseases/hepatitis/slideset/hep_b/slide_3.htm> and <http://www.cdc.gov / ncidod/diseases/hepatitis/slideset/hep_b/slide_4 . htm> [Accessed on 16 Jan. 2008].

Figure 1 shows the curves of serological markers in acute and chronic HBV infections. Table 1 provides interpretations for hepatitis B serologic markers.

HBsAg **anti-HBc** **anti-HBs**	negative negative negative	Susceptible
HBsAg **anti-HBc** **anti-HBs**	negative positive positive	Immune due to natural infection
HBsAg **anti-HBc** **anti-HBs**	negative negative positive	Immune due to hepatitis B vaccination
HBsAg **anti-HBc** **IgM anti-HBc** **anti-HBs**	positive positive positive negative	Acutely infected
HBsAg **anti-HBc** **IgM anti-HBc** **anti-HBs**	positive positive negative negative	Chronically infected
HBsAg **anti-HBc** **anti-HBs**	negative positive negative	Interpretation unclear; four possibilities: 1. Resolved infection (most common) 2. False-positive anti-HBc, thus susceptible 3. "Low level" chronic infection 4. Resolving acute infection

Table 1. Interpretation of hepatitis B serologic test results. Available in <http://www.cdc.gov/hepatitis/HBV/PDFs/SerologicChartv8.pdf> [Accessed on 01 April 2011].

7. Epidemiology of HBV

According to the most recent data of World Health Organization (WHO, 2008), it is estimated that more than 2 billion people worldwide have been infected with HBV. Of these, approximately 360 million suffer from chronic HBV infection, resulting in over

600.000 deaths each year mainly from cirrhosis or liver cancer. The distribution of HBV infection is not uniform around the world. The world areas were classified into high, medium or low endemicity for HBV, depending on the prevalence of the HBV serological marker of active infection, the HBsAg. HBsAg is highly prevalent (8-15 %) in Southeast Asia, China, Philippines, Africa, the Amazon basin and the Middle East. An intermediate prevalence of HBsAg (2-7%) is observed in Eastern Europe, Central Asia, Japan, Israel and Russia, while a low prevalence (<2%) is found in North America, Western Europe, Australia and South America (CDC, 2011) (Figure 2). About 45% of HBV infected people are living in areas where HBsAg prevalence is 8% or higher, with a risk of infection of more than 60%, mostly during the childhood and with a high risk of chronicity. Forty-three percent of worldwide infected people are living in areas of intermediate prevalence with risk of infection of 20-60%, occurring across all age groups. Only the remaining 12% are living in areas of low prevalence with risk of infection of less than 20%, occurring mainly in adulthood (Te&Jensen, 2010). Despite the impressive number of HBV infected people, the worldwide incidence is in decreasing mostly due to the effort toward global prevention of hepatitis B by vaccination. Hepatitis B vaccine has been available since 1982 and at least 1 billion people have been vaccinated worldwide. The efficacy of HBV vaccination in the prevention of HBV infection has been shown to be over 90% in most countries (de Franchis et al., 2003) and universal vaccination is regarded to be the key toward elimination and eradication of HBV (Chen, 2009).

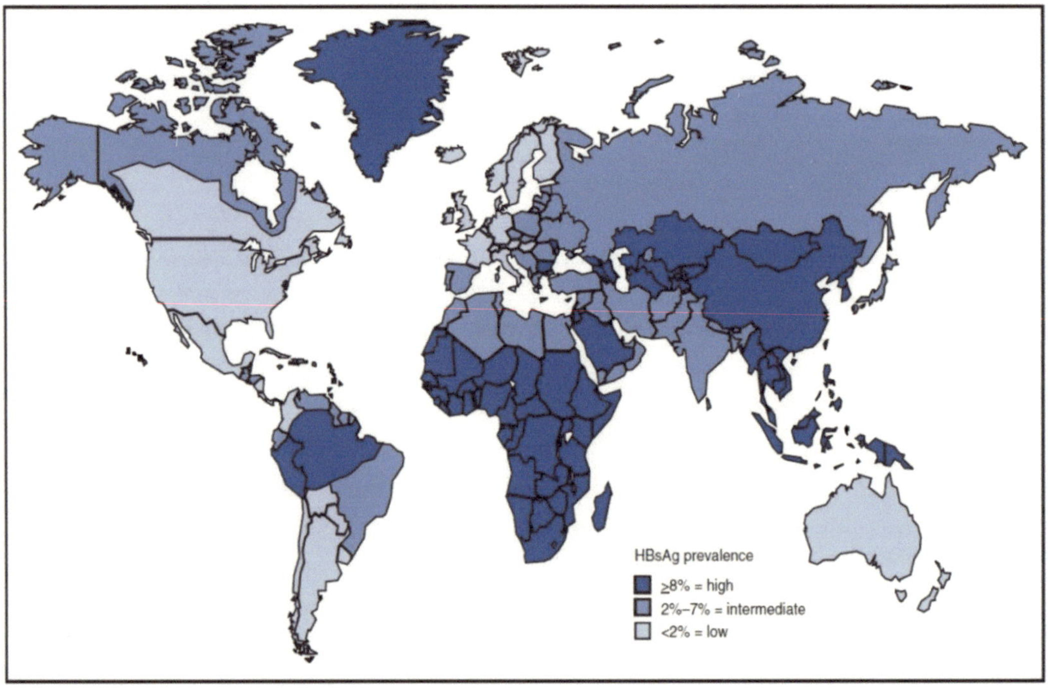

Fig. 2. Geographic distributions of hepatitis B infection worldwide, 2006. (Data from Central Disease Control, available from:
http://www.cdc.gov/hepatitis/HBV/PDFs/HBV_figure3map_08-27-08.pdf

8. Prevention of hepatitis B

The first HBV vaccine was licensed in 1981 and was derived from human plasma of chronic HBV (Heptavax-B, Merck & Co). However, the risk of transmission of other infectious agents present in the plasma, has stimulated the development of recombinant vaccines composed of HBsAg produced by genetic engineering (Engerix-B, Recombivax and SmithKline, Merck & Co). For the production of vaccines, recombinant DNA technology uses expression of HBsAg in yeast (Assad&Francis, 1999). The vaccine has good immunogenicity against HBV, approximately 90% of immunocompetent individuals vaccinated develop an adequate antibody response. Moreover, the vaccine has the potential to reduce the incidence of liver cancer (Blumberg, 1997). The scheme currently recommended to the recombinant vaccines is 3 doses intramuscularly in the deltoid muscle at intervals of one month (between 1st and 2nd dose) and 5 months (between 2nd and 3rd dose) - Schema 0, 1, 6 months (Assad&Francis, 1999). The protective efficacy of HBV vaccine is directly related to the level of anti-HBs produced and it is necessary for protection levels equal or greater than 10 mIU/ml (CDC, 1991). The immunoprophylaxis through the use of specific hyperimmune globulin (HBIG) is used to give immediate passive protection to individuals who have been recently exposed to HBV, for example, after an accidental puncture, sexual contact with a carrier or, during delivery of newborns of HBsAg positive mothers (Perrillo et al., 1984).

9. Treatment of chronic hepatitis B infection

The main goal of treatment for chronic hepatitis B is to suppress viral replication and reducing liver damage, preventing the progression to cirrhosis and hepatocellular carcinoma. Parameters of response to treatment to be considered are: 1) seroconversion of HBeAg to anti-HBe, 2) disappearance of HBV DNA from serum, 3) normalization of ALT level, and 4) improvement of liver histology. Two therapeutic approaches have been used in the treatment of HBV chronic infections: immune modulators and antiviral agents in the form of analogues of nucleos(t)ides. In the first category, conventional or pegylated interferon alpha (IFN-α) is the unique option. Approximately 20% of HBeAg positive patients treated with IFN seroconverted to anti-HBe (Karayiannis, 2004). Treatment with IFN has advantages such as a short duration (six months to one year) of treatment, absence of antiviral resistance and excellent quality and duration of response. Its disadvantages are mainly the side effects such as flu-like symptoms and hematologic, neuropsychiatric, dermatological, endocrine, respiratory, ophthalmic and cardiovascular reactions (Fattovich et al., 1996). The second class of antiviral agents for the treatment of chronic hepatitis B is the analogs of nucleos(t)ides. Today five drugs, lamivudine, adefovir dipivoxil, entecavir, telbivudine, and tenofovir have been approved in many parts of the world (Dienstag, 2008). These agents inhibit reverse transcription of the HBV polymerase and are well tolerated. However the occurrence of drug resistant viral isolates has been the main factor limiting the effectiveness of these drugs. These analogs of nucleos(t)ides are also used as part of the highly active antiretroviral therapy to treat HIV infection. HBV clinical trials and concurrent improvements in diagnostic technology may ensure that treatment options and expert opinion on patient management will continue to evolve. HBV genotyping and phenotyping of resistant isolates helps to delineate patterns of resistance and cross-resistance. These data may help to maximize the benefits of antiviral agents and improve the design of new therapeutic strategies (Zoulim&Locarnini, 2009).

10. Geographic distribution of HBV genotypes in the general population

HBV is a unique enveloped double-stranded DNA virus that employs the error-prone polymerase reverse transcriptase as part of its replication process. This has resulted in a large genetic variability over the years of virus evolution within its hosts. Based on sequence divergence in the entire genome of 8% or more, HBV isolates are classified into eight genotypes, designated A to H, with a distinct geographical distribution (Arauz-Ruiz et al., 2002; Norder et al., 2004; Norder et al., 1994; Stuyver et al., 2000). Genotype A circulates in Europe, India, Africa, and North and South Americas. Isolates belonging to genotypes B and C have been observed in Southeast Asia and the Far East. Genotype D is widespread, with a high prevalence in the Mediterranean area and in the Middle East region. Genotype G is infrequent and has mainly been found in Europe, Mexico, and USA, while genotype E is native from West Africa and genotypes F and H are considered indigenous to Latin America (Figure 3). Recently, two novel genotypes, I and J, the former described in Laos and Vietnam (Olinger et al., 2008; Tran et al., 2008), and the latter in Japan (Tatematsu et al., 2009), have been proposed, but their designation as new genotypes is still controversial. There is a great deal of diversity within the genotypes and this has led to the division of some genotypes into different subgenotypes, such as A1–A6 in HBV of genotype A (HBV/A), B1–B8 in HBV/B, C1–C10 in HBV/C, D1–D7 in HBV/D, and F1-F4 in HBV/F (Huy et al., 2006; Kramvis et al., 2008; Lusida et al., 2008; Meldal et al., 2009; Mulyanto et al., 2009; Norder et al., 2004; Nurainy et al., 2008; Pourkarim et al., 2010; Sakamoto et al., 2006; Utsumi et al., 2009; Wang et al., 2007).

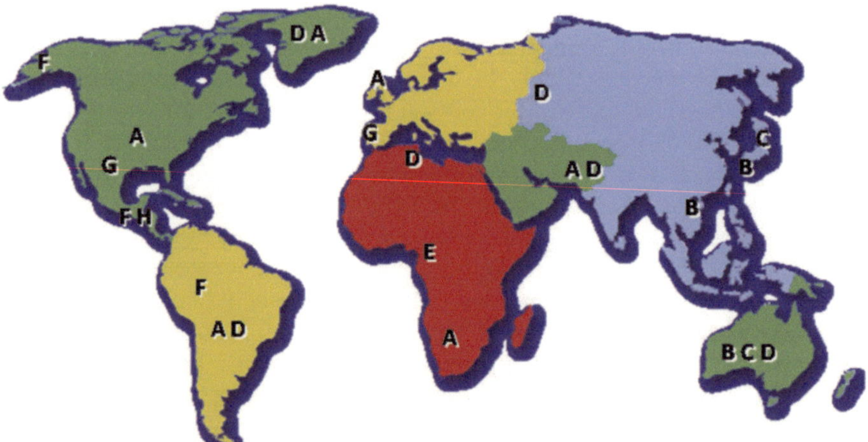

Fig. 3. Worldwide distribution of HBV genotypes. Adapted from <http://web.ucsf.edu/sfhbc/elective/2005/fall/Virology_Bass.ppt> [Date of access: 21 June 2008].

11. HBV and hemodialysis

It is well known that hemodialysis patients are at high risk of acquiring parenterally transmitted infections, not only because of the large number of blood transfusions that they receive, and the invasive procedures that they undergo, but also because of their immunosuppressed state. The prevalence of HBV infection in patients on maintenance hemodialysis is usually higher compared with rates from the general population. Recent data from Mexico showed that prevalence of HBV infection in patients on maintenance hemodialysis was about 7%, 35 times higher than in the general population (Paniagua et al., 2010). In dialysis units both patient-to-patient and patient-to-staff transmission of HBV have been recognized since the 1960s. Controlling the spread of HBV infection in dialysis units has been a major advance in the management of patients with chronic kidney diseases. Before the advent of vaccination, some success in limiting the spread of HBV was achieved by dialysing seropositive patients separately from those who were seronegative. This followed the publication in the UK of the Rosenheim Report in 1972 (RosenheimAdvisoryGroup, 1972), which set out a code of practice for reducing transmission of hepatitis among dialysis patients. Before adoption of the universal infection control practices and HBV vaccination, high prevalence rates of HBV serological markers were found in hemodialysis patients globally. In addition to epidemiologic issues, management of HBV infection in dialysis population has evolved because of advances in antiviral therapy and improvements in diagnostic techniques (Fabrizi et al., 2008).

The rate of de novo HBV infection in patients undergoing regular hemodialysis in the developed world is currently low (Finelli et al., 2005). In developed countries, where the infection control procedures have been implemented, HBV infection declined significantly, reaching HBsAg rates lower than 1.0% (Alter et al., 1986; Tokars et al., 2002). However, outbreaks of HBV infection continue to be reported occasionally in dialysis units in the developed world with some cases of fulminating hepatitis and even death (Inoue et al., 2006; Kondili et al., 2006). In the less-developed world, where the hemodialysis infection control practices and hepatitis B vaccination have been implemented lately, there are reports with rates of chronic HBsAg carriers ranging between 2% and 20% (Boulaajaj et al., 2005; Busek et al., 2002; Chattopadhyay et al., 2005; Covic et al., 1999; Fabrizi et al., 2008; Teles et al., 2002; Vladutiu et al., 2000). The higher HBV infection rates within dialysis units in the developing world can be attributed to several factors, an important one being the higher background prevalence of HBV in the general population. Also playing a prominent role are difficulties following infection control strategies against HBV such as, routine hemodialysis precautions, separating HBsAg-positive patients by rooms, machines, and staff, vaccination against HBV, and blood screening, attributable, at least in part, to a lack of financial and other resources (CDC, 2001).

12. Occult HBV infection in hemodialysis patients

HBsAg is the established serological marker for the diagnosis of acute or chronic HBV infection, and the absence of HBsAg in serum has been used as a surrogate marker for the absence of DNA and active viral replication. However, the development of highly sensitive molecular biology techniques has allowed detection of low levels of HBV DNA in the serum and/or liver of patients without detectable HBsAg (Coursaget et al., 1991; Gomes et al., 1996; Hu, 2002; Jeantet et al., 2002). This peculiar form of chronic viral infection has been termed occult HBV infection (Hu, 2002; Raimondo et al., 2007; Torbenson&Thomas, 2002). Individuals with occult HBV infection usually have serological evidence of previous exposure to the virus, mainly antibodies to core antigen (anti-HBc), although the absence of any serological marker related to HBV has also been described (Villa et al., 1995). Several possible explanations for HBV DNA persistence in the absence of HBsAg have been proposed. Low rate of HBV replication due to host's immune response or co-infection with other infectious agents may account for occult status in the majority of the cases (Raimondo et al., 2007). However, occult HBV infection may also be due to mutations that inhibit HBsAg expression (Chaudhuri et al., 2004) or change HBsAg antigenicity, thus preventing detection by commercial assays (Araujo et al., 2008; Carman et al., 1997; Jeantet et al., 2004; Yamamoto et al., 1994).

The prevalence of occult HBV infection is variable in different populations and depends on the general prevalence of HBV (Allain, 2004; Hu, 2002). The apparent prevalence also depends on the relative sensitivity of HBsAg and HBV DNA assays (Brechot et al., 2001; Conjeevaram&Lok, 2001). Occult HBV infection has been documented in a variety of clinical situations, most commonly among patients with hepatitis C virus (HCV) infection, in which the highest prevalence of occult HBV has been observed, especially in those who are positive for anti-HBc (Chemin&Trepo, 2005; Torbenson&Thomas, 2002). It is now established that occult HBV infection among non-HCV patients suffering from chronic hepatitis ranges from 20–30% in Europe and, in the context of HCV infection, ranges from 20% in France to 80% in Japan (Chemin&Trepo, 2005). Individuals at high risk of parenterally transmitted infections also have a high prevalence of occult HBV infection. Therefore, hemodialysis patients are at increased risk of occult HBV infection. Parenteral exposure also favors contamination by HCV (Dai et al., 2001).

The studies performed up to now on hemodialysis patients provide widely divergent results, reporting a prevalence of occult HBV that ranges from 0% to 36% (Besisik et al., 2003; Fabrizi et al., 2005; Goral et al., 2006; Kanbay et al., 2006; Minuk et al., 2004; Motta et al., 2010; Siagris et al., 2006). These apparent discrepancies may be explained by significant differences in the prevalence of HBV infection in different geographic regions and/or by the detection limits of different HBV-DNA assays. In this context, it is of note that several authors consider occult HBV as a possible source of virus spread in hemodialysis units, thus representing a risk of infection for both patients and staff, and suggest some precautions including HBV DNA screening for all hemodialysis patients (Minuk et al., 2004).

13. HBV variants in the general population vs. among hemodialysis patients

In this topic, we will discuss the flow of contamination of different HBV genotypes in hemodialysis centers. We will address the circulation of HBV variants in the general population and among hemodialysis patients. Are some genotypes more disseminated in the hemodialysis environment? How to trace nosocomial transmission?

HBV itself is not a directly cytotoxic virus. Instead, it destroys liver cells indirectly by stimulating the immune response. When the body fails to produce a sufficiently vigorous immune response to HBV during initial infection, chronic infection develops. This persistent but ineffective response results in progressive liver damage and fibrosis (Lindh et al., 1999). Although the host's immune response to HBV infection determines the extent of liver injury, evidence of an association between HBV genotypes and clinical outcomes, activity of liver disease, HBV replication, and treatment responses, is growing (Chu&Lok, 2002; Kao, 2002;

Mayerat et al., 1999; McMahon, 2009; Schaefer, 2005). An association between genotype A and a chronic outcome of HBV infection has been proposed (Mayerat et al., 1999; Ozasa et al., 2006). It has been demonstrated that the replication capacity of HBV in transfected hepatoma cells varied among HBV genotypes, with genotype A having the lowest replication capacity (Sugiyama et al., 2006). Therefore, it is probable that the propensity of HBV genotype A infections to lead to chronicity would be due to less intensive immune responses because of its slow viral dynamics (Ozasa et al., 2006). In addition, the analysis of the level of cellular stress induced by transfection with distinct HBV genotypes revealed that the lowest level was achieved with genotype A (Sugiyama et al., 2006). On the other hand, the majority of cross-sectional and prospective studies show that individuals infected with HBV genotype C have an increased and earlier risk of liver inflammation, liver fibrosis, cirrhosis and liver cancer than those infected with other genotypes, including genotype B that co-exists in the same geographic area, suggesting that genotype C may be the most virulent of the HBV genotypes (Chan et al., 2004; Chen et al., 2004; Kao, 2002). People infected with HBV genotype C clearly have higher levels of HBV DNA, as evidenced by prolonged HBeAg positivity, than those infected with other genotypes. As a result, they experience prolonged viremia throughout much of their lives, giving more time for HBV integration to occur and more opportunity for liver inflammation and fibrosis. Additionally, certain mutations such as the basal core promoter mutation, that independently may be associated with a higher risk of liver cancer, appear to occur more frequently in those infected with genotype C (McMahon, 2009).

Antiviral resistance to nucleos(t)ides analogs used for hepatitis B treatment has been associated with the genetic variability of HBV (Kramvis&Kew, 2005; Liu&Kao, 2008; Wiegand et al., 2008). Among the five nucleos(t)ides analogs licensed for treatment (see Topic 9), primary resistance mutations have been identified for lamivudine (Allen et al., 1998), telbivudine (Yang et al., 2005), entecavir (Colonno et al., 2006) and adefovir (Angus et al., 2003). Only tenofovir is not certain to cause resistance. All drug resistant mutations are confined to eight (169, 180, 181, 184, 202, 204, 236 and 250) aminoacid positions of the reverse transcriptase domain of pol gene (Locarnini, 2008). Lamivudine, also known as 3TC, was the first nucleoside analog to be licensed by the FDA for use in the treatment of chronic HBV infection in 1998 (Karayiannis, 2004). Primary lamivudine resistance associated changes result in amino acid changes within the tyrosine-methionine-aspartate-aspartate (YMDD) motif - rtM204V/I (methionine to valine or isoleucine substitution at codon 204). These changes cause a greater than 100-fold decrease in susceptibility to lamivudine in phenotypic assays. The compensatory mutations associated with lamivudine resistance, rtV173L (valine to leucine substitution), and rtL180M (leucine to methionine substitution) restore replication fitness of HBV polymerase that harbors the rtM204V/I mutation (Ono et al., 2001).

The genetic variability of HBV strains circulating in hemodialysis units has been an important matter of study worldwide. One of the most extensive studies of HBV contamination and nonequivalent, genotype-specific spread in hemodialysis centers was conducted in Goiania city, located at the Central-West region of Brazil (Teles et al., 2002). Brazil, a country with a highly miscegenated population, exhibits an HBV genotype circulation pattern that is distinct from the distribution found in other Latin American countries. In Brazil, genotypes A, D and F co-circulate. Of these, subgenotype A1, the African subgenotype of genotype A (Bowyer et al., 1997; Kramvis et al., 2002), is the most prevalent among Brazilian HBV carriers (Araujo et al., 2004; Mello et al., 2007). The distribution of HBV genotypes A and D in Brazil exhibit a gradient from northern to southern regions, reflecting the influence of Caucasian, African, and native Indian populations. North, Northeast and Southeast regions show a higher prevalence of genotype A. The high rate of genotype D isolates in the South region could be related to the influx of immigrants from Central Europe (especially Germany and Italy) that occurred in that region at the beginning of the 20th century. The balanced distribution of genotypes A and D in the Central-West region could be explained by the delayed occupation of that area by population migration flows from South, Southeast and Northeast regions (Mello et al., 2007). According to the study of Teles and cols. (Teles et al., 2002), in 1995, HBsAg prevalence among hemodialysis patients was approximately 10%, and genotypes A (50%) and D (46.2%) were almost detected equally in hemodialysis units from Goiania city. A survey of hemodialysis units in this city from 1995 to 1999 indicated that all newly infected patients harbored genotype D. By 1999, this resulted in a shift to genotype D being the predominant genotype (65.5%) (Teles et al., 2002). These data suggest that genotype D would be more likely to disseminate in the hemodialysis environment. In fact, although genotype A is the most prevalent genotype in Brazil, HBV genotype D strains have been involved frequently in hepatitis B outbreaks in dialysis units (Castro-Figueiredo et al., 1986; De Castro et al., 2000; Lewis-Ximenez et al., 2001; Roll et al., 1995), and in some of these cases they were probably more efficiently transmitted than genotype A (Castro-Figueiredo et al., 1986; De Castro et al., 2000; Teles et al., 2002). Additionally, several studies have shown a significant association of HBV genotype D and injection drug use (Fisker et al., 2004; Panessa et al., 2009; Swenson et al., 2001), reinforcing the idea that genotype D could be a blood-borne genotype. Other studies focusing on the molecular analysis of HBV isolates have been reported a high prevalence of genotype H and genotype B among hemodialysis patients from Mexico (Alvarado-Esquivel et al., 2006) and Indonesia (Lusida et al., 2003), respectively.

Nosocomial transmission in the dialysis setting has been reported as a result of reusing multi-dose vials, staff shortages and subsequent need to care simultaneously for HBV infected and uninfected individuals, and contamination of equipment and environmental surfaces (Wreghitt, 1999). To confirm a common source of infection, it is necessary to demonstrate that patients have been infected with the same strain of virus. A nosocomial transmission of hepatitis B genotype E in UK has been recently reported (Ramalingam et al., 2007). In this study, it was likely that two independent transmission events occurred in the ward and/or in the theatre recovery area. Both patients 1 and 2 with acute hepatitis B, and patient 3, an anti-HBe positive carrier had genotype E infections. The phylogenetic analyses demonstrated that the HBV strain infecting the three patients were identical in both the surface and core regions (Ramalingam et al., 2007). De Castro and cols. investigated the genetic variability of HBV strains circulating in two hemodialysis units by RFLP analysis (De Castro et al., 2000). Comparison between RFLP patterns of HBV strains was thus used to assess the nosocomial spread of HBV infection in each hemodialysis center. In this study, viral isolates of 27 HBsAg positive hemodialysis patients and 39 HBV-positive unrelated control patients, were grouped according to their RFLP patterns. In hemodialysis unit A, 14 HBV isolates were grouped into five different RFLP patterns: A1, A2 and A3 (for genotype A strains), and, D3 and D4 (for genotype D). Pattern A2, present at a relatively low prevalence (18%) in the control group, was observed in the majority (53%) of the hemodialysis patients. Notably, all five patients who seroconverted to HBsAg positivity in 1995 carried the strain of RFLP pattern A2. In hemodialysis unit B, where an outbreak of

HBV infection occurred in 1996–1997, RFLP analysis showed that all 13 patients who seroconverted to HBsAg were infected with HBV isolates of genotype D. Coinfection with strains of RFLP pattern A1 was detected in seven of them (De Castro et al., 2000).
There are concerns about HBV variants detected in cases of occult infection, if they may be transmitted to other hemodialysis patients and whether or not they may cause liver disease. Interesting, two studies, one performed in Turkey (Besisik et al., 2003) and other in Brazil (Motta et al., 2010), reported high prevalence of lamivudine resistant mutations in a significant proportion of hemodialysis patients with occult HBV infection, who had not previously received lamivudine treatment. It has been demonstrated that rtM204V/I mutants have a markedly decreased replication phenotype compared with wild-type HBV (Melegari et al., 1998), whereas both rtV173L and rtL180M substitutions act as compensatory changes that partially restore the replication fitness of the virus (Delaney et al., 2003; Ono et al., 2001). The triple lamivudine resistance mutation causes the concomitant amino acid substitutions E164D and I195M in the HBsAg as a result of the overlapping reading frames of the envelope and polymerase genes (Locarnini, 1998). It has been shown that both E164D and I195M substitutions reduce in vitro affinity of HBsAg to anti-HBs antibodies, similar to the HBV vaccine escape mutant G145R (Torresi et al., 2002). The HBsAg Y100C substitution is also frequently found among occult HBV infection carriers. Y100C has been found in cases of occult HBV infection among Venezuelan blood donors (Gutierrez et al., 2004), individuals from an Afro-Brazilian community (Motta-Castro et al., 2008) and HIV-HBV co-infected patients (Araujo et al., 2008). Among hemodialysis patients with occult HBV infection, the Y100C mutation has been also frequently found (Motta et al., 2010). Due to these observations, the role of Y100C substitution in reducing
amount of HBsAg or changing HBsAg affinity by commercial antibodies was recently investigated by Mello and cols. (Mello et al., 2011). This study compared the levels of HBsAg detected by ELISA after transfection assays using recombinant plasmids with or without Y100C substitution. The results indicated that Y100C substitution alone did not negatively affect the detection and/or secretion of HBsAg. However, further studies analyzing the complete genome of HBV strains with the Y100C substitution may elucidate whether this mutation affects HBV replication or if there are mutations in other HBV genomic region that could explain the association of these variants with occult hepatitis B infection (Mello et al., 2011).

14. Conclusions

Hepatitis B remains a major health issue in dialysis patients. Despite the introduction of effective infection control measures to minimize patient-to-patient transmission, occasional outbreaks occur in dialysis units, usually because of lapses in practice. Although the importance of occult HBV infection in the pathogenesis of hepatic disease has not yet been established, an increase number of studies have indicated a need to survey this group of patients. Occult HBV infection has been frequently observed among hemodialysis patients and could be a source of viral spread within hemodialysis units, representing a risk of infection for both patients and staff. YMDD variants are a common accompaniment and require further investigations with regard to clinical implications, once lamivudine treatment of possible HBV relapse in these patients might be accompanied by fast-viral resistance formation. Therefore, further studies with genome sequencing may provide more detail information on the molecular epidemiology of HBV infection, which may be helpful in understanding the HBV transmission in the hemodialysis population.

15. References

Alberti, A., F. Tremolada, G. Fattovich, F. Bortolotti, and G. Realdi. (1983). Virus replication and liver disease in chronic hepatitis B virus infection. *Dig Dis Sci*, 28 (11):961-966.

Allain, J. P. (2004). Occult hepatitis B virus infection. *Transfus Clin Biol*, 11 (1):18-25.

Allen, M. I., M. Deslauriers, C. W. Andrews, G. A. Tipples, K. A. Walters, D. L. Tyrrell, N. Brown, and L. D. Condreay. (1998). Identification and characterization of mutations in hepatitis B virus resistant to lamivudine. Lamivudine Clinical Investigation Group. *Hepatology*, 27 (6):1670-1677.

Alter, H. J., R. H. Purcell, J. L. Gerin, W. T. London, P. M. Kaplan, V. J. McAuliffe, J. Wagner, and P. V. Holland. (1977). Transmission of hepatitis B to chimpanzees by hepatitis B surface antigen-positive saliva and semen. *Infect Immun*, 16 (3):928-933.

Alter, M. J. (1993). Community acquired viral hepatitis B and C in the United States. *Gut*, 34 (2 Suppl):S17-19.

Alter, M. J., M. S. Favero, and J. E. Maynard. (1986). Impact of infection control strategies on the incidence of dialysis-associated hepatitis in the United States. *J Infect Dis*, 153 (6):1149-1151.

Alvarado-Esquivel, C., E. Sablon, C. J. Conde-Gonzalez, L. Juarez-Figueroa, L. Ruiz-Maya, and S. Aguilar-Benavides. (2006). Molecular analysis of hepatitis B virus isolates in Mexico: predominant circulation of hepatitis B virus genotype H. *World J Gastroenterol*, 12 (40):6540-6545.

Angus, P., R. Vaughan, S. Xiong, H. Yang, W. Delaney, C. Gibbs, C. Brosgart, D. Colledge, R. Edwards, A. Ayres, A. Bartholomeusz, and S. Locarnini. (2003). Resistance to adefovir dipivoxil therapy associated with the selection of a novel mutation in the HBV polymerase. *Gastroenterology*, 125 (2):292-297.

Araujo, N. M., M. Branco-Vieira, A. C. Silva, J. H. Pilotto, B. Grinsztejn, A. J. de Almeida, C. Trepo, and S. A. Gomes. (2008). Occult hepatitis B virus infection in HIV-infected patients: Evaluation of biochemical, virological and molecular parameters. *Hepatol Res*, 38 (12):1194-1203.

Araujo, N. M., F. C. Mello, C. F. Yoshida, C. Niel, and S. A. Gomes. (2004). High proportion of subgroup A' (genotype A) among Brazilian isolates of Hepatitis B virus. *Arch Virol*, 149 (7):1383-1395.

Arauz-Ruiz, P., H. Norder, B. H. Robertson, and L. O. Magnius. (2002). Genotype H: a new Amerindian genotype of hepatitis B virus revealed in Central America. *J Gen Virol*, 83 (Pt 8):2059-2073.

Assad, S., and A. Francis. (1999). Over a decade of experience with a yeast recombinant hepatitis B vaccine. *Vaccine*, 18 (1-2):57-67.

Bayer, M. E., B. S. Blumberg, and B. Werner. (1968). Particles associated with Australia antigen in the sera of patients with leukaemia, Down's Syndrome and hepatitis. *Nature*, 218 (5146):1057-1059.

Beltrami, E. M., I. T. Williams, C. N. Shapiro, and M. E. Chamberland. (2000). Risk and management of blood-borne infections in health care workers. *Clin Microbiol Rev*, 13 (3):385-407.

Besisik, F., C. Karaca, F. Akyuz, S. Horosanli, D. Onel, S. Badur, M. S. Sever, A. Danalioglu, K. Demir, S. Kaymakoglu, Y. Cakaloglu, and A. Okten. (2003). Occult HBV infection and YMDD variants in hemodialysis patients with chronic HCV infection. *J Hepatol*, 38 (4):506-510.

Blumberg, B. S. (1997). Hepatitis B virus, the vaccine, and the control of primary cancer of the liver. *Proc Natl Acad Sci U S A*, 94 (14):7121-7125.

Blumberg, B. S., B. J. Gerstley, D. A. Hungerford, W. T. London, and A. I. Sutnick. (1967). A serum antigen (Australia antigen) in Down's syndrome, leukemia, and hepatitis. *Ann Intern Med*, 66 (5):924-931.

Boulaajaj, K., Y. Elomari, B. Elmaliki, B. Madkouri, D. Zaid, and N. Benchemsi. (2005). [Prevalence of hepatitis C, hepatitis B and HIV infection among haemodialysis patients in Ibn-Rochd university hospital, Casablanca]. *Nephrol Ther*, 1 (5):274-284.

Bowyer, S. M., L. van Staden, M. C. Kew, and J. G. Sim. (1997). A unique segment of the hepatitis B virus group A genotype identified in isolates from South Africa. *J Gen Virol*, 78 (Pt 7):1719-1729.

Brechot, C., V. Thiers, D. Kremsdorf, B. Nalpas, S. Pol, and P. Paterlini-Brechot. (2001). Persistent hepatitis B virus infection in subjects without hepatitis B surface antigen: clinically significant or purely "occult"? *Hepatology*, 34 (1):194-203.

Busek, S. U., E. H. Baba, H. A. Tavares Filho, L. Pimenta, A. Salomao, R. Correa-Oliveira, and G. C. Oliveira. (2002). Hepatitis C and hepatitis B virus infection in different hemodialysis units in Belo Horizonte, Minas Gerais, Brazil. *Mem Inst Oswaldo Cruz*, 97 (6):775-778.

Canero-Velasco, M. C., J. E. Mutti, J. E. Gonzalez, A. Alonso, L. Otegui, M. Adragna, M. Antonuccio, M. Laso, M. Montenegro, L. Repetto, M. Brandi, J. Canepa, and E. Baimberg. (1998). [HCV and HBV prevalence in hemodialyzed pediatric patients. Multicenter study]. *Acta Gastroenterol Latinoam*, 28 (3):265-268.

Carman, W. F., F. J. Van Deursen, L. T. Mimms, D. Hardie, R. Coppola, R. Decker, and R. Sanders. (1997). The prevalence of surface antigen variants of hepatitis B virus in Papua New Guinea, South Africa, and Sardinia. *Hepatology*, 26 (6):1658-1666.

Castro-Figueiredo, J. F., M. Moyses-Neto, U. A. Gomes, A. Spalini-Ferraz, M. E. Nardin-Batista, A. M. Coimbra-Gaspar, and C. F. Tachibana-Yoshida. (1986). Hepatitis B virus infection in hemodialysis units: clinical features, epidemiological markers and general control measures. *Braz J Med Biol Res*, 19 (6):735-742.

CDC. (1991). Hepatitis B virus: a comprehensive strategy for eliminating transmission in the United States through universal childhood vaccination. Recommendations of the Immunization Practices Advisory Committee (ACIP). *MMWR Recomm Rep*, 40 (RR-13):1-25.

CDC. (2001). Recommendations for preventing transmission of infections among chronic hemodialysis patients. *MMWR Recomm Rep*, 50 (RR-5):1-43.

CDC. *Hepatitis B FAQs for Health Professionals* 2011 [cited. Available from <http://www.cdc.gov/hepatitis/HBV/HBVfaq.htm>

Chan, H. L., A. Y. Hui, M. L. Wong, A. M. Tse, L. C. Hung, V. W. Wong, and J. J. Sung. (2004). Genotype C hepatitis B virus infection is associated with an increased risk of hepatocellular carcinoma. *Gut*, 53 (10):1494-1498.

Chattopadhyay, S., S. Rao, B. C. Das, N. P. Singh, and P. Kar. (2005). Prevalence of transfusion-transmitted virus infection in patients on maintenance hemodialysis from New Delhi, India. *Hemodial Int*, 9 (4):362-366.

Chaudhuri, V., R. Tayal, B. Nayak, S. K. Acharya, and S. K. Panda. (2004). Occult hepatitis B virus infection in chronic liver disease: full-length genome and analysis of mutant surface promoter. *Gastroenterology*, 127 (5):1356-1371.

Chemin, I., and C. Trepo. (2005). Clinical impact of occult HBV infections. *J Clin Virol*, 34 Suppl 1:S15-21.

Chen, C. H., H. L. Eng, C. M. Lee, F. Y. Kuo, S. N. Lu, C. M. Huang, H. D. Tung, C. L. Chen, and C. S. Changchien. (2004). Correlations between hepatitis B virus genotype and cirrhotic or non-cirrhotic hepatoma. *Hepatogastroenterology*, 51 (56):552-555.

Chen, D. S. (2009). Hepatitis B vaccination: The key towards elimination and eradication of hepatitis B. *J Hepatol*, 50 (4):805-816.

Chu, C. J., and A. S. Lok. (2002). Clinical significance of hepatitis B virus genotypes. *Hepatology*, 35 (5):1274-1276.

Colonno, R. J., R. Rose, C. J. Baldick, S. Levine, K. Pokornowski, C. F. Yu, A. Walsh, J. Fang, M. Hsu, C. Mazzucco, B. Eggers, S. Zhang, M. Plym, K. Klesczewski, and D. J. Tenney. (2006). Entecavir resistance is rare in nucleoside naive patients with hepatitis B. *Hepatology*, 44 (6):1656-1665.

Conjeevaram, H. S., and A. S. Lok. (2001). Occult hepatitis B virus infection: a hidden menace? *Hepatology*, 34 (1):204-206.

Coursaget, P., P. Le Cann, D. Leboulleux, M. T. Diop, O. Bao, and A. M. Coll. (1991). Detection of hepatitis B virus DNA by polymerase chain reaction in HBsAg negative Senegalese patients suffering from cirrhosis or primary liver cancer. *FEMS Microbiol Lett*, 67 (1):35-38.

Covic, A., L. Iancu, C. Apetrei, D. Scripcaru, C. Volovat, I. Mititiuc, and M. Covic. (1999). Hepatitis virus infection in haemodialysis patients from Moldavia. *Nephrol Dial Transplant*, 14 (1):40-45.

Dai, C. Y., M. L. Yu, W. L. Chuang, Z. Y. Lin, S. C. Chen, M. Y. Hsieh, L. Y. Wang, J. F. Tsai, and W. Y. Chang. (2001). Influence of hepatitis C virus on the profiles of patients with chronic hepatitis B virus infection. *J Gastroenterol Hepatol*, 16 (6):636-640.

Dane, D. S., C. H. Cameron, and M. Briggs. (1970). Virus-like particles in serum of patients with Australia-antigen-associated hepatitis. *Lancet*, 1 (7649):695-698.

Davison, F., G. J. Alexander, R. Trowbridge, E. A. Fagan, and R. Williams. (1987). Detection of hepatitis B virus DNA in spermatozoa, urine, saliva and leucocytes, of chronic HBsAg carriers. A lack of relationship with serum markers of replication. *J Hepatol*, 4 (1):37-44.

De Castro, L., N. M. Araujo, R. R. Sabino, F. Alvarenga, C. F. Yoshida, and S. A. Gomes. (2000). Nosocomial spread of hepatitis B virus in two hemodialysis units, investigated by restriction fragment length polymorphism analysis. *Eur J Clin Microbiol Infect Dis*, 19 (7):531-537.

de Franchis, R., A. Hadengue, G. Lau, D. Lavanchy, A. Lok, N. McIntyre, A. Mele, G. Paumgartner, A. Pietrangelo, J. Rodes, W. Rosenberg, and D. Valla. (2003). EASL International Consensus Conference on Hepatitis B. 13-14 September, 2002 Geneva, Switzerland. Consensus statement (long version). *J Hepatol*, 39 Suppl 1:S3-25.

Delaney, W. E. t., H. Yang, C. E. Westland, K. Das, E. Arnold, C. S. Gibbs, M. D. Miller, and S. Xiong. (2003). The hepatitis B virus polymerase mutation rtV173L is selected during lamivudine therapy and enhances viral replication in vitro. *J Virol*, 77 (21):11833-11841.

Dienstag, J. L. (2008). Hepatitis B virus infection. *N Engl J Med*, 359 (14):1486-1500.

Fabrizi, F., P. Messa, and P. Martin. (2008). Hepatitis B virus infection and the dialysis patient. *Semin Dial*, 21 (5):440-446.

Fabrizi, F., P. G. Messa, G. Lunghi, F. Aucella, S. Bisegna, S. Mangano, M. Villa, F. Barbisoni, E. Rusconi, and P. Martin. (2005). Occult hepatitis B virus infection in dialysis patients: a multicentre survey. *Aliment Pharmacol Ther*, 21 (11):1341-1347.

Fattovich, G., G. Giustina, S. Favarato, and A. Ruol. (1996). A survey of adverse events in 11,241 patients with chronic viral hepatitis treated with alfa interferon. *J Hepatol*, 24 (1):38-47.

Finelli, L., J. T. Miller, J. I. Tokars, M. J. Alter, and M. J. Arduino. (2005). National surveillance of dialysis-associated diseases in the United States, 2002. *Semin Dial*, 18 (1):52-61.

Fisker, N., C. Pedersen, M. Lange, N. T. Nguyen, K. T. Nguyen, J. Georgsen, and P. B. Christensen. (2004). Molecular epidemiology of hepatitis B virus infections in Denmark. *J Clin Virol*, 31 (1):46-52.

Ganem, D., and H. E. Varmus. (1987). The molecular biology of the hepatitis B viruses. *Annu Rev Biochem*, 56:651-693.

Gomes, S. A., C. F. Yoshida, and C. Niel. (1996). Detection of hepatitis B virus DNA in hepatitis B surface antigen-negative serum by polymerase chain reaction: evaluation of different primer pairs and conditions. *Acta Virol*, 40 (3):133-138.

Goral, V., H. Ozkul, S. Tekes, D. Sit, and A. K. Kadiroglu. (2006). Prevalence of occult HBV infection in haemodialysis patients with chronic HCV. *World J Gastroenterol*, 12 (21):3420-3424.

Gutierrez, C., M. Devesa, C. L. Loureiro, G. Leon, F. Liprandi, and F. H. Pujol. (2004). Molecular and serological evaluation of surface antigen negative hepatitis B virus infection in blood donors from Venezuela. *J Med Virol*, 73 (2):200-207.

Ho, D. D., T. Moudgil, and M. Alam. (1989). Quantitation of human immunodeficiency virus type 1 in the blood of infected persons. *N Engl J Med*, 321 (24):1621-1625.

Hollinger, F. 1991. Hepatitis B virus. In *Viral Hepatitis*. New York: Raven Press 1-37

Hollinger, F. B., and T. J. Liang, eds. 2001. *Hepatitis B Virus*. Edited by D. M. Knipe and P. M. Howley. 4 ed. Philadelphia: Lippincott Williams & Wilkins.

Hu, K. Q. (2002). Occult hepatitis B virus infection and its clinical implications. *J Viral Hepat*, 9 (4):243-257.

Huy, T. T., H. Ushijima, T. Sata, and K. Abe. (2006). Genomic characterization of HBV genotype F in Bolivia: genotype F subgenotypes correlate with geographic distribution and T(1858) variant. *Arch Virol*, 151 (3):589-597.

Inoue, K., O. Ogawa, M. Yamada, T. Watanabe, H. Okamoto, and M. Yoshiba. (2006). Possible association of vigorous hepatitis B virus replication with the development of fulminant hepatitis. *J Gastroenterol*, 41 (4):383-387.

Jeantet, D., I. Chemin, B. Mandrand, A. Tran, F. Zoulim, P. Merle, C. Trepo, and A. Kay. (2004). Cloning and expression of surface antigens from occult chronic hepatitis B virus infections and their recognition by commercial detection assays. *J Med Virol*, 73 (4):508-515.

Jeantet, D., I. Chemin, B. Mandrand, F. Zoulim, C. Trepo, and A. Kay. (2002). Characterization of two hepatitis B virus populations isolated from a hepatitis B surface antigen-negative patient. *Hepatology*, 35 (5):1215-1224.

Kanbay, M., G. Gur, A. Akcay, H. Selcuk, U. Yilmaz, H. Arslan, S. Boyacioglu, and F. N. Ozdemir. (2006). Is hepatitis C virus positivity a contributing factor to occult hepatitis B virus infection in hemodialysis patients? *Dig Dis Sci*, 51 (11):1962-1966.

Kao, J. H. (2002). Clinical relevance of hepatitis B viral genotypes: a case of deja vu? *J Gastroenterol Hepatol*, 17 (2):113-115.

Karayiannis, P. (2004). Current therapies for chronic hepatitis B virus infection. *Expert Rev Anti Infect Ther*, 2 (5):745-760.

Kondili, L. A., D. Genovese, C. Argentini, P. Chionne, P. Toscani, R. Fabro, R. Cocconi, and M. Rapicetta. (2006). Nosocomial transmission in simultaneous outbreaks of hepatitis C and B virus infections in a hemodialysis center. *Eur J Clin Microbiol Infect Dis*, 25 (8):527-531.

Kramvis, A., K. Arakawa, M. C. Yu, R. Nogueira, D. O. Stram, and M. C. Kew. (2008). Relationship of serological subtype, basic core promoter and precore mutations to genotypes/subgenotypes of hepatitis B virus. *J Med Virol*, 80 (1):27-46.

Kramvis, A., and M. C. Kew. (2005). Relationship of genotypes of hepatitis B virus to mutations, disease progression and response to antiviral therapy. *J Viral Hepat*, 12 (5):456-464.

Kramvis, A., L. Weitzmann, W. K. Owiredu, and M. C. Kew. (2002). Analysis of the complete genome of subgroup A' hepatitis B virus isolates from South Africa. *J Gen Virol*, 83 (Pt 4):835-839.

Krugman, S. (1989). Hepatitis B: historical aspects. *Am J Infect Control*, 17 (3):165-167.

Lewis-Ximenez, L. L., J. M. Oliveira, L. A. Mercadante, L. De Castro, W. Santa Catharina, S. Stuver, and C. F. Yoshida. (2001). Serological and vaccination profile of hemodialysis patients during an outbreak of hepatitis B virus infection. *Nephron*, 87 (1):19-26.

Lindh, M., C. Hannoun, A. P. Dhillon, G. Norkrans, and P. Horal. (1999). Core promoter mutations and genotypes in relation to viral replication and liver damage in East Asian hepatitis B virus carriers. *J Infect Dis*, 179 (4):775-782.

Liu, C. J., and J. H. Kao. (2008). Genetic variability of hepatitis B virus and response to antiviral therapy. *Antivir Ther*, 13 (5):613-624.

Locarnini, S. (2008). Primary resistance, multidrug resistance, and cross-resistance pathways in HBV as a consequence of treatment failure. *Hepatol Int*, 2 (2):147-151.

Locarnini, S. A. (1998). Hepatitis B virus surface antigen and polymerase gene variants: potential virological and clinical significance. *Hepatology*, 27 (1):294-297.

Lurman, A. (1885). Eine icterusepidemic. *Berl Klin Wochenschr*, 22:20-23.

Lusida, M. I., V. E. Nugrahaputra, Soetjipto, R. Handajani, M. Nagano-Fujii, M. Sasayama, T. Utsumi, and H. Hotta. (2008). Novel subgenotypes of hepatitis B virus genotypes C and D in Papua, Indonesia. *J Clin Microbiol*, 46 (7):2160-2166.

Lusida, M. I., Surayah, H. Sakugawa, M. Nagano-Fujii, Soetjipto, Mulyanto, R. Handajani, Boediwarsono, P. B. Setiawan, C. A. Nidom, S. Ohgimoto, and H. Hotta. (2003). Genotype and subtype analyses of hepatitis B virus (HBV) and possible co-infection of HBV and hepatitis C virus (HCV) or hepatitis D virus (HDV) in blood donors, patients with chronic liver disease and patients on hemodialysis in Surabaya, Indonesia. *Microbiol Immunol*, 47 (12):969-975.

Margolis, H. S., M. J. Alter, and S. C. Hadler. (1991). Hepatitis B: evolving epidemiology and implications for control. *Semin Liver Dis*, 11 (2):84-92.

Mayerat, C., A. Mantegani, and P. C. Frei. (1999). Does hepatitis B virus (HBV) genotype influence the clinical outcome of HBV infection? *J Viral Hepat*, 6 (4):299-304.

McIntyre, N. (1990). Clinical presentation of acute viral hepatitis. *Br Med Bull*, 46 (2):533-547.

McMahon, B. J. (2009). The influence of hepatitis B virus genotype and subgenotype on the natural history of chronic hepatitis B. *Hepatol Int*, 3 (2):334-342.

Meldal, B. H., N. M. Moula, I. H. Barnes, K. Boukef, and J. P. Allain. (2009). A novel hepatitis B virus subgenotype, D7, in Tunisian blood donors. *J Gen Virol*, 90 (Pt 7):1622-1628.

Melegari, M., P. P. Scaglioni, and J. R. Wands. (1998). Hepatitis B virus mutants associated with 3TC and famciclovir administration are replication defective. *Hepatology*, 27 (2):628-633.

Mello, F. C., N. Martel, S. A. Gomes, and N. M. Araujo. (2011). Expression of Hepatitis B Virus Surface Antigen Containing Y100C Variant Frequently Detected in Occult HBV Infection. *Hepat Res Treat*, 2011:695859.

Mello, F. C., F. J. Souto, L. C. Nabuco, C. A. Villela-Nogueira, H. S. Coelho, H. C. Franz, J. C. Saraiva, H. A. Virgolino, A. R. Motta-Castro, M. M. Melo, R. M. Martins, and S. A. Gomes. (2007). Hepatitis B virus genotypes circulating in Brazil: molecular characterization of genotype F isolates. *BMC Microbiol*, 7:103.

Minuk, G. Y., D. F. Sun, R. Greenberg, M. Zhang, K. Hawkins, J. Uhanova, A. Gutkin, K. Bernstein, A. Giulivi, and C. Osiowy. (2004). Occult hepatitis B virus infection in a North American adult hemodialysis patient population. *Hepatology*, 40 (5):1072-1077.

Motta-Castro, A. R., R. M. Martins, N. M. Araujo, C. Niel, G. B. Facholi, B. V. Lago, F. C. Mello, and S. A. Gomes. (2008). Molecular epidemiology of hepatitis B virus in an isolated Afro-Brazilian community. *Arch Virol*, 153 (12):2197-2205.

Motta, J. S., F. C. Mello, B. V. Lago, R. M. Perez, S. A. Gomes, and F. F. Figueiredo. (2010). Occult hepatitis B virus infection and lamivudine-resistant mutations in isolates from renal patients undergoing hemodialysis. *J Gastroenterol Hepatol*, 25 (1):101-106.

Mulyanto, S. N. Depamede, K. Surayah, F. Tsuda, K. Ichiyama, M. Takahashi, and H. Okamoto. (2009). A nationwide molecular epidemiological study on hepatitis B virus in Indonesia: identification of two novel subgenotypes, B8 and C7. *Arch Virol*, 154 (7):1047-1059.

Norder, H., A. M. Courouce, P. Coursaget, J. M. Echevarria, S. D. Lee, I. K. Mushahwar, B. H. Robertson, S. Locarnini, and L. O. Magnius. (2004). Genetic diversity of hepatitis B virus strains derived worldwide: genotypes, subgenotypes, and HBsAg subtypes. *Intervirology*, 47 (6):289-309.

Norder, H., A. M. Courouce, and L. O. Magnius. (1994). Complete genomes, phylogenetic relatedness, and structural proteins of six strains of the hepatitis B virus, four of which represent two new genotypes. *Virology*, 198 (2):489-503.

Nurainy, N., D. H. Muljono, H. Sudoyo, and S. Marzuki. (2008). Genetic study of hepatitis B virus in Indonesia reveals a new subgenotype of genotype B in east Nusa Tenggara. *Arch Virol*, 153 (6):1057-1065.

Okochi, K., and S. Murakami. (1968). Observations on Australia antigen in Japanese. *Vox Sang*, 15 (5):374-385.

Olinger, C. M., P. Jutavijittum, J. M. Hubschen, A. Yousukh, B. Samountry, T. Thammavong, K. Toriyama, and C. P. Muller. (2008). Possible new hepatitis B virus genotype, southeast Asia. *Emerg Infect Dis*, 14 (11):1777-1780.

Oliveira, M. L., F. I. Bastos, P. R. Telles, C. F. Yoshida, H. G. Schatzmayr, U. Paetzold, G. Pauli, and E. Schreier. (1999). Prevalence and risk factors for HBV, HCV and HDV infections among injecting drug users from Rio de Janeiro, Brazil. *Braz J Med Biol Res*, 32 (9):1107-1114.

Ono, S. K., N. Kato, Y. Shiratori, J. Kato, T. Goto, R. F. Schinazi, F. J. Carrilho, and M. Omata. (2001). The polymerase L528M mutation cooperates with nucleotide binding-site mutations, increasing hepatitis B virus replication and drug resistance. *J Clin Invest*, 107 (4):449-455.

Ozasa, A., Y. Tanaka, E. Orito, M. Sugiyama, J. H. Kang, S. Hige, T. Kuramitsu, K. Suzuki, E. Tanaka, S. Okada, H. Tokita, Y. Asahina, K. Inoue, S. Kakumu, T. Okanoue, Y. Murawaki, K. Hino, M. Onji, H. Yatsuhashi, H. Sakugawa, Y. Miyakawa, R. Ueda, and M. Mizokami. (2006). Influence of genotypes and precore mutations on fulminant or chronic outcome of acute hepatitis B virus infection. *Hepatology*, 44 (2):326-334.

Panessa, C., W. D. Hill, E. Giles, A. Yu, S. Harvard, G. Butt, A. Andonov, M. Krajden, and C. Osiowy. (2009). Genotype D amongst injection drug users with acute hepatitis B virus infection in British Columbia. *J Viral Hepat*, 16 (1):64-73.

Paniagua, R., A. Villasis-Keever, C. Prado-Uribe Mdel, M. D. Ventura-Garcia, G. Alcantara-Ortega, S. R. Ponce de Leon, N. Cure-Bolt, and S. Rangel-Frausto. (2010). Elevated prevalence of hepatitis B in Mexican hemodialysis patients. A multicentric survey. *Arch Med Res*, 41 (4):251-254.

Perrillo, R. P., C. R. Campbell, S. Strang, C. J. Bodicky, and D. J. Costigan. (1984). Immune globulin and hepatitis B immune globulin. Prophylactic measures for intimate contacts exposed to acute type B hepatitis. *Arch Intern Med*, 144 (1):81-85.

Piot, P., C. Goilav, and E. Kegels. (1990). Hepatitis B: transmission by sexual contact and needle sharing. *Vaccine*, 8 Suppl:S37-40; discussion S41-33.

Pourkarim, M. R., P. Lemey, S. Amini-Bavil-Olyaee, P. Maes, and M. Van Ranst. (2010). Novel hepatitis B virus subgenotype A6 in African-Belgian patients. *J Clin Virol*, 47 (1):93-96.

Prince, A. M. (1968). An antigen detected in the blood during the incubation period of serum hepatitis. *Proc Natl Acad Sci U S A*, 60 (3):814-821.

Raimondo, G., T. Pollicino, I. Cacciola, and G. Squadrito. (2007). Occult hepatitis B virus infection. *J Hepatol*, 46 (1):160-170.

Ramalingam, S., T. Leung, H. Cairns, P. Sibley, M. Smith, S. Ijaz, R. Tedder, and M. Zuckerman. (2007). Transmission of hepatitis B virus (genotype E) in a haemodialysis unit. *J Clin Virol*, 40 (2):105-109.

Roll, M., H. Norder, L. O. Magnius, L. Grillner, and V. Lindgren. (1995). Nosocomial spread of hepatitis B virus (HBV) in a haemodialysis unit confirmed by HBV DNA sequencing. *J Hosp Infect*, 30 (1):57-63.

RosenheimAdvisoryGroup. 1972. Hepatitis and the Treatment of Chronic Renal Failure, edited by D. o. H. a. S. Security. London.

Sakamoto, T., Y. Tanaka, E. Orito, J. Co, J. Clavio, F. Sugauchi, K. Ito, A. Ozasa, A. Quino, R. Ueda, J. Sollano, and M. Mizokami. (2006). Novel subtypes (subgenotypes) of hepatitis B virus genotypes B and C among chronic liver disease patients in the Philippines. *J Gen Virol*, 87 (Pt 7):1873-1882.

Schaefer, S. (2005). Hepatitis B virus: significance of genotypes. *J Viral Hepat*, 12 (2):111-124.

Siagris, D., M. Christofidou, K. Triga, N. Pagoni, G. J. Theocharis, D. Goumenos, A. Lekkou, K. Thomopoulos, A. C. Tsamandas, J. Vlachojannis, and C. Labropoulou-Karatza. (2006). Occult hepatitis B virus infection in hemodialysis patients with chronic HCV infection. *J Nephrol*, 19 (3):327-333.

Simonsen, L., A. Kane, J. Lloyd, M. Zaffran, and M. Kane. (1999). Unsafe injections in the developing world and transmission of bloodborne pathogens: a review. *Bull World Health Organ*, 77 (10):789-800.

Sjogren, M. H. (1994). Serologic diagnosis of viral hepatitis. *Gastroenterol Clin North Am*, 23 (3):457-477.

Stuyver, L., S. De Gendt, C. Van Geyt, F. Zoulim, M. Fried, R. F. Schinazi, and R. Rossau. (2000). A new genotype of hepatitis B virus: complete genome and phylogenetic relatedness. *J Gen Virol*, 81 (Pt 1):67-74.

Sugiyama, M., Y. Tanaka, T. Kato, E. Orito, K. Ito, S. K. Acharya, R. G. Gish, A. Kramvis, T. Shimada, N. Izumi, M. Kaito, Y. Miyakawa, and M. Mizokami. (2006). Influence of hepatitis B virus genotypes on the intra- and extracellular expression of viral DNA and antigens. *Hepatology*, 44 (4):915-924.

Swenson, P. D., C. Van Geyt, E. R. Alexander, H. Hagan, J. M. Freitag-Koontz, S. Wilson, H. Norder, L. O. Magnius, and L. Stuyver. (2001). Hepatitis B virus genotypes and HBsAg subtypes in refugees and injection drug users in the United States determined by LiPA and monoclonal EIA. *J Med Virol*, 64 (3):305-311.

Tatematsu, K., Y. Tanaka, F. Kurbanov, F. Sugauchi, S. Mano, T. Maeshiro, T. Nakayoshi, M. Wakuta, Y. Miyakawa, and M. Mizokami. (2009). A genetic variant of hepatitis B virus divergent from known human and ape genotypes isolated from a Japanese patient and provisionally assigned to new genotype J. *J Virol*, 83 (20):10538-10547.

Te, H. S., and D. M. Jensen. (2010). Epidemiology of hepatitis B and C viruses: a global overview. *Clin Liver Dis*, 14 (1):1-21, vii.

Teles, S. A., R. M. Martins, S. A. Gomes, A. M. Gaspar, N. M. Araujo, K. P. Souza, M. A. Carneiro, and C. F. Yoshida. (2002). Hepatitis B virus transmission in Brazilian hemodialysis units: serological and molecular follow-up. *J Med Virol*, 68 (1):41-49.

Tokars, J. I., M. Frank, M. J. Alter, and M. J. Arduino. (2002). National surveillance of dialysis-associated diseases in the United States, 2000. *Semin Dial*, 15 (3):162-171.

Torbenson, M., and D. L. Thomas. (2002). Occult hepatitis B. *Lancet Infect Dis*, 2 (8):479-486.

Torresi, J., L. Earnest-Silveira, G. Deliyannis, K. Edgtton, H. Zhuang, S. A. Locarnini, J. Fyfe, T. Sozzi, and D. C. Jackson. (2002). Reduced antigenicity of the hepatitis B virus HBsAg protein arising as a consequence of sequence changes in the overlapping polymerase gene that are selected by lamivudine therapy. *Virology*, 293 (2):305-313.

Tran, T. T., T. N. Trinh, and K. Abe. (2008). New complex recombinant genotype of hepatitis B virus identified in Vietnam. *J Virol*, 82 (11):5657-5663.

Utsumi, T., M. I. Lusida, Y. Yano, V. E. Nugrahaputra, M. Amin, Juniastuti, Soetjipto, Y. Hayashi, and H. Hotta. (2009). Complete genome sequence and phylogenetic relatedness of hepatitis B virus isolates in Papua, Indonesia. *J Clin Microbiol*, 47 (6):1842-1847.

Villa, E., A. Grottola, P. Buttafoco, P. Trande, A. Merighi, N. Fratti, Y. Seium, G. Cioni, and F. Manenti. (1995). Evidence for hepatitis B virus infection in patients with chronic hepatitis C with and without serological markers of hepatitis B. *Dig Dis Sci*, 40 (1):8-13.

Vladutiu, D. S., A. Cosa, A. Neamtu, D. State, M. Braila, M. Gherman, I. M. Patiu, and I. Dulau-Florea. (2000). Infections with hepatitis B and C viruses in patients on maintenance dialysis in Romania and in former communist countries: yellow spots on a blank map? *J Viral Hepat*, 7 (4):313-319.

Wang, Z., Y. Huang, S. Wen, B. Zhou, and J. Hou. (2007). Hepatitis B virus genotypes and subgenotypes in China. *Hepatol Res*, 37 (s1):S36-41.

WHO. *Hepatitis B. World Health Organization Fact Sheet* 2008 [cited. Available from http://www.who.int/mediacentre/factsheets/fs204/en/index.html.

Wiegand, J., D. Hasenclever, and H. L. Tillmann. (2008). Should treatment of hepatitis B depend on hepatitis B virus genotypes? A hypothesis generated from an explorative analysis of published evidence. *Antivir Ther*, 13 (2):211-220.

Wreghitt, T. G. (1999). Blood-borne virus infections in dialysis units--a review. *Rev Med Virol*, 9 (2):101-109.

Yamamoto, K., M. Horikita, F. Tsuda, K. Itoh, Y. Akahane, S. Yotsumoto, H. Okamoto, Y. Miyakawa, and M. Mayumi. (1994). Naturally occurring escape mutants of hepatitis B virus with various mutations in the S gene in carriers seropositive for antibody to hepatitis B surface antigen. *J Virol*, 68 (4):2671-2676.

Yang, H., X. Qi, A. Sabogal, M. Miller, S. Xiong, and W. E. t. Delaney. (2005). Cross-resistance testing of next-generation nucleoside and nucleotide analogues against lamivudine-resistant HBV. *Antivir Ther*, 10 (5):625-633.

Zoulim, F., and S. Locarnini. (2009). Hepatitis B virus resistance to nucleos(t)ide analogues. *Gastroenterology*, 137 (5):1593-1608 e1591-1592.

3

Resistance to Recombinant Human Erythropoietin Therapy in Haemodialysis Patients

Elísio Costa[1,2], Luís Belo[2,3] and Alice Santos-Silva[2,3]
[1]*Instituto de Ciências da Saúde da Universidade Católica Portuguesa;*
[2]*Instituto de Biologia Molecular e Celular da Universidade do Porto;*
[3]*Faculdade de Farmácia da Universidade do Porto,*
Portugal

1. Introduction

The involvement of a humoral factor (named as haemopoietin) in the regulation of haematopoiesis, was firstly described in literature in 1906 (Carnot & Deflandre, 1906). However, only 40 years later a linkage between erythropoietin (EPO) and erythropoiesis was described (Bondsdorff & Jalavisto, 1948), and only in the 1950s was established that the kidney is the main site of production of EPO (Jacobson, 1957). In 1977, EPO was purified from urine collected from patients suffering from aplastic anaemia (Miyake, 1977). The nucleotide sequence of human EPO gene was determined in 1985 and the cloning and expression of the gene led to the production of recombinant human EPO (rhEPO) (Lin, 1985; Jacobs, 1985).

EPO is an endogenous cytokine that is essential in erythropoiesis regulation. This glycoprotein has a molecular mass of 30-35 kDa, 165 amino acids and is heavily glycosylated, with the carbohydrate moiety comprising approximately 40% of its weight. There are three N-terminal glycosylation sites at aspartate residues 24, 38 and 83, and one O-linked acidic oligonucleotide side-chain at serine 126. Human EPO has two disulphide bridges, between cysteines 7 and 161, and between cysteines 29 and 33, which are important in maintaining its *in vivo* bioactivity and the correct shape for binding to the EPO receptor (EPOR) (Lai, 1986).

The regulation of EPO gene expression occurs essentially at the transcriptional level by DNA-dependent mRNA synthesis and gene activation. In kidneys, hypoxia gives rise to increased EPO expression, stimulated by the DNA binding protein, hypoxia inducible factor, which binds to the 3´ flanking region of EPO gene (Wang & Semenza, 1993). EPO is secreted into the plasma and, within the bone marrow, binds to EPOR in the surface of erythroid progenitor cells. EPOR activation follows a sequential dimerization activation mechanism involving the Janus kinase 2 (JAK2), and phosphorylation and nuclear translocation of signal transducer and activator of transcription 5 (STAT5) pathways (Fig. 1).

The first clinical trial using rhEPO in the treatment of the anaemia of end-stage renal failure was published in 1987 (Eschbach, 1987), and, nowadays, rhEPO is currently used for the treatment of that anaemia in haemodialysis (HD) patients (Kimel, 2008; Obladen, 2000), as well as for a variety of other clinical situations associated with anaemia.

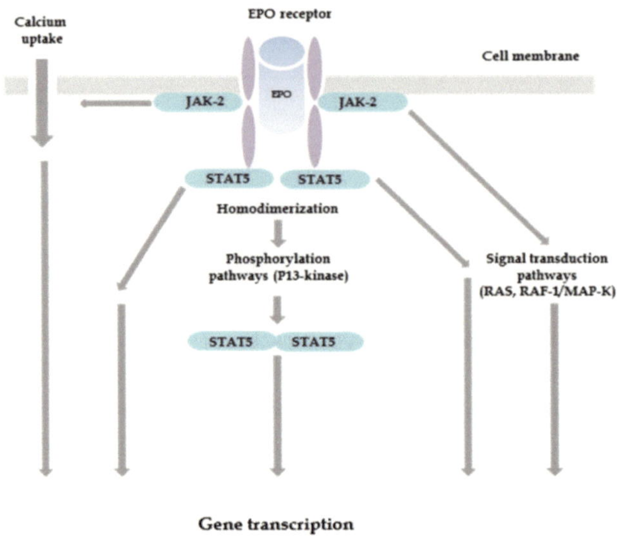

Fig. 1. Schematic diagram showing signalling pathways activated by EPO receptors (adapted from Marsden, 2006).

Anaemia is a common complication that contributes to the burden of HD patients. It has also a negative impact on cardiovascular system, cognitive function, exercise capacity and quality of life, resulting in a significant morbidity and mortality in these patients. The introduction of rhEPO therapy for treatment of anaemia of HD patients led to a significant reduction in anaemia and to an improvement in patients' quality of life (Locatti, 1998; Bárány, 2001; Locatelli, 2004a; Smrzova, 2005). There is, however, a marked variability in the sensitivity to rhEPO, with up to 10-fold variability in dose requirements to achieve correction of the anaemia. Furthermore, around 5-10% of the patients show a marked resistance to rhEPO therapy (Bárány, 2001; Macdougall, 2002a; Schindler, 2002; Smrzova, 2005). The European Best Practice Guidelines define "resistance to rhEPO therapy" as a failure to achieve target haemoglobin levels (between 11 and 12 g/dL) with maintained doses of rhEPO higher than 300 IU/Kg/week of epoetin or of higher doses than 1.5 µg/Kg/week of darbopoietin-alfa (Locatelli, 2004b).
Resistance to rhEPO has been reported as an independent risk factor for mortality in HD patients, due to both the inability to achieve the target haemoglobin levels and to the administration of high rhEPO doses, which have been associated with increased risk of myocardial infarction, congestive heart failure and stroke.
The reasons for the variability in rhEPO response are unclear (Foley, 1996; Spittle, 2001; Drueke, 2002; Cooper, 2003; Himmelfard, 2004; Smrzova, 2005). There are several conditions reported as associated with rhEPO resistance, namely, inflammation, oxidative stress and iron deficiency, as major causes (Foley, 1996; Gunnell, 1999; Spittle, 2001; Drueke, 2002; Cooper, 2003; Himmelfard, 2004; Pupim, 2004; Smrzova, 2005), and blood loss, hyperparathyroidism, aluminium toxicity and vitamin B12 or folate deficiencies, as minor causes. However, exclusion of these factors does not eliminate the marked variability in sensitivity to rhEPO (Macdougall, 2002b). In this chapter, a revision of the mechanisms proposed to underlie the resistance to rhEPO therapy will be performed, with particular emphasis on the role of inflammatory cytokines, neutrophil activation, iron status, and erythrocyte damage.

2. Inflammatory cytokines

Inflammation is the physiological response to a variety of noxious stimuli, such as tissue injury caused by infection or physical damage. It is a complex process that involves the participation of several cells and molecules, and may present different intensities and duration.

Inflammation usually refers to a localised process. However, if the noxious stimulus is severe enough, distant systemic changes may also occur, and these changes are referred as "acute phase response", which is accompanied by signs and symptoms such as fever, anorexia, and somnolence. This acute phase response may include neuroendocrine, metabolic and haematopoietic changes, as well as changes in non-protein plasma constituents (Ceciliani, 2002). The haematopoietic response includes leukocytosis and leukocyte activation, thrombocytosis, and anaemia secondary to erythrocyte damage and/or decreased erythropoiesis (Trey & Kushner, 1995).

Inflammatory stimuli induces the release of cytokines, including tumour necrosis factor (TNF)-α, interleukin (IL) -1, IL-6, and interferon (IFN)-γ, which may be produced by several cells, including leukocytes, fibroblasts and endothelial cells (Kushner, 1999). This release of cytokines causes many systemic changes, including increased synthesis and release of positive acute-phase proteins, such as C-reactive protein (CRP) and fibrinogen, as well as the suppression of negative acute-phase proteins, such as albumin and transferrin (Mcdougall, 1995; Cooper, 2003; Smrzova, 2005).

The causes for the inflammatory response in HD patients are not well clarified. There are several potential sources, including bacterial contamination of the dialyser, incompatibility with the dialyser membrane and infection of the vascular access. However, the dialysis procedure may only be partially responsible for the inflammatory response, because even patients with renal insufficiency who are not yet on dialysis present raised inflammatory markers, which rise further after starting regular HD treatment, suggesting that the disease *per se* triggers an inflammatory response (Gunnel, 1999; Schindler, 2002; Macdougall, 2002b).

The exact mechanisms by which the effects of inflammation on erythropoiesis occur are still to be determined. However, along an inflammatory response (Fig. 2), the iron from the erythropoiesis traffic is mobilised to storage sites within the reticuloendothelial system, inhibiting erythroid progenitor proliferation and differentiation, and blunting, therefore, the response to EPO (endogenous and/or exogenous). An erythropoiesis-suppressing effect has been also attributed to increased activity of pro-inflammatory cytokines reported in association with inflammatory conditions, and this relationship has been proposed as a potential factor associated to rhEPO therapy resistance (Gunnel, 1999; Schindler, 2002; Macdougall, 2002b; cooper, 2003). Actually, some studies have shown that genetic variations in some pro-inflammatory cytokines leading to increased levels of the cytokines, may play an important role in the pathogenesis of the anaemia (Maury, 2004). Recently, it was proposed that the c.511C>T polymorphism in the gene encoding for IL-1β, which is associated with increased serum levels of IL-1β, is linked to increased needs of rhEPO to correct anemia (Jeong, 2008).

It was reported that pro-inflammatory cytokines, such as IL-1, IL-2, IL-4, IL-6, TNF-α and INF-γ diminish BFU-E and CFU-E cells, resulting in suppression of erythropoiesis (Macdougall, 2002a). In fact, some of these cytokines, such as IL-1, IL-6, TNF-α, IFN-γ, and C-reactive protein (CRP), have been reported to play an important role in rhEPO resistance (Panichi, 2000; Pecoits-Filho, 2003; Cooper, 2003). Moreover, it was reported (Macdougall,

2002a) that serum derived from HD patients suppresses erythroid colony-forming response to rhEPO, in a manner that can be inhibited by antibodies against TNF-α and INF-γ. These data also strongly suggest a key role in the rhEPO response for these inflammatory mediators (Waltzer, 1984; Foley, 1996; Meier, 2002; Cooper, 2003).

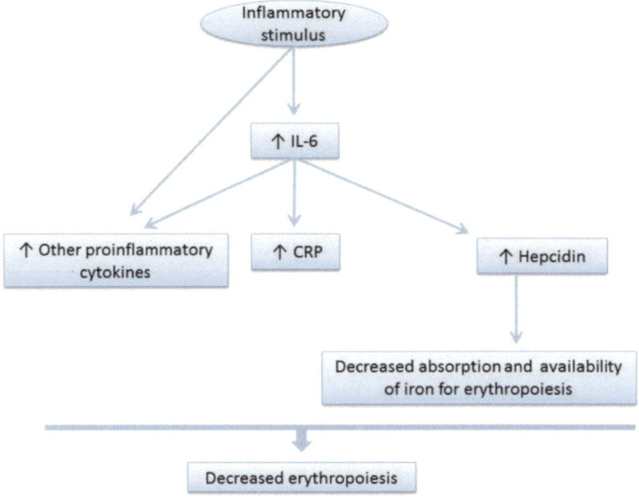

Fig. 2. Inflammatory stimulus is associated to a decrease in erythropoiesis. Interleukin-6 (IL-6) and hepcidin have a critical role in the association between inflammation and erythropoiesis.

Recently, our group demonstrated that non-responders patients, as compared to responders, presented higher CRP and neutrophil/lymphocyte ratio, and lower albumin serum levels (Costa, 2008a), suggesting a relationship between resistance to rhEPO therapy and the inflammatory response. Moreover, we observed a CD4+ lymphopenia associated with increased IL-7 serum levels (Costa, 2008b), an activation stage of T-cells and an enhanced ability of these cells to produce Th1 related cytokines (IL-2, INF-γ and TNF-α) after short term *in vitro* stimulation. This increased capacity of T-cells to produce Th1 cytokines could justify, at least in part, the anaemia found in HD patients.

These results, published by our group and by others, show that raised inflammatory cytokines are a consistent finding associated with resistance to rhEPO therapy, by acting directly in erythropoiesis and/or indirectly, by decreasing iron availability for erythropoiesis.

3. Neutrophil activation

Leukocytosis and recruitment of circulating leukocytes into the affected areas are hallmarks of inflammation. Leukocytes are chimio-attracted to inflammatory regions and their transmigration from blood to the injured tissue is primarily mediated by the expression of cell-adhesion molecules in the endothelium, which interact with surface receptors on leukocytes (Muller, 1999; Sullivan, 2000). This leukocyte-endothelial interaction is regulated by a cascade of molecular steps that correspond to the morphological changes that accompany adhesion. At the inflammatory site, leukocytes release their granular content and may exert their phagocytic capacities.

In acute inflammation, the leukocyte infiltration is predominantly of neutrophils, whereas in chronic inflammation a mononuclear cell infiltration (predominantly macrophages and lymphocytes) is observed. Although leukocyte-endothelial cell interaction is important for leukocyte extravasation and trafficking in physiological situations, there is increasing evidence that altered leukocyte-endothelial interactions are implicated in the pathogenesis of diseases associated with inflammation, possibly by damaging the endothelium or altering endothelial function (Harlan, 1985; Ley, 2007).

Leukocytosis is essential as the primary host defence, and neutrophils, the major leukocyte population of blood in adults, play a primordial role. It is well known that neutrophils have mechanisms that are used to destroy invading microorganisms. These cells use an extraordinary array of oxygen-dependent and oxygen-independent microbicidal weapons to destroy and remove infectious agents (Witko-Sarsat, 2000). Oxygen-dependent mechanisms involve the production of reactive oxygen species (ROS), which can be microbicidal (Roos, 2003), and lead to the development of oxidative stress. Oxygen-independent mechanisms include chemotaxis, phagocytosis and degranulation. The generation of microbicidal oxidants by neutrophils results from the activation of a multiprotein enzyme complex known as the reduced nicotinamide adenine dinucleotide phosphate oxidase, which catalyzes the formation of superoxide anion ($O_2^{\cdot-}$). Activated neutrophils also undergo degranulation, with the release of several components, namely, proteases (such as elastase) and cationic proteins (such as lactoferrin).

Elastase is a member of the chymotrypsin superfamily of serine proteinases, expressed in monocytes and mast cells, but mainly expressed by neutrophils, where it is compartmentalized in the primary azurophil granules. The intracellular function of this enzyme is the degradation of foreign microorganisms that are phagocytosed by the neutrophil (Brinkmann, 2004). Elastase can also degrade local extracellular matrix proteins (such as elastin), remodel damaged tissue, and facilitate neutrophil migration into or through tissues. Moreover, elastase also modulates cytokine expression at epithelial and endothelial surfaces, up-regulating the production of cytokines, such as IL-6, IL-8, transforming growth factor β (TGF-β) and granulocyte-macrophage colony-stimulating factor (GM-CSF); it also promotes the degradation of cytokines, such as IL-1, TNF-α and IL-2. There is evidence in literature that high levels of elastase are one of the major pathological factors in the development of several chronic inflammatory lung conditions (Fitch, 2006).

Few data exists in literature about a possible correlation between leukocyte activation, particularly with neutrophil activation, and resistance to rhEPO therapy. In a recent study, we found that patients under HD, particularly those who were non-responders to rh-EPO therapy, presented a decreased expression of the CXCR1 neutrophil surface markers (Pereira, 2010) and higher elastase plasma levels (tables 1 and 2).

	Controls (n=18)	**Responders (n=26)**	**Non-Responders (n=8)**
CXCR1 (MFI)	308.40 ± 76.3	261.30 ± 45.74*	222.85 ± 29.01*§
CD11b (MFI)	236.3±81.9	223.33 ± 73.99	207.96 ± 86.50

Table 1. Neutrophil activation markers for controls and for responders and non-responders HD patients.*p<0.05 *vs* controls; § p<0.05 *vs* Responders. MFI: mean fluorescence intensity. * Data are presented as the mean fluorescence intensity of each cell marker (MFI) ± two standard deviations. Adapted from Pereira, 2010.

	Controls (n=26)	Responders (n=32)	Non-responders (n=31)
Hb (g/dL)	13.90 (13.2-15.00)	11.70 (10.83-12.68)*	10.4 (9.00-11.30) *§
White cell counts (x 10^9/L)	5.78 ± 1.59	6.42 ± 1.96	6.04 ± 2.26
Lymphocytes (x 10^9/L)	2.35 ± 0.75	1.58 ± 0.49*	1.36 ± 0.69 *§
Monocytes (x 10^9/L)	0.25 ± 0.08	0.40 ± 0.13*	0.35 ± 0.17*
Neutrophils (x 10^9/L)	3.03 ± 1.02	4.17 ± 1.87*	4.11 ± 1.73*
Albumin (g/dL)	ND	4.0 ± 0.4	3.7 ± 0.4§
CRP (mg/dL)	1.75 (0.76-4.70)	3.20 (1.73-7.23)*	10.14 (3.82-38.99)*§
Elastase (µg/L)	28.29 (26.03-34.74)	34.13 (28.76-39.16)*	39.75 (31.15-64.84)*§
Elastase/Neutrophil ratio	10.86 (7.44-12.12)	8.70 (7.32-11.42)	10.25 (7.56-17.41)

Table 2. Haematological data and neutrophil activation markers, for controls and for responders and non-responders HD patients.* $p<0.05$, *vs* controls; § $p<0.05$, *vs* responders. NM: not done. Results are presented as mean ± standard deviation and as median (interquartile ranges). Hb: Haemoglobin; CRP: C-reactive protein. Adapted from Costa, 2008c.

CXCR1 is a receptor that recognizes CXC chemokines, particularly the pro-inflammatory IL-8 (Pay, 2006; Sherry, 2008). The decreased expression of this receptor in neutrophil surface is associated to the release of components of neutrophil granules and reflects the need for inotropic support. Recently, it was shown that the levels of the neutrophil chemoattractant receptor, CXCR1, are mildly diminished in pediatric patients, as a consequence of end stage renal disease itself, and that recurrent serial bacterial infection markedly exacerbated the loss of CXCR1 by neutrophils (Sherry, 2008). This loss of CXCR1 on neutrophils can be due to the uremic state, to changes in leukocyte adhesion molecule expression or membrane microvilli and/or to cross-desensitization of this receptor, due to prior exposure to several unrelated chemoattractants, including N-formylated peptides and the complement cleavage product C5a. Chronic exposure of circulating inflammatory cells to these mediators may lead also to loss of this chemokine receptor expression and/or function via cross-desensitization.

The HD procedure, itself, seems to lead to neutrophil activation found in HD patients (Costa, 2008c). However, the rise in neutrophil activation products observed after the HD procedure does not explain the higher neutrophil activation found in non-responders patients. Actually, a significant positive correlation between elastase levels and CRP, suggests that the rise in neutrophil activation is part of the inflammatory process found in HD patients, which is particularly enhanced in non-responders. The statistically significant correlation that we found between elastase levels and the weekly rhEPO doses also strengthens this hypothesis; in fact, non-responders to rhEPO therapy patients, requiring higher weekly rhEPO doses to achieve target hemoglobin levels, present an increased inflammatory process (Costa, 2008c).

4. Iron status

Iron is an essential trace element that is required for growth and development of living organisms, but excess of free iron is toxic for the cell (Arth, 1999; Atanasio, 2006). Mammals lack a regulatory pathway for iron excretion, and iron balance is maintained by the tight regulation of iron absorption from the intestine (Park, 2001; Atanasio, 2006). The intestinal

iron absorption is regulated by the level of body iron stores and by the amount of iron needed for erythropoiesis (Arth, 1999; Park, 2001; Atanasio, 2006; Nemeth, 2003).
In HD patients, iron absorption is similar to that found in healthy individuals; however, when under rhEPO therapy, the absorption of iron increases as much as 5 times (Skikne, 1992). This increased iron absorption is not sufficient to compensate for the iron lost during the HD procedure, and with the frequent blood draws performed on these patients. For this reason, and because the association of rhEPO with iron therapy achieves a better erythropoietic response, intravenous iron administration has become a standard therapy for most patients receiving rhEPO. To avoid iron overload, with potentially harmful consequences, there is a need to monitor iron therapy by performing regular blood tests reflecting body's iron stores. However, analytical and intra-individual variability of classical iron markers, limits its value. For instance, in case of inflammation, several parameters (transferrin and ferritin) used to study iron status, are misleading. This, triggered the search for more useful new markers to monitor patients with disturbances in iron status. One of these new markers is the soluble transferrin receptor (sTfR), which reflects the iron needs of the erythroid cells and is independent of an on-going inflammatory process. More recently, a complex regulatory network that governs iron traffic emerged, and points to hepcidin as a major evolutionary conserved regulator of iron distribution (Nicolas, 2002; Kemma, 2005; Nemeth, 2006). This small hormone produced by the mammalian liver has been proposed as a central mediator of dietary iron absorption, due to its inhibitory effect in iron uptake from the small intestine, and in iron release from macrophages and hepatocytes, leading to decreased iron availability for erythropoiesis; a decreased placental iron transport was also observed (Kulaksiz, 2004). The synthesis of hepcidin is regulated by anemia/hypoxia, inflammation and iron overload.
The *in vitro* stimulation of fresh human hepatocytes by pro-inflammatory IL-6 showed a strong induction of hepcidin mRNA, indicating that this cytokine is an important mediator of hepcidin induction, in inflammation (Fleming, 2001; Dallilio, 2003; Hsu, 2006; Domenico, 2007). Moreover, it was shown that hepcidin expression is also regulated by other hepatic proteins, including the hereditary hemacromatosis protein (HFE), transferrin receptor 2, hemojuvelin, bone morphogenic proteins, transferrin and EPO (Fig. 3).
Hepcidin is synthesized as preprohepcidin, a protein with 84 amino acids. This peptide is cleaved, leading to prohepcidin with 60 aminoacids, which is further processed, giving rise to the 25 aminoacids protein, hepcidin (Dallilio, 2003; Hsu, 2006). Hepcidin was reported to bind to the transmembrane iron exporter ferroportin, which is present on macrophages, on the basolateral site of enterocytes, and also on hepatocytes. *In vitro* studies showed that hepcidin induces the internalization and degradation of ferroportin, crucial for cellular iron export (Domenico, 2007). By diminishing the effective number of iron exporters on the membrane of the enterocytes and of the macrophages, hepcidin inhibits iron uptake and release, respectively. This is the phenotype of ferroportin disease, in which the deficiency in ferroportin leads to iron accumulation, mainly in macrophages, and, usually, to anaemia (Njajou, 2002).
Increased hepcidin expression along an inflammatory process, explains sequestration of iron in the macrophages and inhibition of intestinal iron absorption, the two hallmarks of the anaemia of inflammation, which is normocytic or microcytic iron-refractory (Nicolas, 2002; Kulaksiz, 2004; Hsu, 2006). This decreased availability in iron may be a host defence mechanism against invading microorganisms.

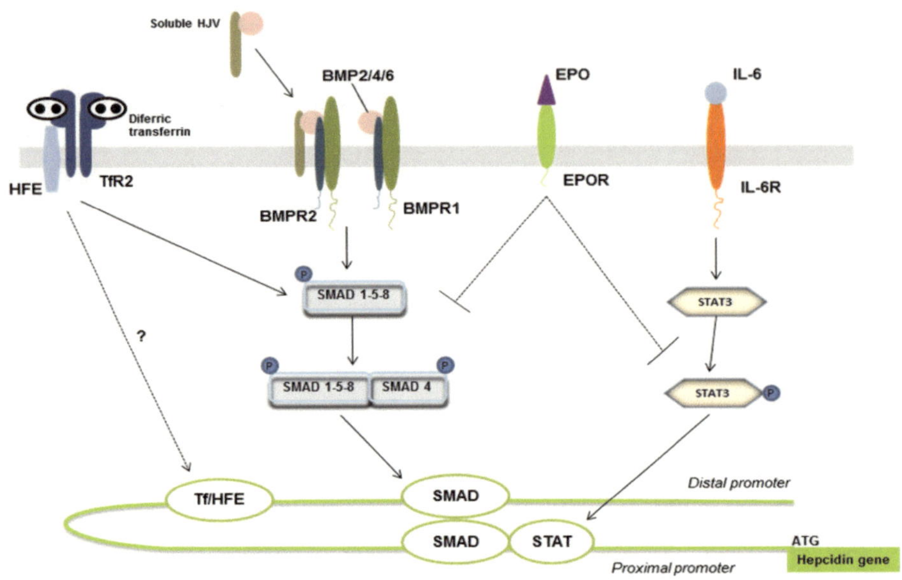

Fig. 3. Schematic pathways involved in hepcidin gene expression. Interleukin (IL)- 6 stimulates hepcidin synthesis via STAT activation; bone morphogenic proteins (BMP) stimulate hepcidin gene expression in a pathway dependent on hemojuvelin (HJV), BMP receptors (BMPR1 and BMPR2), and SMAD activation; transferrin also stimulates hepcidin gene expression in a pathway dependent on transferrin receptor 2 (TfR2), HFE protein, and SMAD activation. Erythropoietin (EPO) has an inhibitory effect in hepcidin expression in a pathway dependent on EPO receptor (EPOR), and STAT and SMAD inhibition. For simplicity, only some factors associated with hepcidin expression are shown.

The resistance to rhEPO therapy has been associated with disturbances in iron metabolism. Actually, the main cause for rhEPO resistance described in literature in HD patients, is iron deficiency, which persists in some patients, even after iron supplementation (Drueke, 2001). This iron deficiency can be absolute, with serum ferritin concentration less than 100 mg/dL, or functional.

We recently reported that HD patient's non-responders to rhEPO therapy present a mild to moderate anaemia, even with the administration of higher rhEPO doses (Costa, 2008d). This anaemia is hypochromic (decreased mean cell haemoglobin and mean cell haemoglobin concentration), and presents with a more accentuated anisocytosis than in HD patients that are good responders to rhEPO therapy. The haematological changes in non-responders seem to reflect a "functional" iron deficiency, as they presented adequate iron stores, as defined by conventional criteria, and an apparent inability to mobilize the iron needed to adequately support erythropoiesis. Actually, no statistically significant differences were found in serum iron status markers between responders and non-responders HD patients, except for the soluble transferrin receptor (s-TfR), which was significantly higher in non-responders (Table 3). The levels of this soluble receptor may be increased in two clinical settings, in case of increased erythropoietic activity and of iron deficiency (Atanasio, 2006; Deicher, 2006). We observed in our HD patients a positive and significant correlation between s-TfR and the weekly rhEPO/Kg doses, suggesting that s-TfR was an indicator of the erythropoietic stimuli of the administrated rhEPO, and not an indicator of iron body deficiency. Moreover, no differences were found for transferrin saturation, between responders and non-responders HD patients, excluding, therefore, iron deficiency as the principal cause of the elevated s-TfR found in HD patients non-responders to rhEPO therapy.

	Controls (n=25)	Responders (n=25)	Non-responders (n=25)
Iron (µg/dL)	73.42 ± 25.24	60.24 ± 22.97	50.40 ± 29.27*
Ferritin (ng/mL)	85.10 (37.88-123.95)	380.30 (252.30-543.75)*	452.00 (163.00-674.50)*
Transferrin (mg/dL)	231.50 (205.00-268.00)	173.00 (152.50-186.00)*	161.00 (139.00-211.00)*
TS (%)	21.83 ± 7.97	25.05 ± 9.69	20.73 ± 12.09
s-TfR (nmol/L)	20.85 ± 8.56	19.56 ± 6.83	34.13 ± 11.4§
Prohepcidin (ng/mL)	92.11 ± 18.28	165.72 ± 36.69*	137.77 ± 46.03*§
CRP (mg/dL)	1.75 (0.76-4.70)	3.20 (1.73-7.23)*	10.14 (3.82-38.99)*§
s-IL2R (nmol/L)	758.83 ± 234.95	4005.71 ± 1835.70*	4394.17 ± 1701.80*
IL-6 (pg/mL)	1.90 (0-3.75)	5.75 (3.83-13.95)*	8.80 (4.55 – 21.30)*

Table 3. Serum markers of iron status and of inflammation, for controls, responders and non-responders HD patients.* $p<0.05$, *vs* controls; § $p<0.05$, *vs* responders. Results are presented as mean ± standard deviation and as median (interquartile ranges). TS: Transferrin saturation; CRP: C-reactive protein; s-IL2R: Soluble interleukin-2 receptor; IL-6: Interleukin-6. Adapted from Costa, 2008d.

Inverse correlations between CRP and mean cell volume, mean cell haemoglobin, serum iron and transferrin saturation were also found in non-responders patients, suggesting that the "functional" iron deficiency may be related with the enhanced chronic inflammation found in these patients. Actually, as previously referred hepcidin may have an import key role in "anaemia of inflammation" by limiting iron availability for erythropoiesis and, in that way provides a direct link between inflammation and iron metabolism.

In literature there is evidence that HD patients present increased serum levels of prohepcidin and hepcidin (Costa, 2008d; Costa, 2009). As non-responders patients present high inflammatory markers, it would be expected that prohepcidin and hepcidin serum levels were increased in non-responders patients. However, in our studies, we found that non-responders patients present lower prohepcidin, and a trend to lower hepcidin serum levels, when compared with responder's patients (Fig. 4). These findings might result from the downregulation of liver hepcidin expression induced by high doses of rhEPO, acting, therefore, as a hepcidin inhibitory hormone. Since non-responders were treated with much higher doses of rhEPO, as compared with responders, the lower prohepcidin and hepcidin levels among non-responders could be explained by this inhibitory effect of rhEPO.

Our data suggest that hepcidin serum levels are dependent on the degree of the inflammatory stimuli and of the therapeutic doses of rhEPO. In addition, the use of high doses of rhEPO, may induce increased iron utilization by the bone marrow, that may lead to depletion of iron stores and to a decrease in iron availability for erythroid cells, which will trigger a decrease in prohepcidin and hepcidin levels, in order to favour iron absorption (Costa, 2008d; Costa, 2009).

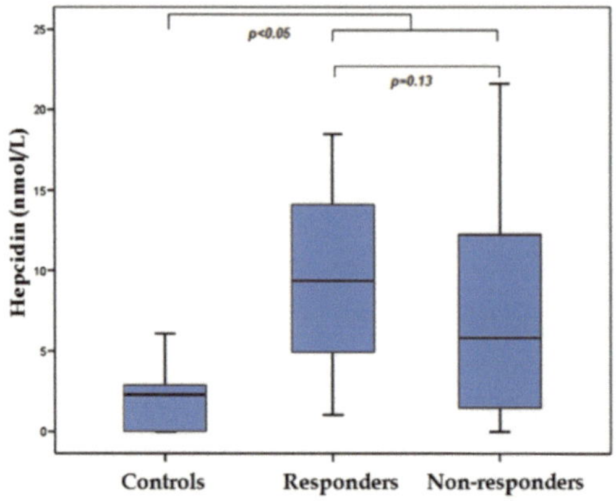

Fig. 4. Serum hepcidin levels for controls and for HD patients, responders and non-responders to rhEPO therapy. Boxplot shows median value (horizontal line in box) and first and third quartiles (inferior and superior line of the box, respectively). Adapted from Costa, 2009.

There is evidence in literature of a close interaction between inflammation, iron status and hepcidin serum levels, which, ultimately, regulates intracellular iron absorption and availability. It is also accepted that hepcidin plays a significant role in anaemia of HD patients; however, we wonder it is useful as a marker of resistance to rhEPO therapy, considering the overlap of the hepcidin levels between responders and non-responders HD patients, and the several influences and interrelations with other substances.

Clearly, more work is required for a better understanding about the role of iron metabolism in the development of resistance to rhEPO therapy and to provide useful therapeutic biomarkers of resistance.

5. Erythrocyte damage

The erythrocyte membrane is a complex structure comprising a lipidic bilayer, integral proteins and the skeleton. Spectrin is the major protein of the cytoskeleton, and, therefore, the major responsible for erythrocyte shape, integrity and deformability. It links the cytoskeleton to the lipid bilayer, by vertical protein interactions with the transmembrane proteins, band 3 and glicophorin A (Lucchi, 2000). In the vertical protein interaction of spectrin with band 3 are also involved ankyrin (known as band 2.1) and protein 4.2. A normal linkage of spectrin with the other proteins of the cytoskeleton assures normal horizontal protein interactions.

In HD patients, the erythrocytes are physically stressed during the HD procedure, metabolically stressed by the unfavourable plasmatic environment, due to metabolite accumulation, and by the high rate of haemoglobin autoxidation, due to the increase in haemoglobin turnover, a physiologic compensation mechanism triggered in case of anaemia (Lucchi, 2000; Stoya, 2002). The erythrocytes are, therefore, continuously challenged to sustain haemoglobin in its reduced functional form, as well as to maintain the integrity and deformability of the membrane.

When haemoglobin is denatured, it links to the cytoplasmic pole of band 3, triggering its aggregation and leading to the formation of strictly lipidic portions of the membrane, poorly linked to the cytoskeleton. These cells are, probably, more prone to undergo vesiculation (loss of poorly linked membrane portions) whenever they have to circulate through the HD membranes or the microvasculature. Vesiculation may, therefore, lead to modifications in the erythrocyte membrane of HD patients (Reliene, 2002; Rocha, 2005).

Erythrocytes that develop intracellular defects earlier during their life span are removed prematurely from circulation (Santos-Silva, 1998; Rocha-Pereira, 2004). The removal of senescent or damaged erythrocytes seems to involve the development of a senescent neoantigen on the membrane surface, marking the cell for death. This neoantigen is immunologically related to band 3 (Kay, 1994). The deterioration of the erythrocyte metabolism and/or of its antioxidant defences may lead to the development of oxidative stress within the cell, allowing oxidation and linkage of denatured haemoglobin to the cytoplasmatic domain of band 3, promoting its aggregation, the binding of natural antiband 3 autoantibodies and complement activation, marking the erythrocyte for death. The band 3 profile [high molecular weight aggregates (HMWAg), band 3 monomer and proteolytic fragments (Pfrag)], differs between younger, damaged and/or senescent erythrocytes. Older and damaged erythrocytes present with higher HMWAg and lower Pfrag. Younger erythrocytes show reduced HMWAg and higher Pfrag (Santos-Silva, 1998). Several diseases, known as inflammatory conditions, present an abnormal band 3 profile, suggestive of oxidative stress development (Santos-Silva, 1998; Belo, 2002; Rocha-Pereira, 2004).

Leukocyte activation is part of an inflammatory response, and is an important source of ROS and proteases, both of which may impose oxidative and proteolytic damages to erythrocyte and plasma constituents. Actually, oxidative stress has been reported to occur in HD patients and has been proposed as a significant factor in HD-related shortened erythrocyte survival.

Erythrocyte membrane protein studies performed in HD patients, using cuprophane and polyacrylonitrile dialysis membranes, showed a reduction in spectrin and band 3, and an isolated reduction in band 3, respectively (Delmas-Beauvieux, 1995).

As referred, we hypothesized that non-responders patients to rhEPO therapy could have an enhanced erythrocyte damage and/or senescence; we, actually, found an altered erythrocyte membrane band 3 profile in HD patients, with a decrease in HMWAg, Pfrag and in Pfrag/band 3 monomer and HMWAg/band 3 monomer ratios, as compared to control. This profile presents changes reflecting the co-existance of an increased number of younger and damaged erythrocytes. Non-responders patients also showed a decrease in Pfrag and in Pfrag/band 3 monomer ratio (Fig. 5), suggesting that they present a higher number of damaged erythrocytes that may result from an even more adverse plasmatic microenvironment (Costa, 2008e).

We also found some changes in erythrocyte membrane protein composition of HD patients using high-flux polysulfone FX-class dialysers of Fresenius, being the decrease in spectrin the most significant change. This reduction in spectrin may account for a poor linkage of the cytoskeleton to the membrane, favoring membrane vesiculation, and, probably, a reduction in the erythrocyte lifespan of these patients (Reliene, 2002). Significant increases in protein bands 6 and 7 were also observed, which may further reflect an altered membrane protein interaction and destabilization of membrane structure. This membrane destabilization was further strengthened by the significant changes observed for spectrin/band 3 ratio (table 4). In non-responders HD patients these changes were more accentuated than in responders, presenting a trend to lower values for spectrin (table 4) and significantly lower value for ankyrin/band 3 and spectrin/ankyrin ratios (Costa, 2008f; Costa, 2008g). These enhanced alterations may be due to a higher erythrocyte metabolic stress and/or to changes resulting from the HD procedure *per se*.

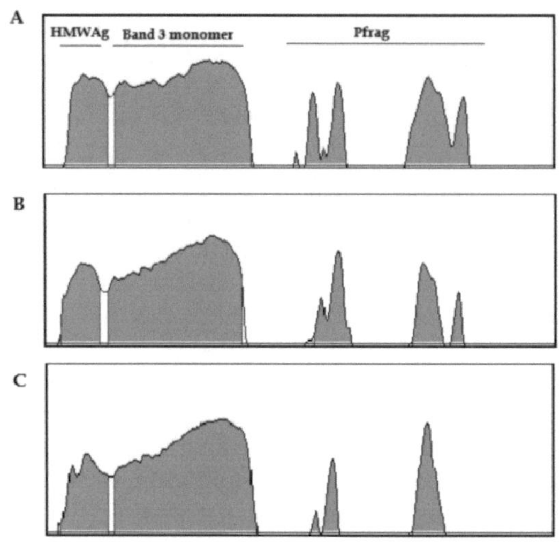

Fig. 5. Examples of densitometer tracing of immunoblots for band 3 profile. A- Control; B- Responder HD patient; C- Non-responder HD patient.

	Controls (n=26)	Responders (n=32)	Non-responders (n=31)
Spectrin (%)	27.63 (26.41-28.79)	24.75 (22.38-26.63)*	22.35 (18.95-25.92)*
Ankyrin (%)	6.97±1.62	6.09±2.07	6.97±1.60§)
Band 3 (%)	38.57 ± 3.99	39.92±4.03	38.65±3.70
Protein 4.1 (%)	7.56±1.45	7.18±1.33	7.31 ±1.63
Protein 4.2 (%)	5.51±0.72	5.54±1.57	5.35±1.29
Band 5 (%)	6.82±0.86	6.70±1.02	7.04±1.00
Band 6 (%)	5.19±1.04	6.61±1.30*	7.37±1.32*
Band 7 (%)	2.20±0.65	3.16±0.98*	3.49±1.43*
Protein 4.1/Spectrin	0.276 ± 0.624	0.310 ± 0.105	0.340 ± 0.130*
Protein 4.1/Band 3	0.192 (0.154–0.227)	0.183 (0.154-0.208)	0.183 (0.159-0.205)
Protein 4.2/Band 3	0.149 (0.125-0.162)	0.135 (0.110-0.169)	0.142 (0.110-0.161)
Spectrin/Band 3	0.707 (0.649-0.822)	0.572 (0.541-0.685)*	0.544 (0.486 -0.687)*
Ankyrin/Band 3	0.185 ± 0.585	0.155 ± 0.060	0.183 ± 0.052§
Spectrin/Ankirin	4.18 ± 1.07	4.44 ± 2.25	3.10 ± 0.94*§

Table 4. Erythrocyte membrane protein profile for controls, responders and non-responders HD patients.* $p<0.05$, *vs* controls; § $p<0.05$, *vs* responders. Results are presented as mean ± standard deviation and as median (interquartile ranges). Adapted from Costa, 2008f.

Although HD procedure seems to have an important role in these alterations in erythrocyte membrane protein composition, their exact origin(s) are not fully understood. We hypothesized that the increased plasma levels of elastase found in HD patients could induce alterations in erythrocyte membrane proteins, leading to a decrease in erythrocyte lifespan in HD patients, particularly enhanced in non-responders, and, consequently, to an increase in the degree of the anaemia, in these patients (Fig. 6).

To establish the value of elastase in the erythrocyte membrane changes observed in HD patients, we performed in a more recent study (unpublished data), some *in vitro* assays using erythrocytes from 18 HD patients (10 responders and 8 non-responders) and from 8 healthy controls; erythrocyte suspensions in phosphate buffered saline, pH 7.4, were incubated at 37° C, under gentle rotation, in the presence of 0.03, 0.1 and 0.5 μg/mL of neutrophil elastase. These assays used erythrocytes collected before and immediately after HD procedure. Before the HD procedure, the erythrocytes from responders and non-responders HD patients are more susceptible to the proteolytic action of elastase than the erythrocytes from the controls, and this susceptibility is more pronounced for the erythrocytes from non-responders. As after the HD procedure the composition of the erythrocyte membrane from both responders and non-responders did not change, it seems that the more susceptible erythrocytes are removed during the HD procedure.

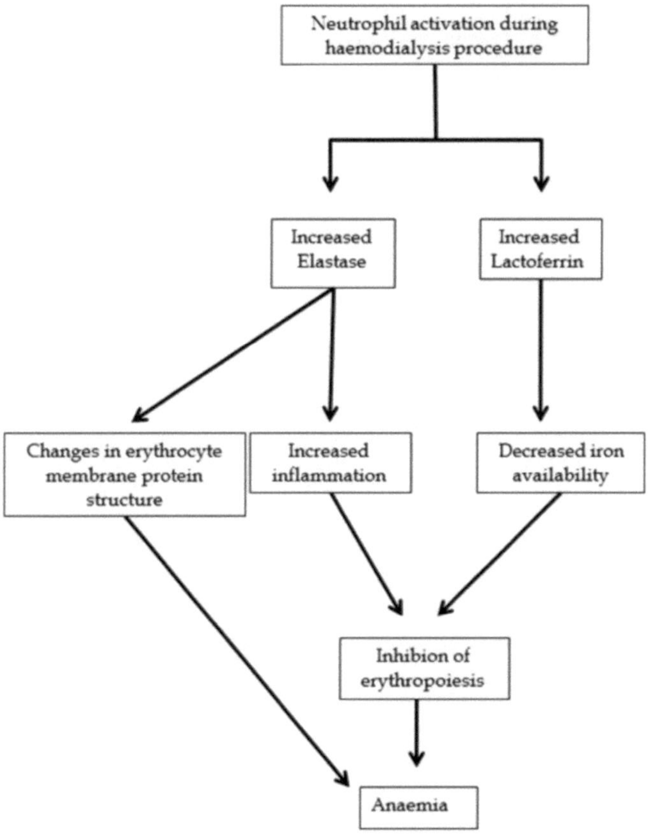

Fig. 6. In HD patients, the increased plasma levels of elastase can induce changes in erythrocyte membrane proteins, leading to a decrease in the erythrocyte lifespan and, consequently, to increase the degree of anaemia in these patients. Moreover, the increased levels of elastase might exacerbate the inflammatory process that has an inhibitory effect on erythropoiesis. The release of lactoferrin during the HD procedure may contribute to decrease iron availability for erythropoisis. These changes are enhanced in non-responders HD patients.

5. Conclusions

Although the etiology of resistance to rhEPO therapy is still unknown, inflammation seems to have an important role in its pathophysiology. Resistance to rhEPO therapy is also associated with "functional" iron deficiency, neutrophil activation, and with changes in erythrocyte membrane protein structure.

The exact origins of the inflammatory process remain unclear. We wonder if the release of elastase during the HD procedure could amplify the inflammatory process in HD patients, particularly in non-responders, and if this elastase release has a role in the alterations observed in the erythrocyte membrane protein structure, further contributing to worsening of anaemia (Fig 6). The inflammatory process, the rhEPO doses administrated, and the lactoferrin release during the haemodialysis procedure, seem to play an important role in iron uptake from the small intestine, in the release of iron from macrophages and, finally, in the availability of iron for erythropoiesis.

Further studies are needed to better understand the rise in inflammation and the associated need for higher doses of rhEPO and reduced iron availability. It is also important to clarify the effect of higher levels of elastase in the inflammatory process, and in the alterations in the erythrocyte membrane protein composition and in the band 3 profile.

New therapeutic options, in order to decrease rhEPO doses, are currently under investigation, namely the protein product of the growth arrest-specific gene 6, the mixture of herbal extracts - jusen-taiho-to, the growth hormone, the insulin-like growth factors-1, and the development of an inhibitor of hepcidin.

6. Acknowledgments

This work was supported by national funds-"Fundacao Portuguesa para a Ciencia e Tecnologia" (FCT:PIC/IC/83221/2007) and co-financed by FEDER (FCOMP-01-0124-FEDER-008468).

7. References

Allen, D.A.; Breen, C.; Yaqoob, M.M. & Macdougall, I.C. (1999). Inhibition of CFU-E colony formation in uremic patients with inflammatory disease: role of INF-γ and TNF- α. *J Invest Med*, Vol. 47, pp. 204-11, ISSN 0021-9738

Arth, R.H. (1999). Iron metabolism in end-stage renal disease. *Seminars in Dialysis*, vol. 12, pp. 224-230, ISSN 0894-0959

Atanasio, V.; Manolescu, B. & Stoian, I. (2006). Hepcidin – central regulator. *Eur J Haematol*, vol. 78, pp. 1-10, ISSN 0902- 4441

Bárány, P. (2001). Inflammation, serum C-reactive protein, and erythropoietin resistance. *Nephrol Dial transplant*, vol. 16, pp. 224-227, ISSN 0931- 0509

Belo, L.; Rebelo, I.; Castro, E.M.B.; Catarino, C.; Pereira-Leite, L.; Quintanilha, A. & Santos-Silva, A. (2002). Band 3 as a marker of erythrocyte changes in pregnancy. *Eur J Haematol*, vol. 69, pp. 145-151, ISSN 0902- 4441

Bondsdorff, E. & Jalavisto E. (1948). A humoral mechanism in anoxic erythrocytosis. *Acta Physiol Scand*, vol. 16, pp.150-170, ISSN 1365-201X

Brinkmann, V.; Reichard, U.; Goosmann, C.; Fauler, B.; Uhlemann, Y.; Weiss, D.S.; Weinrauch, Y. & Zychlinsky, A. (2004). Neutrophil extracellular traps kill bacteria. *Science*, vol. 303, pp.1532-1535, ISSN 0036-8075

Carnot, P. & Deflandre C. (1906). Sur l´activite hemopoietique du serum au cours de la regeneration du sang. *C R Acad Sci (Paris)*, vol.143,pp.384-386, ISSN 1287-4620

Ceciliani, F.; Giordano, A. & Spagnolo, V. (2002). The systemic reaction during inflammation: the acute-phase proteins. *Curr Pharm Des*, vol. 9, pp. 211-223, ISSN 1381-6128

Cooper, A.C.; Breen, C.P.; Vyas, B.; Ochola, J.; Kemeny, D.M. & Macdougall, I.C. (2003). Poor response to recombinant erythropoitin is associated with loss of T-lymphocyte CD28 expression and altered interleukin-10 production. *Nephrol Dial Transplant*, vol. 18, pp. 133-40, ISSN 0931- 0509

Cooper, A.C.; Mikhail, A.; Lethbridge, M.W.; Kemeny, D.M. & Macdougall, I.C. (2003). Increased expression of erythropoiesis inhibiting cytokines (IFN-γ, TNF-α, IL-10, and IL-13) by T cells in patients exhibiting a poor response to erythropoietin therapy. *J Am Soc Nephrol*, vol. 14, pp. 1776- 1784, ISSN 1046-6673

Costa, E.; Lima, M.; Alves, J.M.; Rocha, S.; Rocha-Pereira, P.; Castro, E.; Miranda, V.; Faria, M.S.; Loureiro, A.; Quintanilha, A.; Belo, L. & Santos-Silva A. (2008a). Inflammation, T-cell phenotype, and inflammatory cytokines in chronic kidney disease patients under hemodialysis and its relationship to resistance to recombinant human erythropoietin therapy. *J Clin Immunol*, vol. 28, pp. 268-275, ISSN 0271-9142

Costa, E.; Lima, M.; Rocha, S.; Rocha-Pereira, P.; Castro, E.; Miranda, V.; Faria, M.S.; Loureiro, A.; Quintanilha, A.; Belo, L. & Santos-Silva, A. (2008b). IL-7 serum levels and lymphopenia in hemodialysis patients, non-responders to recombinant human erythropoietin therapy. *Blood Cells Mol Dis*, vol. 4, pp. 134-1355, ISSN 1079- 9796

Costa, E.; Rocha, S.; Rocha-Pereira, P.; Nascimento, H.; Castro, E.; Miranda, V.; Faria, M.S.; Loureiro, A.; Quintanilha, A.; Belo, L. & Santos-Silva, A. (2008c). Neutrophil activation and resistance to recombinant human erythropoietin therapy in hemodialysis patients. *Am J Nephrol*, vol. 28, pp. 935-940, ISSN 1046-6673

Costa, E.; Pereira, B.J.G.; Rocha-Pereira, P.; Rocha, S.; Reis, F.; Castro, E.; Teixeira, F.; Miranda, V.; Sameiro- Faria, M.; Loureiro, A.; Quintanilha, A.; Belo, L. & Santos-Silva, A. (2008d). Role of prohepcidin, inflammatory markers and iron status in resistance to rhEPO therapy in hemodialysis patients. *Am J Nephrol*, vol. 28, pp. 677-683, ISSN 1046-6673

Costa, E.; Rocha, S.; Rocha-Pereira, P.; Castro, E.; Miranda, V.; Sameiro-Faria, M.; Loureiro, A.; Quintanilha, A.; Belo, L. & Santos-Silva, A. (2008e). Band profile as a marker of erythrocyte changes in chronic kidney disease patients. *The Open Clinical Chemistry Journal*, vol. 1, pp. 57-63, ISSN 1874-2416

Costa, E.; Rocha, S.; Rocha-Pereira, P.; Castro, E.; Miranda, V.; Sameiro-Faria, M.; Loureiro, A.; Quintanilha, A.; Belo, L. & Santos-Silva, A. (2008f). Alterated erythrocyte membrane protein composition in chronic kidney disease stage 5 patients under haemodialysis and recombinant human erythropoietin therapy. *Blood Purif*, vol. 26, pp. 267-273, ISSN 0253-5068

Costa, E.; Rocha, S.; Rocha-Pereira, P.; Castro, E.; Miranda, V.; Sameiro-Faria, M.; Loureiro, A.; Quintanilha, A.; Belo, L. & Santos-Silva, A. (2008g). Changes in red blood cells membrane protein composition during hemodialysis procedure. *Ren Fail*, vol. 30, pp. 971-975, ISSN 0886- 022

Costa, E.; Swinkels, D.W.; Laarakkers, C.M.; Rocha-Pereira, P.; Rocha, S.; Reis, F.; Teixeira, F.; Miranda, V.; Sameiro-Faria, M.; Loureiro, A.; Quintanilha, A.; Belo, L. & Santos-Silva, A. (2009). Hepcidin serum levels and resistance to recombinant human erythropoietin therapy in haemodialysis patients. *Acta Haematol*, vol. 122, pp. 226-229, ISSN 0001-5792

Dallalio, G.; Fleury, T. & Means, R.T. (2003). Serum hepcidin in clinical specimens. *Br J Haematol*, vol. 122, pp. 996-1000, ISSN 0007-1048

Deicher, R. & Horl, W.H. (2006). New insights into the regulation of iron homeostasis. *European J Clin Invest*, vol. 36, pp. 301-309, ISSN: 0014-2972

Delmas-Beauvieux, M.C.; Combe, C.; Peuchant, E.; Carbonneau, M.A.; Dubourg, L.; de Précigout, V.; Aparicio, M.; Clerc, M. (1995). Evaluation of red blood cell lipoperoxidation in hemodialysed patients during erythropoietin therapy supplemented or not with iron. *Nephron*, vol. 69, pp. 404-410, ISSN 0028-2766

Domenico, I.; Ward, D.M.; Langelier, C.; Vaughn, M.B.; Nemeth, E.; Sundquist, W.I.; Ganz, T.; Musci, G. & Kaplan, J. (2007). The molecular mechanism of hepcidin-mediated ferroportin down-regulation. *Mol Biol Cell*, vol. 18, pp. 2569-2578, ISSN 1059-1524

Drueke, T. (2001). Hyporesponsiveness to recombinant human erythropoietin. *Nephrol Dial Transplant*, vol. 16, pp. 25–28 ISSN 0931- 0509

Drueke, T.B. & Eckardt, K.U. (2002). Role of secondary hyperparathyroidism in erythropoietin resistance of chronic renal failure patients. *Nephrol Dial Transplant*, vol. 17, suppl 5, pp. 28-31, ISSN 0931- 0509

Eschbach, J.W.; Egrie, J.C.; Downing, M.R.; Browne, J.K. & Adamson, J.W. (1987). Correction of the anemia of end-stage renal disease with recombinant human erythropoietin. Results of a combined phase I and II clinical trial. *N Engl J Med*, vol. 316, pp. 73-78, ISSN 0028-4793

Fitch, P.M.; Roghanian, A.; Howie, S.E.M. & Sallenave, J.M. (2006). Human neutrophil elastase inhibitors in innate and adaptive immunity. *Biochemical Society Transactions*, vol. 34, pp. 279-282, ISSN 0300-5127

Fleming, R.E. & Sly, W.S. (2001). Hepcidin: a putative iron-regulatory hormone relevant to hereditary hemochromatosis and the anemia of chronic disease. *Proc Natl Acad USA*, vol. 98, pp. 8160-8162, ISSN 0027-8424

Foley, R.N.; Parfrey, P.S.; Harnett, J.D.; Kent, G.M.; Murray, D.C. & Barre, P.E. (1996). The impact of anemia on cardiomyopathy morbidity and mortality in endstage renal disease. *Am J Kidney Dis*, vol. 28, pp. 53-61, ISSN 0272-6386

Gunnell, J.; Yeun, J.Y.; Depner, T.A. & Kaysen G.A. (1999). Acute-phase response predicts erythropoietin resistance in hemodialysis and peritoneal dialysis patients. *Am J Kidney Dis*, vol. 33, pp. 63-72, ISSN 0272-6386

Harlan, J.M. (1985). Leukocyte-endothelial interactions. *Blood*, vol. 65, pp. 513- 525, ISSN 0006-4971

Himmelfarb, J. (2004). Linking oxidative stress and inflammation in kidney disease: which is the chicken and which is the egg? *Seminars in Dialysis*, vol. 17, pp. 449-454, ISSN 0894-0959

Hsu, S.P.; Ching, C.K.; Chien, C.T. & Hung, K.Y. (2006). Plasma Prohepcidin positively correlates with haematocrit in chronic hemodialysis patients. *Blood Purif*, vol. 24, pp. 311-316, ISSN 0253-5068

Jacobson, L.O.; Goldwasser, E.; Fried, W. & Ptzak L. (1957). Role of the kidney in erythropoiesis. *Nature*, vol. 179, pp.633-634, ISSN 0028-0836

Jeong, K.; Lee, T.; Lee, S. & Moon, J. Polymorphisms in two genes, IL-1B and ACE, are associated with erythropoietin resistance in Korean patients on maintenance hemodialysis. *Exp Mol Med*, vol. 40, pp. 161-166, ISSN 1226-3613

Kay, M.M.; Wyant, T. & Goodman, J. (1994). Autoantibodies to band 3 during aging and disease and aging interventions. *Ann N Y Acad Sci*, vol. 719, pp. 419- 447, ISSN 0077-8923

Kemma, E.; Tjalsma, H.; Laarakkers, C.; Nemeth, E.; Willems, H. & Swinkels, D. (2005). Novel urine hepcidin assay by mass spectrometry. *Blood*, vol. 106, pp. 3268-3270, ISSN 0006-4971

Kimel, M.; Leidy, N.K.; Mannix, S. & Dixon, J. (2008). Does epoetin alfa improve health-related quality of life in chronically ill patients with anemia? Summary of trials of cancer, HIV/AIDS, and chronic kidney disease. *Value Health*, vol. 11, pp. 57-75, ISSN 1524-4733

Kulaksiz, H.; Gehrke, S.G.; Janetzko, A.; Rost, D.; Bruckner, T.; Kallinowski, B. & Stremmel, W. (2004). Pro-hepcidin: expression and cell specific localization in the liver and its regulation in hereditary haemochromatosis, chronic renal insufficiency, and renal anemia. *Gut*, vol. 53, pp. 735-743, ISSN 0017-5749

Kushner, I. & Rzewnicki, D. (1999). Acute phase response, In: *Inflammation: basic principles and clinical correlates*, Gallin, J.I.; Snyderman, R.; Fearon, D.T.; Haynes, B.F. & Nathan C. (Ed.), 317-293, Lippincott Williams and Wilkins, ISBN 978-039-7517-59-6, Philadelphia, USA

Lai, P.H.; Everett, R.; Wang, F.F.; Arakawa, T. & Goldwasser E. (1986). Structural characterization of human erythropoietin. *J Biol Chem*, Vol. 261, pp.3116-3121, ISSN 0021-9258

Ley, K.; Laudanna, C.; Cybulsky, M.I. & Nourshargh, S. (2007). Getting to the site of inflammation: the leukocyte adhesion cascade updated. *Nature Reviews Immunology*, vol. 7, pp. 678-689, ISSN 1474-1733

Lin, K.; Suggs, S.; Lin, C.; Browne, J.; Smalling, R.; Egrie, J.C.; Chen, K.K.; Fox, G.M.; Martin, F.; Stabinsky, Z.; Badrawi, S.M.; Lai, P. & Goldwassert E. (1985). Cloning and expression of the human erythropoietin gene. *Proc Natl Acad Sci USA*, vol. 82, pp. 7580-4, ISSN 0027-8424

Locatelli, F.; Aljama, P.; Barany, P.; Canaud, B.; Carrera, F.; Eckardt, K.U.; Horl, W.H.; Macdougal, I.C.; Macleod, A.; Wiecek, A. & Cameron, S. (2004a). European Best Practice Guidelines Working Group. Revised European best practice guidelines for the management of anemia in patients with chronic renal failure. *Nephrol Dial Transplant*, vol. 19, Suppl 2, pp. ii1-ii47, ISSN 0931- 0509

Locatelli, F.; Pisoni, R.L.; Combe, C.; Bommer, J.; Andreucci, V.E.; Piera, L.; Greenwood, R.; Feldman, H.I.; Port, F.K. & Held, P.J. (2004b). Anaemia in haemodialysis patients of five European countries: association with morbidity and mortality in the Dialysis Outcomes and Practice Patterns Study (DOPPS). *Nephrol Dial Transplant*, vol. 19, pp. 121-132, ISSN 0931- 0509

Locatelli, F.; Conte, F. & Marcelli, D. (1998). The impact of hematocrit levels and erythropoietin treatment on overall and cardiovascular mortality and morbidity –

the experience of the Lombardy dialysis registry. *Nephrol Dial Transplant*, vol. 13, pp. 1642-1644, ISSN 0931- 0509

Lucchi, L.; Bergamini, S.; Botti, B.; Rapanà, R.; Ciuffreda, A.; Ruggiero, P.; Ballestri, M.; Tomasi, A. & Albertazzi, A. (2000). Influence of different hemodialysis membrane on red blood cell susceptibility of oxidative stress. *Artif Organs*, vol. 24, pp. 1-6, ISSN 1525-1594

Macdougal, I.C. (1995). Poor response to erythropoietin: practical guidelines on investigation and management. *Nephrol Dial Transplant*, vol. 10, pp. 607-614, ISSN 0931- 0509

Macdougall, I.C. & Cooper, A.C. (2002a). Erythropoietin resistance: the role of inflammation and pro-inflammatory cytokines. *Nephrol Dial Transplant*, vol. 17, Suppl 11, pp. 39-43, ISSN 0931- 0509

Macdougall, I.C. & Cooper, A.C. (2002b). Erythropoietin resistance: the role of inflammation and pro-inflammatory cytokines. *Nephrol Dial Transplant*, vol. 17, suppl 11, pp. 39-43, ISSN 0931- 0509

Marsden, J.T. (2006). Erythropoietin - measurement and clinical applications. *Ann Clin Biochem*, vol. 43, pp.97-104, ISSN 0004-5632

Maury, C.P.J.; Liljestrom, M.; Laiho, K.; Tiitinen, S.; Kaarela, K. & Hurme, H. (2004). Anaemia of chronic didease in AA amyloidosis is associated with allele 2 of the interleukin-1β-511 promoter gene and raised levels of interleukin-1β and interleukin-18. *J Int Med*, vol. 256, pp. 145-152, ISSN 0884-8734

Means, R.T. & Krantz, S.B. (1996). Inhibition of human erythroid colony forming units by interferons α and β: differing mechanisms despite shared receptor. *Exp Haematol*, vol. 24, pp. 204-208, ISSN 1127-0020

Meier, P.; Dayer, E.; Blanc, E. & Wauters, J.P. (2002). Early T cell activation correlates with expression of apoptosis markers in patients with end stage renal disease. *J Am Soc Nephol*, vol. 13, pp. 204-212, ISSN 1046-6673

Miyake, T.; Kung, C. & Goldwasser, E. (1977). Purification of human erythropoietin. *J Biol Chem*, vol. 252, pp. 5558-5564, ISSN 0021-9258

Muller, W.A. (1999). Leukocyte-endothelial cell adhesion molecules in transendothelial migration, pp. 585-592, In: *Inflammation: basic principles and clinical correlates*, Gallin, J.I.; Snyderman, R.; Fearon, D.T.; Haynes, B.F. & Nathan C. (Ed.), 585-592, Lippincott Williams and Wilkins, ISBN 978-039-7517-59-6, Philadelphia, USA

Nemeth, E.; Valore, E.V.; Territo, M.; Schiller, G.; Lichtenstein, A. & Ganz, T. (2003). Hepcidin, a putative mediator of anemia of inflammation, is type II acute-phase protein. *Blood*, vol. 101, pp. 2461-2463, ISSN 0006-4971

Nemeth, E.; Preza, G.C.; Jun, C.L.; Kaplan, J.; Waring, A.J. & Ganz, T. (2006). The N terminus of hepcidin is essential for its interation with ferroportin: struture-function study. *Blood*, vol. 107, pp. 328-333, ISSN 0006-4971

Nicolas, G.; Chauvet, C.; Viatteb, L.; Danan, J.L.; Bigard, X.; Devaux, I.; Beaumont, C.; Kahn, A. & Vaulont, S. (2002). The gene encoding the iron regulatory peptide hepcidin is regulated by anemia, hypoxia, and inflammation. *J Clin Invest*, vol. 110, pp. 1037-1044, ISSN 0021-9738

Njajou, O.T.; Jong, G.; Berghuis, B.; Vaessen, N.; Snijders, P.J.; Goossens, J.P.; Wilson, J.H.; Breuning, M.H.; Oostra, B.A.; Heutink, P.; Sandkuijl, L.A. & van Duijn, C.M. (2002).

Dominant hemochromatosis due to N144H mutation of SLC11A3: clinical and biological characteristics. *Blood Cells Mol Dis*, vol. 29, pp. 439-443, ISSN 1079- 9796

Obladen, M.; Diepold, K. & Maier, R.F. (2000). Venous and arterial hematologic profiles of very low birth weight infants. European Multicenter rhEPO Study Group. *Pediatrics*, vol. 106, pp. 707-711, ISSN 0031 4005

Panichi, V.; Migliori, M.; Pietro, S.; Taccola, D.; Bianchi, A.M.; Norpoth, M.; Giovannini, L.; Palla, R. & Tetta, C. (2000). Plasma C-reactive protein in hemodialysis patients: a cross-sectional, longitudinal clinical survey. *Blood Purif*, vol.18, pp. 30–36, ISSN 0253-5068

Park, C.H.; Valore, A.J.; Waring, A.J. & Ganz, T. (2001). Hepcidin, a urinary antimicrobial peptide synthesized in the liver. *J Biol Chem*, vol. 276, pp. 7806-10, ISSN 0021-9258

Pay, S.; Musabak, U.; Simşek, I.; Pekel, A.; Erdem, H.; Dinç, A. & Sengül, A. (2006). Expression of CXCR-1 and CXCR-2 chemokine receptors on synovial neutrophils in inflammatory arthritides: does persistent or increasing expression of CXCR-2 contribute to the chronic inflammation or erosive changes? *Joint Bone Spine*, vol. 73, pp. 691-6, ISSN 1778-7254

Pecoits-Filho, R.; Heimburger, O.; Barany, P.; Suliman, M.; Fehrman- Ekholm, I.; Lindholm, B. & Stenvinkel, P. (2003). Associations between circulating inflammatory markers and residual renal function in CRF patients. *Am J Kidney Dis*, vol. 41, pp. 1212–1218, ISSN 0272-6386

Pereira, R.; Costa, E.; Gonçalves, M.; Miranda, V.; Sameiro-Faria, M.; Quintanilha, A.; Belo, L.; Lima, M. & Santos-Silva, A. (2010). Neutrophil and monocyte activation in chronic kidney disease patients under hemodialysis and its relationship with resistance to recombinant human erythropoietin and to the hemodialysis procedure. *Hemodial Int*, vol. 14, pp. 295-301, ISSN 1492-7535

Pupim, L.B.; Himmelfarb, J.; McMonagle, E.; Shyr, Y. & Ikizler, T.A. (2004). Influence of initiation of maintenance hemodialysis on biomarkers of inflammation and oxidative stress. *Kidney International*, vol. 65, pp. 2371- 2379, ISSN 0085-2538

Reliene, R.; Marini, M.; Zanella, A.; Reinhart, W.H.; Ribeiro, M.L.; del Giudice, E.M.; Perrotta, S.; Ionoscon, A.; Eber, S. & Lutz, H.U. (2002). Splenectomy prolongs in vivo survival of erythrocytes differently in spectrin/ankyrin- and band 3-deficient hereditary spherocytosis. *Blood*, vol. 100, pp. 2208-2215, ISSN 0006-4971

Rocha, S.; Rebelo, I.; Costa, E.; Catarino, C.; Belo, L.; Castro, E.M.B.; Cabeda, J.M.; Barbot, J.; Quintanilha, A. & Santos-Silva, A. (2005). Protein deficiency balance as a predictor of clinical outcome in hereditary spherocytosis. *Eur J Haematol*, vol. 74, pp. 374-80, ISSN 0902- 4441

Rocha-Pereira, P.; Santos-Silva, A.; Rebelo, I.; Figueiredo, A.; Quintanilha, A. & Teixeira, F. (2004). Erythrocyte damage in mild and severe psoriasis. *Br J Dermatology*, vol. 150, pp. 232–44, ISSN 0007-0963

Roos, D.; Van Bruggen, R. & Meischl, C. (2003). Oxidative killing of microbes by neutrophils. *Microbes Infect*, vol. 5, pp. 1307–1315, ISSN 1286-4579

Santos-Silva, A.; Castro, E.M.B.; Teixeira, N.A.; Guerra, F.C. & Quintanilha, A. (1998). Erythrocyte membrane band 3 profile imposed by cellular aging, by activated neutrophils and by neutrophilic elastase. *Clin Chim Acta*, vol. 275, pp.185–196, ISSN 0009-8981

Schindler, R.; Senf, R. & Frei U. (2002). Influencing the inflammatory response of hemodialysis patients by cytokine elimination using large-pore membranes. *Nephrol Dial Transplant*, vol. 17, pp. 17-19, ISSN 0931- 0509

Sherry, B.; Dai, W.W.; Lesser, M.L. & Trachtman, H. (2008). Dysregulated chemokine receptor expression and chemokine-mediated cell trafficking in pediatric patients with ESRD. *Clin J Am Soc Nephrol*, vol. 3, pp. 397-406, ISSN 1555-9041

Skikne, B.S. & Cook, J.D. (1992). Effect of enhanced erythropoiesis on iron absortion. *J Lab Clin Med*, vol. 120, pp. 746-751, ISSN 0022-2143

Smrzova, J.; Balla, J. & Bárány, P. (2005). Inflammation and resistance to erythropoiesis-stimulating agents--what do we know and what needs to be clarified? *Nephrol Dial Transplant*, vol. 20, Suppl 8, pp. viii2-7, ISSN 0931- 0509

Spittle, M.A.; Hoenich, N.A.; Handelman, G.J.; Adhikarla, R.; Homel, P. & Levin, N.W. (2001). Oxidative stress and inflammation in hemodialysis patients. *Am J Kidney Diseases*, vol. 38, pp. 1408-1413, ISSN 0272-6386

Stoya, G.; Klemm, A.; Baumann, E.; Vogelsang, H.; Ott, U.; Linss, W. & Stein, G. (2002). Determination of autofluorescence of red blood cells (RBCs) in uremic patients as a marker of oxidative damage. *Clin Nephrol*, vol. 58, pp.198-204, ISSN 0301- 0430

Sullivan, G.W.; Sarembock, I.J. & Linden, J. (2000). The role of inflammation in vascular diseases. *J Leukoc Biol*, vol. 67, pp. 591-602, ISSN 0741-5400

Trey, J.E. & Kushner, I. (1995). The acute phase response and the hematopoietic system: the role of cytokines. *Crit Rev Oncol Hematol*, vol. 21, pp. 1-18, ISSN 1040-8428

Waltzer, W.C.; Bachvaroff, R.J.; Raisbeck, A.P.; Egelandsdal, B.; Pullis, C.; Shen, L. & Rapaport, F.T. (1984). Immunological monitoring in patients with endstage renal disease. *J Clin Immunol*, vol. 4, pp. 364-368, ISSN 0271-9142

Wang, G.L. & Semenza, G.L. (1993). General involvement of hypoxia-inducible factor 1 in transcriptional response to hypoxia. *Proc Natl Acad Sci USA,* vol. 90, pp. 4304-4308, ISSN 0027-8424

Witko-Sarsat, V.; Rieu, P.; Descamps-Latscha, B.; Lesavre, P. & Halbwachs-Mecarelli, L. (2000). Neutrophils: molecules, functions and pathophysiological aspects. *Lab Invest*, vol. 80, pp. 617–653, ISSN 0023-6837

4

Blood Pressure and Hemodialysis

Robert Ekart[1], Sebastjan Bevc[1] and Radovan Hojs[2]
Clinic for Internal Medicine,
[1]Department of Dialysis and
[2]Department of Nephrology,
University Medical Centre Maribor,
Slovenia

1. Introduction

Hypertension is common in patients with advanced stages of chronic kidney disease (CKD) and its prevalence remain very high in patients with end stage renal disease (ESRD) treated with hemodialysis. Using various definitions of hypertension, the prevalence of hypertension in hemodialysis patients is up to 90%. The diagnosis of hypertension in hemodialysis patients is often complicated especially because there are large swings in blood pressure with dialysis and it is difficult to accurately ascertain the blood pressure in the interdialytic period.

The pathogenesis of hypertension in hemodialysis patients is multilayered and at present still not completely elucidated. One or more of the factors play a role in a individual patient - hypervolemia, increased sympathetic activity, erythropoietin, altered endotelial cell function and many others.

Poorly controlled hypertension is a risk factor for cardiovascular disease, congestive heart failure, and cerebrovascular disease in the general population. The influence of hypertension on cardiovascular outcomes in hemodialysis patients is less clear, and complicated because of the high prevalence of comorbid conditions in these patients. The management of hypertension is difficult in hemodialysis patients, because there is a significant difference in blood pressure between the pre-, post- and interdialytic period. The best timing and method of blood pressure measurement in hemodialysis patients is still uncertain. The blood pressure variability and extreme changes of the volemic state make it difficult to obtain a truly representative value of blood pressure in hemodialysis patients if based only on an isolated blood pressure measurements in dialysis center. There are many differences related to technique of blood pressure measurement, timing of measurement in relation to hemodialysis session, and reliance on the use of home blood pressure measurements or ambulatory blood pressure monitoring (ABPM). Casual conventional sphygmomanometry blood pressure measurements at home and in dialysis center are far from being ideal to reflect blood pressure levels precisely in hemodialysis patients and adjusting antihypertensive treatment according to casual blood pressure measurements may cause an inadequate blood pressure control.

ABPM is the most reproducible method of blood pressure measurement in hemodialysis patients, and most would argue that it should be used as the gold standard for the definition

of hypertension in ESRD. ABPM has also been used to better define the relationship between blood pressure, target organ damage, and outcomes in patients with CKD and ESRD. ABPM has been shown to predict cardiovascular events better than conventional blood pressure measurement in patients with essential hypertension. Although many patients received antihypertensive drugs, only small percent have adequately controlled blood pressure. There are many reasons for this problem.
The purpose of this chapter is to discuss about the pathogenesis of hypertension, definition of hypertension, optimal time and target blood pressure, different methods of blood pressure measurements, discuss the relationship between blood pressure and cardiovascular outcomes and - finally outline the therapies to control blood pressure in hemodialysis population.

2. Pathogenesis of hypertension in end stage renal disease

Several of the generally accepted pathogenetic factors that may be involved in the development of hypertension in ESRD and CKD are listed in Table 1. These will be discussed separatelly.

2.1 Sodium and volume excess

The normal physiologic response to intravascular volume expansion in the healthy person is to increase glomerular filtration via a rise in cardiac output, enhance urinary sodium excretion by supression of the renin-angiotensin-aldosterone system, and increase natriuresis as a result of the effects of atrial natriuretic peptide and an endogenous digitalis-like factor. The result of these physiologic adaptations is natriuresis and diuresis, and restoration of normal plasma volume. In contrast, excess extracellular fluid volume and increases in total body exchangeable sodium are common in patients with ESRD, because of diminished sodium and fluid excretory capacity. It has been shown that normotensive patients have significantly less total body water than hypertensive hemodialysis patients, demonstrating the importance of intravascular volume in the pathogenesis of hypertension in patients with ESRD (Lins et al, 1997).

Sodium and volume excess
Increased sympathetic activity
Activation of the renin - angiotensin - aldosterone system due to primary vascular disease or regional ischemia induced by scarring
Erythropoietin administration
An increase in endothelium-derived vasoconstrictors (endothelin) or a reduction of endothelium-derived vasodilators (nitric oxide)
Parathyroid hormone excess secretion
Renal vascular disease
Worsening of preexisting essential hypertension
Reduced production of prostaglandins/bradykinins

Table 1. Putative Pathogenetic Mechanisms of Hypertension in ESRD patients.

Overhydration and sodium retention plays a role not only by volume overload, but also by nonhemodynamic direct effects on the left ventricle and vascular system. The patients at greatest risk in a vicious cycle (fluid overload → problems in removing fluid → further fluid overload) are those who begin dialysis with low predialysis blood pressures as the result of severe cardiac failure. The prognosis of these patients is very poor because fluid can be removed only very slowly in such patients. To further aggravate this situation, dialysis patients often have diastolic dysfunction. In these patients, even a small decrease in filling pressure following dialysis ultrafiltration may result in decreased cardiac output and hypotension. As a result, fluid accumulation progresses inexorably. In addition, autonomic neuropathy complicating uremia and diabetes with inadequate peripheral arteriolar tone reactivity further increases the risk that hypotension occurs when the patient is still fluid overloaded. While the importance of salt regulating fluid balance by dietetic means and avoidance of sodium loading during dialysis has received major emphasis, sodium has also been proposed as a uremic toxin with specific effects stimulating oxidative stress. Possibly related to this is the finding that excess sodium may be stored nonosmotically at concentrations of 180 to 190 mEq/L in skin, connective tissue, cartilage, and bone, possibly bound to glucosoaminoglycans. Under various circumstances, this sodium could be intermittently released into the circulation causing hypervolemia and oxidative stress. Control of volume status can either normalize the blood pressure or make the hypertension easier to control in the great majority of dialysis patients. Volume status of ESRD patients influences both pre- and postdialysis blood pressure. Volume status is perhaps the most important factor in the development and maintenance of hypertension in dialysis patients (Mailloux & Haley, 1998). Volume expansion leads to an elevation in blood pressure through the combination of an increase in cardiac output and an inappropriately high systemic vascular resistance. Numerous authors described a correlation between hypertension and hypervolemia in dialysis patients, since hypervolemia is the cause of hypertension in up to 90% of dialysis patients (De Leeuw, 1994, Katzarski et al, 1997, Kirchner, 1997, Luik et al, 1998, Özkahya et al, 1999, Remuzzi, 1999, Agarwal et al, 2011). Also our study with 86 included hemodialysis patients confirmed this as well (Ekart & Hojs, 2006). Estimation of excess of volume is dependent upon estimation of dry weight. In a dialysis patient, dry weight is that body weight at the end of dialysis at which the patient can remain normotensive until the next dialysis despite the retention of salt water (saline). Dry weight varies over time as lean body mass and body fat change. At dry weight, the extracellular volume is at or near normal but not less than normal (Charra et al, 1996). An incorrect estimation of dry weight will lead either to chronic fluid overload or chronic underhydration. The blood pressure should remain in the normal range during the whole interdialytic period. If the patient remains hypertensive after a dialysis or becomes hypertensive before the next dialysis, he is, by definition, above his dry weight (Charra et al, 1996). The postdialysis body weight should ideally reflect a state of normohydration. The assessment of dry weight is usually based on clinical observations, such as weight gain, blood pressure, jugular venous pressure, presence of edema, congestion, and chest X-ray parameters (Cheriex et al, 1989, Katzarski et al, 1997). These methods are not very reliable, and a more accurate, objective, non-invasive assessment of optimal dry weight is therefore mandatory. The diameter of the inferior vena cava may be used to evaluate the volume state and serve as a guideline for assessing dry weight. Inferior vena cava diameter measured in expiration just below the diaphragm in the hepatic segment in patients lying in a supine position, correlated well with central venous pressure (Figure 1). Inferior vena cava diameter, corrected for body surface area between 8.0 and 11.5 mm/m^2, was considered to represent normovolemia (Cheriex et al, 1989). The collapse index was defined as ({maximal diameter on expiration minus minimal diameter on deep inspiration}divided by maximal diameter on expiration) times 100 (Figure 2 & 3). Hypervolemia (mean right atrial pressure > 7 mmHg) was defined as a collapse index of less than 40% and/or inferior vena cava diameter of above 11.5 mm/m^2. Hypovolemia (mean right atrial pressure < 3 mmHg) was defined as a inferior vena cava diameter of less than 8 mm/m^2 and/or collapse index of more than 75% (Cheriex et al, 1989). In patients with severe valvular and pulmonary disease, and patients in whom there is an increased inthrathoracic or intrabdominal pressure, these measurements are unreliable. Unfortunately, one problem with a reliance upon a clinical assessment of volume status is that volume expansion may persist even among those thought to have attained dry weight. The timing of the postdialysis inferior vena cava diameter measurement is critical. During hemodialysis, ultrafiltrated fluid is primarily removed from the circulating blood volume, which is refilled by fluid from the interstitial space. Since this process does not occur instantaneously, a state of disequilibrium follows hemodialysis, during which refilling continues and blood volume increases until equilibrium is attained; this must be taken into account when using inferior vena cava diameter to assess dry weight. The lowest values of inferior vena cava diameter were found immediately at the end of hemodialysis, followed by an increase during the following 2 hours due to refilling of the plasma volume from the interstitial space (Katzarski et al, 1997). Thus, it seems doubtful that measurements of inferior vena cava diameter within 2 hours after hemodialysis reliably reflect the state of hydration.

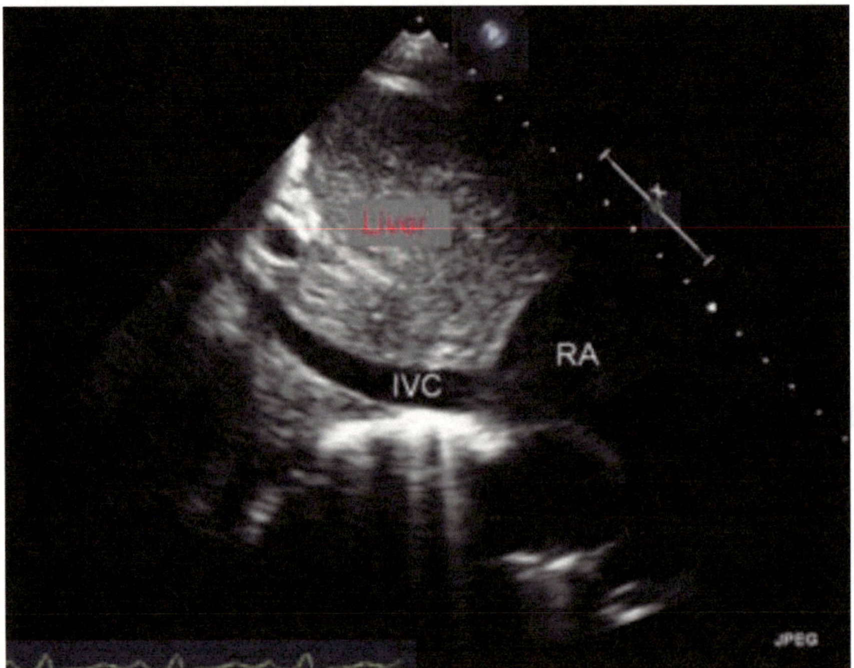

Fig. 1. Ultrasound determination of inferior vena cava (IVC) diameter; RA=right atrium.

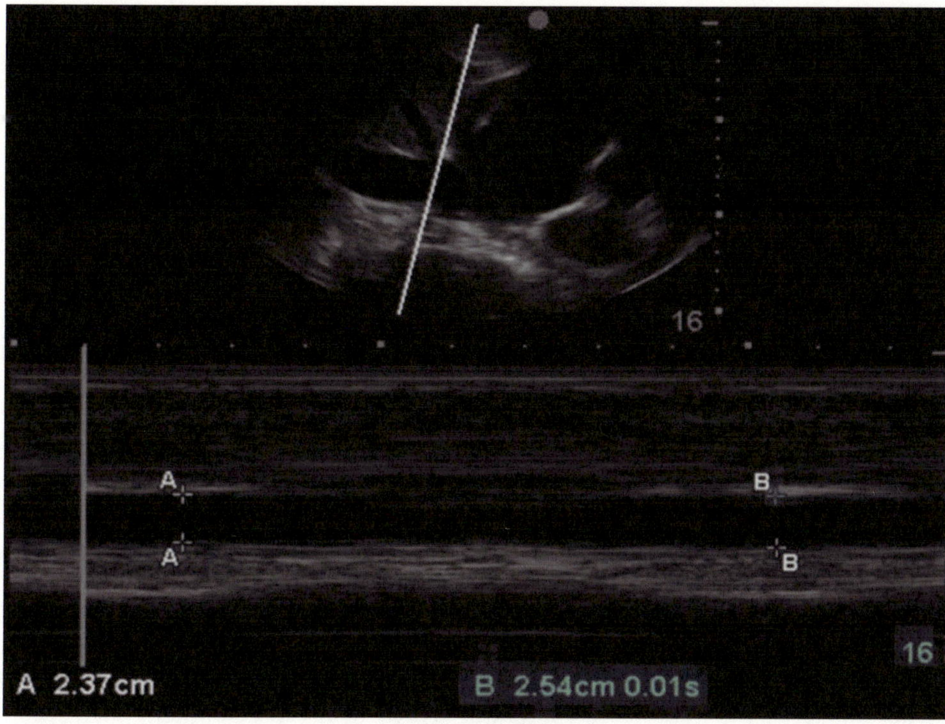

Fig. 2. Inferior vena cava diameter through the respiratory cycle using M mode.

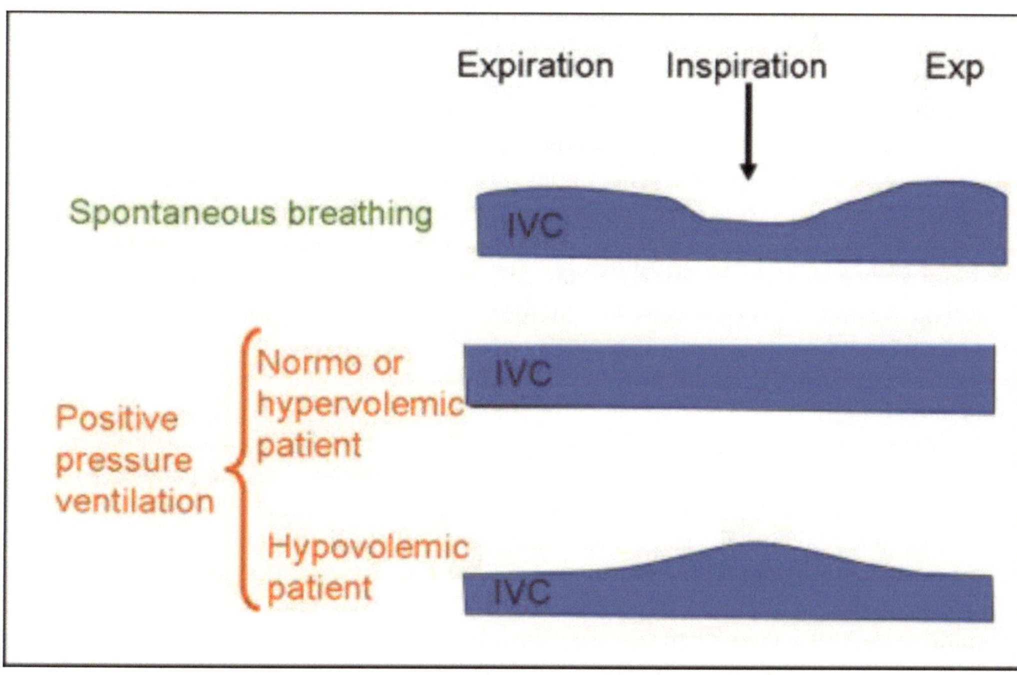

Fig. 3. Inferior vena cava diameter variations with the respiratory cycle.

This is especially true if the duration of hemodialysis is short and the ultrafiltration rate is rapid. It appears that inferior vena cava diameter before hemodialysis may be useful as an indicator of extracellular fluid overload. Inferior vena cava diameter measured at the end or shortly after hemodialysis may be misleading in assessing dry weight (Katzarski et al, 1997). Among hemodialysis patients a period of time must ensue between the attainment of dry weight and adequate control of blood pressure, a property termed the lag phenomen (Charra et al, 1998). In clinical practice, the dry weight is usually established by a progressive decrease in the post-dialysis body weight, usually over a 4-8 week period after the initiation of maintenance hemodialysis (Chazot et al, 1999). Acquired cystic kidney disease (ACKD) and hypertension are frequent complications of CKD. ACKD is a result of CKD, its prevalence and grade depending on the duration of CKD and dialysis treatment. We know that renal cysts are present prior to hemodialysis treatment in approximately one third of all patients. The prevalence of ACKD described in hemodialysis patients lies between 35 and 79% (Ishikawa, 1991). So far the literature offers only few data to clarify whether hypertension is also a possible complication of ACKD. Described are individual clinical cases of hypertension in patients with simple renal cysts. Some studies established a connection between simple renal cysts and hypertension in a large number of patients with normal renal function (Pedersen et al, 1993, 1997, Ekart et al, 2001). The question of whether perhaps ACKD is also involved in the pathogenesis of hypertension in hemodialysis patients and whether hypertension is also a complication of ACKD remains open. Hardly any studies dealing with this specific topic are to be found while the results of available studies do not clarify the likely involvement of ACKD in the development of hypertension in hemodialysis patients. The aim of our published study was to establish the prevalence and the grade of ACKD in patients on renal replacement therapy with hemodialysis, the frequency of hypertension in these patients as well as the possible connection between the presence of ACKD and hypertension in hemodialysis patients (Ekart & Hojs, 2006). In the study 86 hemodialysis patients (46 males and 40 females; mean age 51.3 years; mean duration of hemodialysis treatment 55.3 months) were included. Their native kidneys were examined with an ATL-HDI 3000 ultrasound device (2-4 MHz convex probe). Depending on the number of cysts in the kidney, the manifestations were divided into three grades: grade 0: no cysts; grade 1: less than ten cysts in both kidneys; grade 2: more than ten cysts in both kidneys. Blood pressure was measured 30 minutes before and after hemodialysis. Mean one-month values were analyzed. Hypertension was defined as systolic blood pressure of ≥ 150 mmHg, diastolic blood pressure of ≥ 90 mmHg and/or antihypertensive treatment. The diameter of the inferior vena cava (indicator of dry weight) was measured with the same ultrasound device as the kidneys 3 hours after hemodialysis. ACKD was present in 48 (55.8%) patients, there was no statistically significant difference regarding sex. 24 (50%) patients had grade 1 ACKD and 24 (50%) grade 2 ACKD. 68 (79.1%) patients suffered from hypertension, which was statistically significantly more common in male patients ($p=0.048$). In 68 (79.1%) patients hypertension was detected before hemodialysis and in 54 (62.8%) patients also after hemodialysis. 39 (45.3%) patients suffered simultaneously from ACKD and hypertension; 22 (56.4%) of them were males and 17 (43.6%) females. No statistically significant correlation between hypertension and ACKD was established. The prevalence and grade of ACKD were statistically significantly associated with the duration of dialysis treatment ($p<0.01$). Multiple regression analysis detected a significant correlation only between hypertension and the diameter of the inferior vena cava ($p<0.05$). Prevalence and grade of ACKD increase with the duration of dialysis treatment. ACKD was not associated with hypertension. There was a correlation between the diameter of the inferior vena cava as a factor of circulating fluid volume and hypertension in hemodialysis patients (Ekart & Hojs, 2006).

2.2 Increased sympathetic activity

Sympathetic activity is a common finding in ESRD, correlating with the increase in both vascular resistance and systemic blood pressure (Converse et al, 1992). Investigators have demonstrated that sympathetic activity is increased in those patients on chronic hemodialysis who still have their native kidneys. Sympathetic nerve activity was found to be normal in hemodialysis patients with bilateral nephrectomy, leading to the hypothesis that sympathetic overactivity in uremia is caused by a neurogenic signal (carried by renal afferents) arising in the failing kidney (Augustyniak et al, 2002). This hypothesis is supported by rat studies showing that renal deafferentation abrogates hypertension in the 5/6 nephrectomy model of chronic renal insufficiency. In addition, in patients with chronic renal insufficiency and renin-dependent hypertension, sympathetic overactivity was normalized by chronic angiotensin converting enzyme inhibition but not by calcium channel blockade, implicating a major central neural action of angiotensin II. Factors such as renal ischemia, chronic inflammation, oxidative stress, obesity, nocturnal hypoxia, and elevated plasma levels of asymmetric di-methyl-arginine (ADMA) may contribute to increased sympathetic activity (Levin et al, 2010).

2.3 Activation of the renin – angiotensin - aldosterone system

Although many patients may have plasma renin activity in the normal range, inappropriately increased plasma renin activity in relation to exchangeable sodium has long been recognized in uremic patients with hypertension (Kornerup et al, 1984). That the renin-angiotensin system is activated even in hemodialysis patients is illustrated by the fact that renin is increased with ultrafiltration dialysis (Henrich et al, 1977) and infusion of angiotensin II antagonist, improves blood pressure. Furthermore, patients treated with the angiotensin-converting enzyme inhibitor lisinopril have a dose-dependent increase in plasma renin activity and an improvement in blood pressure (Agarwal et al, 2001). Patients whose blood pressure is not controlled by maintenance of dry weight have increased plasma renin activity and demonstrate a dramatic improvement in hypertension control after interruption of the renin-angiotensin axis by bilateral nephrectomy (Bellinghieri et al, 1999).

2.4 Erythropoietin

Hypertension is a common adverse effect of erythropoietin therapy. It occurs more commonly in those people with preexisting hypertension, a positive family history of hypertension, rapid correction of anemia, or with severe anemia (Ishimitsu et al, 1993, Lebel et al, 1994, Bellinghieri et al, 1999). Nearly one third of renal failure patients treated with erythropoietin develop an increase in blood pressure of 10 mmHg or more (Eschbach et al, 1989). Although the exact mechanism by which erythropoietin increases blood pressure is not known, it may involve reduced nitric oxide activity due to scavenging by hemoglobin, increase in whole blood viscosity (Koppensteiner et al, 1990), and increased vascular reactivity to norepinephrine (Hand et al, 1995) or other mechanisms (Bode-Boger et al, 1996). There also may be more hypertension associated with the intravenous route of administration and larger dose ranges.

2.5 Endothelium – derived factors

The endothelium plays an important role in the regulation of vasomotor tone. Endothelin-1, an endothelium-derived peptide with vasoconstrictive and mitogenic effects on smooth muscles, is involved in vascular tone regulation and in the pathogenesis of atherosclerosis (Stefanidis et al, 2004). Elevated plasma levels of endothelin-1 have been found in uremic patients. The concentrations of other endothelin isoforms also may be increased, but only endothelin-1 has been linked to the high blood pressure. Endothelium-derived nitric oxyde plays a critical role in the maintenance and regulation of vascular tone and modulates key processes mediating vascular disease, including leukocyte adhesion, platelet aggregation, and vascular smooth muscle proliferation (Furchgott, 1996). The endothelium also produces potent vasodilators, such a prostacycline and nitric oxide. Endothelial nitric oxide synthase enzymatically produces nitric oxide from the substrate L-arginine. L-arginine supplementation can partially reverse renal failure - associated endothelial dysfunction. A circulating inhibitor of nitric oxide synthase, ADMA, competes with L-arginine for nitric oxide synthase. In humans with salt-sensitive hypertension, administration of a high-salt diet increases plasma ADMA and blood pressure (Fujiwara et al, 2000). Circulating ADMA is increased in subjects with CKD (Vallance et al, 1992) and ESRD (Mallamaci et al, 2004) and may contribute to endothelial dysfunction and increased blood pressure. In ESRD patients, ADMA is a death predictor (Aucella et al, 2009) and is correlated with increased left ventricular thickness and reduced ejection fraction, consistent with its ability to increase systemic vascular resistence (Zoccali et al, 2002). Oxidative stress leads to the accumulation of ADMA and promotes endothelial dysfunction. Inflammation, increased homocysteine levels, reduced antioxidant defenses, and increased free radicals in ESRD may therefore provide an explanation for the relationship between oxidative stress, endothelial dysfunction, and the generation of hypertension.

2.6 Parathyroid hormone excess secretion

There may be a correlation between an increase in intracellular calcium levels induced by parathyroid hormone excess and hypertension. Calcium entry into smooth muscle cells of the blood vessels can lead to vasoconstrition and hypertension. Some observations linking the correction of hyperparathyroidism by either vitamin D administration or parathyroidectomy in chronic dialysis patients, resulting in a lower blood pressure, have supported this hypothesis. In one small series, administration of alfacalcidiol, a vitamin D analogue, to treat hyperparathyrodism resulted in significant decreases in levels of parathyroid hormone, platelet intracellular calcium, and mean blood pressure (Raine et al, 1993).

2.7 Renal vascular disease

Ischemic renal disease is defined as a clinically important reduction in glomerular filtration rate (GFR) or loss of renal parenchyma caused by hemodynamically significant renal artery stenosis. Many patients with a presumed diagnosis of hypertensive nephrosclerosis actually have undiagnosed ischemic nephropathy as the etiology of their ESRD. It is important for the clinician to identify ischemic renal disease, because ischemic renal disease is a potentially reversible cause of chronic renal failure in a hypertensive patient. Atherosclerotic renal artery disease is common among patients with coronary artery disease and aortic and peripheral vascular disease. Atherosclerotic renal artery disease is a progressive disorder, and its progression is associated with loss of renal mass and functioning (Preston & Epstein, 1997). In a review of hypertension in ESRD patient, the diagnosis of ischemic nephropathy and renal vascular disease should not be overlooked.

2.8 Reduced production of prostaglandins/bradykinins

The kidneys produces several vasodilating substances such as kinins, prostaglandins, or antihypertensive neural renomedullary lipids, and decreased production and activity of these substances could play a role in the pathogenesis of hypertension. Indeed, decreased blood levels of vasodilating prostaglandin PgE_2 have been observed in hypertensive ESRD patients, and a negative correlation between the prostacyclin metabolite 6-keto-PgF1α and blood pressue has been observed in uremic patients.

3. Time of measurement of blood pressure, definition, and meaning of hypertension in hemodialysis patients

3.1 When should blood pressure be measured?

The prevalence of hypertension in hemodialysis patients is very high: in the time of progression from different stages of CKD to ESRD is between 40 and 90% (Salem, 1995, Agarwal & Lewis, 2001, Agarwal, 2002). Despite this high prevalence, there is limited knowledge about how to manage it in hemodialysis patients. Blood pressure variability is present in all people but is particularly prevalent in hemodialysis patients. This greater variability is related to the following: changes in volume status, change of sympathetic activity, hypotensive episodes during hemodialysis, antihypertensive drugs concentration and their dialyzability, erythropoietin, renin-angiotensin-aldosterone system activation, secondary hyperparathyroidism and other factors. Unlike the general population, for which there is a clear consensus of how to measure blood pressure and the blood pressure goal that is needed to reduce risk, this is not the case for people who receive renal replacement therapy. Moreover, in the patient with ESRD, a consensus for how to measure blood pressure has not been reached. In hemodialysis patients we can see blood pressure changes during hemodialysis in the dialysis center and in the interdialytic period. Which blood pressure should be taken to signify hypertension is more pertinent in dialysed individual than in the general population because of their fluctuating fluid status and other factors associated with the hemodialysis session. In the general hypertensive population it is known that the use of single measurements as a reliable indicator of the overall blood pressure control is fraught with difficulty because of transient and persistent elevations of pressure in clinical settings (Mezzeti et al, 1997). The variability of casual measurements in relation to the dialysis cycle confound management decisions and pose a dilemma with regard to the optimum timing and method of blood pressure measurement in this setting. Treatment decisions are mostly based on pre-dialysis blood pressure measurements. However the relevance of these measurements has been questioned. Several options exist for blood pressure measurement in hemodialysis patients, such as pre- or post-dialysis blood pressure, ABPM, and interdialytic home blood pressure. There is a marked difference in blood pressure between the pre-, post- and interdialytic period. It is unclear as to which time of blood pressure measurement best reflects the burden of hypertension and correlates best with cardiovascular outcomes (Rahman, 2005). Pre-dialysis blood pressure often overestimated basal blood pressure while post-dialysis blood pressure underestimated it,

although the latter is closer to the basal blood pressure value. Blood pressure variability pre-dialysis, post-dialysis and in interdialytic period is the reason for different conclusions in the studies - studies concluded, that the most important and representative are pre-dialysis (Conion et al, 1996, Agarwal, 1999), post-dialysis blood pressure measurements (Kooman et al, 1992, Mitra et al, 1999), in other study there were most representative the combination of pre- and post-dialysis blood pressure values (Coomer et al, 1997).
It is well known »white-coat effect«, which is defined as transient rise in blood pressure that occurs in the clinical settings (Myers et al, 1997). ABPM is required for the diagnosis of the white-coat effect. Mitra et al compared interdialytic ABPM with blood pressure obtained in hemodialysis patients at arrival to the dialysis center, after 10 minutes of rest in a quiet room, and at other time points (Mitra et al, 1999). White-coat effect was defined as the rise in blood pressure of > 20/10 mmHg in the reading on attendance to the dialysis center above the daytime ambulatory blood pressure during the 6 hours prior to attending the dialysis center (Mitra et al, 1999). White-coat effect was observed in 41% patients at arrival to dialysis center and this effect did not persist throughout the dialysis session (Mitra et al, 1999). The timing of the dialysis session did not influence the presence of white-coat effect, which persists even in patients on antihypertensive therapy (Mitra et al, 1999). The white-coat effect may be more common in renal patients than in the general hypertensive population perhaps due to an exaggerated sympathetic response conditioned by uremia (Rosansky et al, 1995). The timing of casual pre-dialysis and post-dialysis blood pressure measurement is crucial. Both can be biased by the dialysis procedure itself. The traditional diagnosis of hypertension based solely on pre-dialysis clinic measurements can lead to gross overestimation attributable to a white-coat effect. The best single approximation of interdialytic blood pressure is the 20-min post-dialytic measurement (Mitra et al, 1999). Canella and associates have pointed out that »false normotensive classification to subjects who are actually hypertensive, may possibly cause the link between arterial hypertension and left ventricular hypertrophy to be missed« (Canella et al, 2000). Those patients who have normal blood pressure in the dialysis center, but increased blood pressure outside the dialysis center as assessed by ABPM have »masked hypertension«. In an elderly population of patients with essential hypertension but without kidney disease, 9% were found to have masked hypertension (Bobrie et al, 2004). The cardiovascular prognosis of such patients is similar to that of poorly controlled hypertensives. The causes of masked hypertension in the dialysis population are not known. However, sleep apnea, which commonly occurs in hemodialysis patients, may be an important cause of masked hypertension. Sleep apnea causes a nocturnal increase in blood pressure, the magnitude of which increases with the severity of sleep apnea (Zoccali et al, 1998). The daytime blood pressure in these patients may not be elevated or may not accurately reflect the cardiovascular burden of hypertension; ABPM may be of particular value in assessing cardiovascular risk in such individuals. Hemodialysis blood pressure measurement and ABPM correlation is poor. A recent meta-analysis showed that pre- and post-dialysis blood pressure measurements are imprecise estimates of interdialytic ambulatory blood pressure (Agarwal et al, 2006a). In this meta-analysis median pre-dialysis systolic blood pressure and diastolic blood pressure were 8.6 and 2.6 mmHg higher than ABPM, respectively. In a single-center cross-sectional study, 1-week-averaged home systolic blood pressure was similar to interdialytic ABPM and superior to pre- and post-dialysis blood pressure in predicting left ventricular hypertrophy; diastolic blood pressure was not associated with left ventricular hypertrophy (Agarwal et al,

2009a). In an earlier study, ABPM added minimal information to the prediction of left ventricular hypertrophy, compared with the average of 12 routine pre-dialysis blood pressure measurements (Zocalli et al, 1999). Although a worthy goal, neither measurement of ABPM nor self-measured home blood pressure may be feasible for most patients throughout the world, leaving pre-dialysis and post-dialysis blood pressure measurements to be used, but with caution and with the knowledge that these are inferior (Levin et al, 2010).

3.2 Target blood pressure and what blood pressure level defines hypertension in chronic hemodialysis patients

There is still no consensus about whether to lower increased blood pressure in hemodialysis patients or the level to which blood pressure should be targeted (Agarwal, 2005, Foley & Agarwal, 2007). Hypertension is common and difficult to control and define in ESRD patients undergoing hemodialysis. ESRD patients are most frequently characterized by an increased systolic blood pressure with diastolic blood pressure within the normal range (<90 mm Hg) or even lower, resulting in increased pulse pressure. The increased systolic blood pressure is already found in young hemodialysis population. Diastolic blood pressure is usually higher in younger hemodialysis patients and declined with advancing age. All these changes result in a blood pressure pattern close to that observed in older subjects in general populations, i.e., isolated (or predominant) systolic hypertension, and attributable to »accelerated ageing« in ESRD. The definition of blood pressure targets and normotension in ESRD is not defined and in the absence of prospective controlled interventional studies, values accepted for general populations (<140/90 mm Hg) cannot be extrapolated to uremic patients.

In ESRD patients consensus to which level blood pressure should be reduced has not been reached. For definition and treatment of hypertension in hemodialysis patients, we need to know exactly blood pressure measurements. To evaluate blood pressure fluctuations better over the 2-days period (on the hemodialysis and on interdialytic day), ABPM is the gold standard to define a hemodialysis patient`s blood pressure. ABPM can provide information during sleep and early morning awakening, when blood pressure and cardiovascular risk are highest (Hopkins & Bakris, 2009a). In the general population, ABPM provided a more accurate prediction of cardiovascular outcomes than office blood pressure (Levin et al, 2010). Blood pressure levels defining the presence or absence of hypertension differ with the use of pre-dialysis, post-dialysis, self-measured home blood pressure, and ABPM. The recent National Kidney Foundation Kidney Disease Outcomes Quality Initiative guidelines suggest that pre-dialysis and post-dialysis blood pressure should be <140/90 and <130/80 mmHg, respectively (K/DOQI Workgroup, 2005). These targets were largely based on the expert judgment of the workgroup, applying weak evidence. Future research will decide whether the definition of hypertension on the basis of home blood pressure should be the same as that for the general population, as outlined in the Seventh Report of the Joint Natonal Committee (JNC 7) (Chobanian et al, 2003), with systolic blood pressure > 139 mmHg or diastolic blood pressure > 89 mmHg. In summary, the target goals should be realized upon individual patient. In some younger patients, the target blood pressure may even be set as low as 120/80 mmHg.

4. Blood pressure measurement in hemodialysis patients

In patients with ESRD, routine clinic and dialysis center blood pressure measurements may be poor indicators of blood pressure control. Patients on hemodialysis typically do not have their blood pressure measured under standardized conditions, a source of error in the assessment of their blood pressure. There are some unique sources of error involving interdialytic weight gain, occurence of sleep apnea and consequent nocturnal hypertension, inability to take blood pressure in both arms in patients who have hemodialysis angioaccess in the arm, and the white coat effect in these patients as well (Agarwal, 2002). Although blood pressure is measured frequently in the dialysis treatment enviroment, the technical aspects are often unsatisfactory. The recommendation for measuring blood pressure in the general population includes the patient´s sitting quietly upright in a chair for approximately 5 min with the arm supported at heart level. In addition, an appropriately fitting sphygmomanometer cuff is recognized as vital to accurate readings (Chobanian et al, 2003). Conversely, there remains disagreement concerning the utility and reproducibility of such method in hemodialysis patients. In most studies of ESRD patients, dialysis center measurements were used to explore the relationship between hypertension and cardiovascular events. However, dialysis center measurements fail to accurately characterize blood pressure in ESRD patients on hemodialysis, making it difficult to define the prognostic significance of hypertension in this population (Thompson & Pickering, 2006). ABPM has a better reproducibility than isolated or aggregated pre-dialysis and post-dialysis blood pressure values (Peixoto et al, 2000). Out-of-office blood pressure measurements (home blood pressure or ABPM) are better predictors of target organ damage and mortality in patients with essential hypertension and in patients with kidney disease (Agarwal et al, 2009a). The reproducibility of blood pressure measurements followed the following order: home blood pressure monitoring > ABPM >> pre-dialysis blood pressure > post-dialysis blood pressure (Agarwal et al, 2009b). A substantial number of prospective studies has shown that ABPM predicts cardiovascular events better than clinic-based readings, and also correlates more closely with target organ damage. In many studies a poor correlation was found between dialysis center measurements and ABPM readings obtained in the interdialytic period (Thompson & Pickering, 2006). In a study performed with ABPM in a group of dialysis patients, 44-hour interdialytic ABPM was compared with dialysis center measurements taken by a nurse. In that study, 43% of patients classified as hypertensive by pre-dialysis systolic blood pressure were normotensive on ABPM, whereas 25% of patients classified as normotensive by pre-dialysis systolic blood pressure were hypertensive (Santos et al, 2003). However, other studies found good agreement between average pre-dialysis blood pressure and interdialytic ABPM (Agarwal & Lewis, 2001). Changes that occur in ABPM during the interdialytic period likely account for the discrepancies with dialysis center measurements found in some studies. Conlon et al averaged dialysis center measurements from multiple visits and showed that pre-dialysis blood pressures averaged over 12 treatment sessions showed a strong correlation with ABPM (Conlon et al, 1996). Based on the results of 48-h ABPM in 36 hemodialysis patients, Coomer et al developed a model to predict mean blood pressure based on age, sex, race, and pre- and post-dialysis blood pressure (Coomer et al, 1997). Agarwal and Lewis compared ABPM with a 2-week average of dialysis center measurements in 70 dialysis patients and found that a 2-week average cutoff pre-dialysis blood pressure of 150/80 mmHg or higher had 80% sensitivity and 67% specificity to detect interdialytic hypertension as defined by an average ambulatory blood pressure of 135/85 mmHg or higher (Agarwal & Lewis, 2001).

Although these methods can be used to obtain a better estimate of interdialytic control, they cannot reliably determine blood pressure in any individual patient. Home blood pressure monitoring and standardized predialysis blood pressure measurements can aide in the assessment of blood pressure control. In a prospective cross-sectional study, home blood pressures averaged over one week were shown to be superior to routine dialysis center measurements averaged over 2 weeks in predicting hypertension on 44-h ABPM. Standardized pre-dialysis blood pressure averaged over 2 weeks had similar predictive ability as home measurements (Agarwal et al, 2006b). ABPM is superior to dialysis center blood pressure measurements in predicting target organ damage in patients with ESRD (Thompson & Pickering, 2006). In one of the largest study to date 44-h ABPM and home blood pressure monitoring, although weak determinants of left ventricular hypertrophy, were superior to a 2-week average of standardizes and routine dialysis center measurements in 140 chronic hemodialysis patients (Agarwal et al, 2006c). The correlation between left ventricular hypertrophy and blood pressure was similar using ABPM and an average of 12 standardized pre-dialysis measurements in a study of 35 stable hemodialysis patients (Conlon et al, 1996). In last decade, a few studies have assessed the prognostic power of ABPM and outcomes in hemodialysis patients (Amar et al, 2000, Liu et al, 2003, Tripepi et al, 2005, Agarwal et al, 2007, Moriya et al, 2008, Agarwal, 2010). In all these four studies ABPM contain greater prognostic information compared to blood pressure measurements in the dialysis center. The use of out-of-office blood pressure measurement techniques including self-measured blood pressure and ABPM in the management of hemodialysis patients is increasing. In the general population, blood pressure falls on average by 10-20% during sleep, a phenomen reffered to as »dipping«. In about 25% of healthy subjects, and in certain disease states, however, a loss in diurnal variation in blood pressure has been reported (non-dipping) (Thompson & Pickering, 2006). Non-dipping is particularly common in both children and adults with CKD, and an inverse relationship between GFR and the prevalence of non-dipping has been described (Farmer et al, 1997). Although the reported prevalence of non-dipping in adults with CKD varies, rates of 50% or higher have been observed at the earliest stages of disease, whereas rates of more than 80% have been observed in patients on dialysis (Farmer et al, 1997). A loss of diurnal variation in blood pressure has been associated with a poor renal prognosis and linked to left ventricular hypertrophy, adverse cardiovascular outcomes, and all-cause mortality in patients with ESRD. In a study of 59 hemodialysis patients, a correlation was found between the day/night ratio and left ventricular mass index (Rahman et al, 2005). In a cohort of 80 dialysis patients without a history of congestive heart failure or significant cardiovascular disease, non-dipping status was associated with an increased adjusted hazard ratio for cardiovascular morbidity and mortality (Liu et al, 2003). A study of 57 hypertensive ESRD patients without a history of systolic cardiac disfunction or valvular disease found that after controlling for age, sex, and cardiovascular history, an elevated nocturnal blood systolic blood pressure was associated with increased cardiovascular mortality (Amar et al, 2000). In a study by Tripepi et al, 168 dialysis patients without a history of diabetes, cardiovascular disease, or clinical evidence of heart failure were followed for 38 months. In a multi-regression analysis model not including left ventricular hypertrophy, an association between the highest night/day blood pressure tertile and increased cardiovascular and all-cause mortality was found. In contrast, the predialysis blood pressure averaged over one month did not predict events (Tripepi et al, 2005). Why this loss of nocturnal variation carries such a poor prognosis is unknown. It is possible that the absence of a nocturnal decline in blood pressure is not itself a cause of adverse outcomes, but is instead just a marker of sicker patients. In the meantime, ambulatory or some form of home blood pressure monitoring should be used to obtain a more accurate picture of blood pressure control in patients with ESRD. Clinic blood pressures frequently under- or overestimate the true blood pressure in CKD patients and dialysis center blood pressure measurements, although widely used to guide therapy, are poor indicators of interdialytic blood pressures.

5. Cardiovascular changes in hemodialysis hypertension

The association between uraemia and an increased risk of cardiovascular disease was first documented by Lindner (Lindner et al, 1974). Cardiovascular disease is the leading cause of morbidity and mortality in patients with ESRD (Guerin et al, 2006). Compared to the general population the annual cardiovascular death rate in dialysis patients is higher for all age groups, though particularly for the young whose mortality is up to 100 times greater than the general population. The average life expectancy of patients with ESRD is approximately 5 years, regardless of the modality of dialysis. Most patients with ESRD have a higher prevalence of traditional and also nontraditional cardiovascular disease risk factors when compared to the general population. The associations between traditional cardiovascular disease risk factors and atherosclerosis such as age, diabetes mellitus, hypertension, smoking, obesity, and dyslipidemia have been well described in dialysis patients. Cardiac deaths account for the majority of cardiovascular deaths in dialysis patients. The exact etiologies of these cardiac deaths are often unknown and likely include primary and secondary arrhythmias, cardiomyopathy, and coronary artery disease, and involve complex pathogenes. Although fluid overload, increased afterload from hypertension and vascular calcification, calcified valvular disease, and ischemia are probably important contributory factors, uremia per se seems to be an additional factor. To what extend hyperkalemia and hypokalemia, frequently present in this patients, contribute to the high incidence of sudden death in dialysis patients is not certain, but recent papers suggested the greater danger of hypokalemia (Karnik et al, 2001, Herzog et al, 2008,). Hypertension is a frequent finding in all stages of CKD. Because the pathogenesis of atherosclerosis in patients with CKD is multifactorial, it has been difficult to ascertain the precise role of hypertension in its development. Hypertension increases nearly linearly as renal function falls, and the vast majority of patients with significant renal failure present with high blood pressure. Blood pressure control is of paramount importance in slowing the progression of CKD toward ESRD, and also decreasing cardiovascular risk in these patients. Adequate blood pressure control should be a major objective in the management of patients with CKD in both the earlier and late stages. Uncontrolled hypertension in pre-ESRD patients is an important predictor for cardiovascular mortality during ESRD. More than 80% of patients have a history of hypertension, and more than two-thirds of these are uncontrolled (Agarwal et al, 2003). Foley et al found in a study with 432 hemodialysis patients that high blood pressure during dialysis therapy was associated with several adverse outcomes, including concentric left ventricular hypertrophy, left ventricular dilatation, ischemic heart disease and cardiac failure (Foley et al, 1996). They found an inverse association between average blood pressure level while on dialysis and mortality. Low blood pressure was associated with earlier death independently of age, diabetes, ischemic heart disease, anemia and hypoalbuminemia. There was an inverse relationship between average blood pressure and mortality (Foley et al, 1996). Port et al in a study of 4499 hemodialysis patients found the association of a low pre-dialysis systolic blood pressure with an elevated adjusted mortality risk (relative mortality risk = 1.86 for systolic blood pressure < 110 mmHg, P < 0.0001) (Port et al, 1999). A »U-shaped« curve (Figure 4) exists between blood pressure level and mortality in hemodialysis patients, with higher mortality noted at lower levels of blood pressure <120 mmHg and levels >180 mmHg measured before hemodialysis (Zager et al, 1998, Port et al, 1999, Kalantar-Zadeh et al, 2005, Luther & Golper, 2008, Hopkins & Bakris, 2009b). An analysis based on the CREED study cohort adjusted for Framingham risk factors, background cardiovascular complication, and left ventricular mass and ejection fraction shows that the risk of death is lowest in dialysis patients with a pre-dialysis systolic blood pressure between 100 and 125 mmHg (Zager et al, 1998), whereas systolic blood pressure > 150 mmHg was associated with increased mortality (Zoccali, 2003). Both post-dialysis systolic blood pressure ≥ 180 mmHg and diastolic blood pressure ≥ 90 mmHg were associated with a substantial increase in cardiovascular mortality (Zager et al, 1998). Severe cardiomyopathy modifies the relationship between blood pressure and mortality, and survival is very low in ESRD patients with systolic blood pressure < 115 mmHg (Klassen et al, 2002, Li et al, 2006).

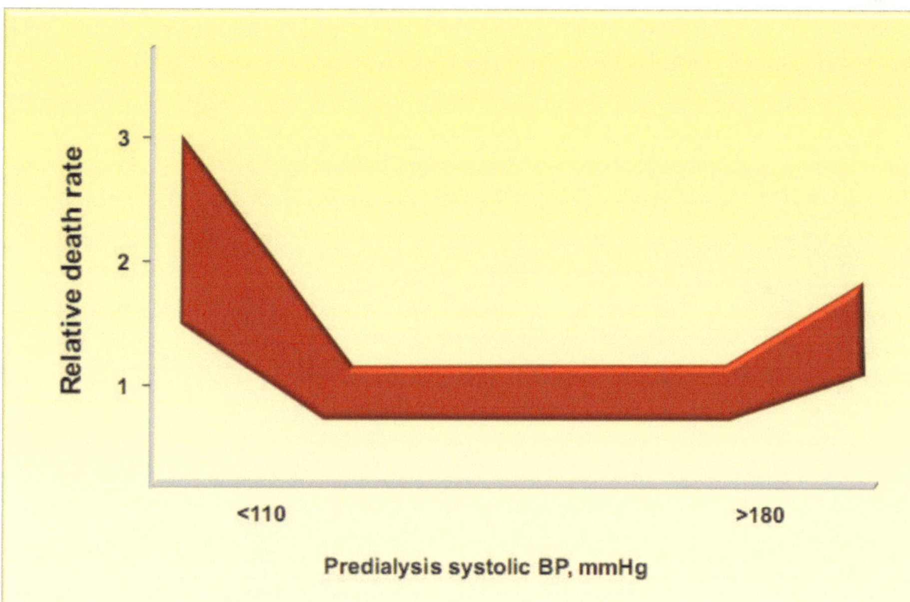

Fig. 4. Basic relationship of blood pressure to mortality in dialysis patients, as obtained from observational studies (Luther & Golper, 2008).

In an observational study in incident hemodialysis patients pre-dialysis systolic blood pressure ≥ 200 mmHg was associated with increased mortality or cardiovascular events (Li et al, 2006). Therefore, pre-dialysis blood pressure above this level should be treated aggressively. It is assumed, that carotid intima media thickness (IMT) is mirror for general atherosclerosis. IMT and plaque occurrence in the carotid arteries are strong predictors for cardiovascular events in the general population (Burke et al, 1995). B-mode ultrasound imaging is a useful and noninvasive tool to directly quantitate the atherosclerotic burden (Kato et al, 2003). Hemodialysis patients are known to have an advanced carotid IMT compared with age- and gender-matched normal controls (Kato et al, 2003). We performed the study in which determined that carotid IMT, measured with high resolution B-mode ultrasound, may be usefully applied for cardiovascular mortality risk stratification in non-diabetic HD patients (Ekart et al, 2005). Ninety-nine non-diabetic hemodialysis patients were included in the study. During a follow-up of 42.4 ± 19.5 months (from 12 to 76 months) 33 patients died, 19 (57.6 %) of them of cardiovascular causes (myocardial infarction, sudden cardiac death, heart failure, cerebrovascular insult). In these patients IMT values of the common carotid arteries was significantly higher (0.89 vs 0.69 mm; P < 0.0001) than in those who survived. Correlation between cardiovascular mortality and IMT was also found (r = 0.433; P < 0.001). Hemodialysis patients were divided in relationship to the tertiles of IMT and the survival rates were analyzed using Kaplan-Meier curves (Figure 5).The risk for cardiovascular death was progressively higher from the first tertile of IMT onward (log rank test; P < 0.0006). In a Cox regression model that included calcium, phosphate, intact parathyroid hormone (iPTH), duration of dialysis treatment, smoking, presence of hypertension, cholesterol (total cholesterol, low-density lipoprotein (LDL) cholesterol, high-density lipoprotein (HDL) cholesterol), triglycerides and lipoprotein (a), IMT turned out to be an independent predictor of cardiovascular death (P < 0.025). Our results suggest that measurement of IMT thickness in patients with ESRD could be a good predictor for the risk of cardiovascular event and also for cardiovascular death (Ekart et al, 2005).

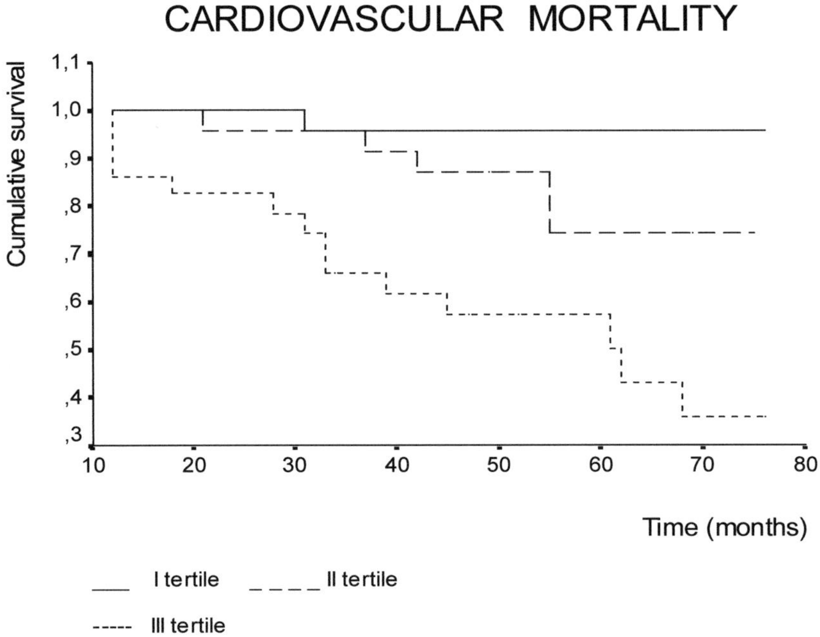

Fig. 5. Hemodialysis patients (N=99) were divided in relationship to the tertiles of IMT: I tertile, <0.65 mm; II tertile, ≥ 0.65 and < 0.8 mm; III tertile, ≥ 0.8 mm. Survival rates were analyzed using Kaplan-Meier curves. (Ekart et al, 2005).

We also performed a cross-sectional study in which we assess the relationship between carotid IMT as a marker of asymptomatic atherosclerosis and blood pressure measurements obtained with a standard mercury sphygmomanometer before and after the hemodialysis session, the average one-monthly values of the routine blood pressure measurements and 24- and 48-hour ABPM (Ekart et al, 2009). Hypertension was defined as systolic blood pressure of 140 mmHg (ABPM ≥ 135 mmHg), diastolic blood pressure of ≥ 90 mmHg (ABPM ≥ 85 mmHg) and/or also lower levels if the patient was taking antihypertensive drugs. In 85 hemodialysis patients we found statistically significant correlation between carotid IMT and average one-monthly pre-hemodialysis diastolic blood pressure ($P<0.05$), diastolic blood pressure on the hemodialysis day ABPM, interdialytic day ABPM and 48-hour ABPM ($P<0.05$). We also found a high prevalence of uncontrolled blood pressure despite treatment with antihypertensive drugs (Figure 6). The possible reason for uncontrolled hypertension in hemodialysis patients is probably bad compliance and withholding antihypertensive drugs on the hemodialysis day. Using multiple regression analysis we found statistically significant correlation only between carotid IMT and diastolic blood pressure on the hemodialysis day ABPM, interdialytic day ABPM and 48-hour ABPM ($P<0.05$). It is important that carotid IMT correlated only with long-term blood pressure measurements (one-monthly, 24- and 48-hour ABPM). Isolated systolic hypertension was more prevalent compared with isolated diastolic hypertension. It was interesting finding about casual connection between carotid IMT and values of diastolic blood pressure on the hemodialysis day ABPM, interdialytic day ABPM and 48-hour diastolic blood pressure values (Ekart et al, 2009).

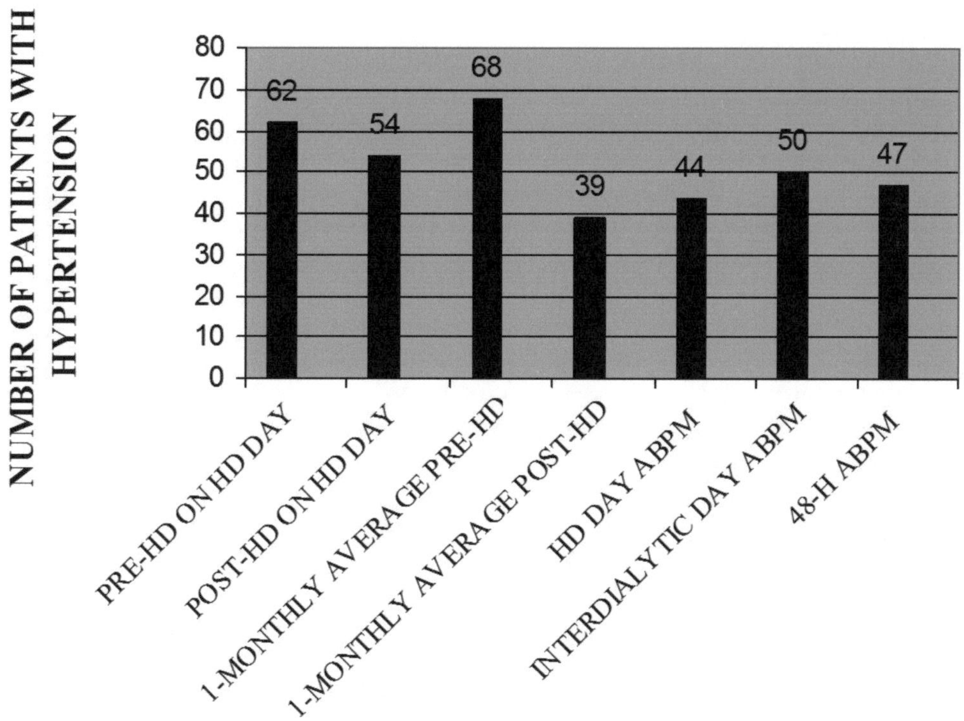

Fig. 6. Prevalence of uncontrolled hypertension in hemodialysis patients (N=85): different blood pressure measurements and not regarding treatment with antihypertensive drugs; HD=hemodialysis; (Ekart et al, 2009).

6. Treatment

The complex pathogenesis of hypertension in hemodialysis patient explains the difficulty of its treatment. Management of blood pressure in hemodialysis population requires both generally applicable plans and individualization in order to determine the blood pressure target and the treatment regimen. For patients with essential hypertension, CKD not yet on dialysis, and those with diabetes mellitus, clear guidelines on blood pressure targets exist. There are no such guidelines for ESRD patients on hemodialysis. The reason is because no randomized controlled trials have been performed in this patients to demonstrate the advantages of a given blood pressure target. Very low blood pressure in these individuals may make them intolerant to the hemodynamic stress of hemodialysis. An ideal blood pressure for a dialysis patient is the lowest that ensures hemodynamic stability during dialysis as well as orthostatic tolerance immediately postdialysis and is associated with good health-related quality of life. Such a blood pressure should also be associated with the lowest cardiovascular morbidity and mortality. A single blood pressure target may not be appropriate for all hemodialysis patients. Those patients who are older, who have vascular disease, and those with underlying diabetes may have different blood pressure goals than those with more pliable circulations and little or no left ventricular hypertrophy. Even though blood pressure targets are not defined for hemodialysis patients, most clinicians agree that treatment of high blood pressure is warranted. It seems that reaching a pre-dialysis blood pressure in the range of 130-160 mmHg/80-100 mmHg is safe and advisable (Peixoto & Santos, 2010).

6.1 Control of volume status

Whatever the target chosen, the strategies should focus first on management of salt and water balance, as control of extracellular fluid volume is associated with better blood pressure control (Katzarski et al, 1999). This includes dietary sodium restriction (Kayikcioglu et al, 2009), increased ultrafiltration and closer attention to the dialysate sodium prescription. The control of overhydration in ESRD patients is also of primary importance. The absolute content of total body water and sodium must be at level that does not cause signs and symptoms of volume overload, including hypertension and signs and symptoms of sodium and water depletion, such as dizziness and hypotension. The primary goal in the treatment of hypertension should be to attain a dry-weight. In the Tassin experience, the »dry weight method«, must be applied and is efficient to correct hypertension in these patients. Avoidance of large weight gains in the interdialytic period is desirable. To achieve this goal, patients should adhere to a restricted salt diet (750-1000 mg os sodium per day), which also helps decrease thirst (Mailloux, 2000, Locatelli et al, 2004). The clinician must define the dry weight and goal blood pressure for each dialysis patients based upon his or her best judgment. In attempting to achieve dry weight, particularly in incident patients starting dialysis, clinicians should me mindful also of the lag in time (from several weeks to months) between correction of extracellular volume and hypertension (Charra et al, 1998). The lag phenomenon reflects the time required to convert the patient from a catabolic to an anabolic state, a period in which extracellular fluid space slowly stabilizes (Charra et al, 1998). Two other factors may limit the degree of fluid removal by predisposing to episodes of hypotension during the hemodialysis procedure: antihypertensive drugs; and rapid fluid removal required by shorter dialysis times. Thus, tapering drug therapy and gradual fluid removal may be beneficial in patients in whom hypotension during dialysis prevents the attainment of dry weight and a normal blood pressure.

6.2 Prolonged and or more frequent hemodialysis

Longer and/or more frequent dialysis results in better blood pressure control both in observational studies and in clinical trials (Walsh et al, 2005, Chan, 2009). In most programs of long daily hemodialysis, 80-95% of patients are normotensive without medications. Patients in a dialysis center in Tassin, France and some home hemodialysis patients undergo long, slow hemodialysis in which the standard regimen is eight hours, three times per week. This regimen is associated with the maintenance of normotension without medications in allmost all patients (Charra et al, 1992, Covic et al, 1999, McGregor et al, 1999). Although these results have been largely attributed to optimal volume control, other factors may also contribute, such as more complete control of uremia (Chazot et al, 1995), which may decrease afferent renal nerve activity and efferent sympathetic activation (Converse et al, 1992). A subset of these patients are normotensive despite the presence of increased extracellular fluid volume while having achieved clinical dry weight (Katzarski et al, 1999). Nocturnal hemodialysis, procedure in which dialysis is performed six or seven nights a week during sleep for a variable amount of time based upon the length of sleep desired (usually 6 to 12 hours in total), is also associated with excellent blood pressure control (Agarwal, 2003). Allmost all patients become normotensive without medications. To achieve this, the »target weight« is progressively decreased until all antihypertensive agents are discontinued (Henrich & Mailloux, 2010). Some studies also suggest that more frequent hemodialysis treatments, via short daily hemodialysis, may also be associated with normotension without medications and with regression of left ventricular hypertrophy (Henrich & Mailloux, 2010). The 2007 European Best Practice Guidelines recommend that the treatment time and/or frequency of dialysis should be increased in patients with hypertension despite optimal volume removal (Tattersall et al, 2007). The prescription of longer and/or more frequent hemodialysis sessions allows the decrease in ultrafiltration rate and reduces the risk of intradialytic complications (Brunet et al, 1996, Laurent & Charra, 1998, Okada et al, 2005).

6.3 Dialysate sodium management

Achievement of adequate extracellular fluid volume requires not only assessment of dry weight and ultrafiltration, but also minimization of exposure to sodium. This occurs by dietary salt restriction and optimization of the dialysate sodium prescription. Most hemodialysis patients have serum sodium levels that are lower than normal and have a relatively fixed set points at these lower levels (Peixoto et al, 2010). Because of these lower serum sodium levels, approximately two-thirds of patients will have a high dialysate-to-plasma sodium gradient if dialyzed against a typical dialysate sodium concentration of 140 mmol/l (Santos & Peixoto, 2008). This unfavorable gradient leads to decreased sodium dialysance, which contributes to sodium overload (Peixoto & Santos, 2010). Use of lower dialysate sodium levels (134-136 mmol/l) results in increased sodium removal (Manlucu et al, 2010) and, in most but not in all studies, better blood pressure control (Thein et al, 2007, Santos & Peixoto, 2010, Manlucu et al, 2010). This effect is the result of a modest (~10%) decrease in the extracellular to intracellular water volume ratio (Manlucu et al, 2010) and a 33% fall in peripheral vascular resistence (Farmer et al, 2000). However, indiscriminate decreases in dialysate sodium may lead to hemodynamic instability and cramping in those patients whose baseline serum sodium is 140 mmol/l or higher. Therefore, individualizing the dialysate prescription to the patient`s own serum sodium is a preferable approach that results in decreased thirst, interdialytic weight gain and blood pressure without causing any increase in dialysis-related symptoms (De Paula et al, 2004). Attention to the prescribed dialysate sodium level is an essential part of achieving volume control in hemodialysis patients. Lowering the dialysate sodium level to match the patient`s own serum sodium is an effective means of accomplishing this goal.

6.4 Antihypertensive drugs

The majority of patients with ESRD on chronic dialysis undergoing standard thrice weekly treatment need antihypertensive drug therapy (Agarwal et al, 2003). Several observational studies have suggested that the use of antihypertensive drugs is associated with improved survival (Salem & Bower, 1996, Zager et al, 1998). Furthermore, among antihypertensive drugs, beta blockers have been reported to be associated with improved outcomes in observational studies (Foley et al, 2002). Therefore it appears that the use of antihypertensive drugs at least does not increase mortality among hemodialysis patients. Drug therapy for hypertension in hemodialysis patients includes all classes of antihypertensive drugs, but only selected patients may benefit from loop diuretic therapy (Hörl & Hörl, 2004). In addition to their antihypertensive effects, some drugs are variably cardioprotective, which may be independent of their blood pressure-lowering effects. The meta-analysis by Agarwal and Sinha showed a cardiovascular benefit for hypertensive hemodialysis patients from blood pressure lowering unlike what is suggested by observational studies (Agarwal & Sinha, 2009). However, the possibility that the benefits of antihypertensive drugs used in hemodialysis patients were because of non-hemodynamic actions is not ruled out. Pharmacokinetics of antihypertensive and putative cardioprotective drugs are altered by both impaired kidney excretion of the drugs and by their dializability. The multitude of drugs that these patients usually take reduces compliance, because of tolerability, interactions with other drugs, side effects, and financial costs (Schmid et al, 2009). Pharmacotherapy to lower blood pressure may cause additional problems that are unique to dialysis patients, such as intradialytic hypotension and vascular access thrombosis. The selection of antihypertensive drugs should be guided by considering their comorbidities, pharmacokinetics, and hemodynamic effects. For example, in patients with left ventricular hypertrophy, angiotensin converting enzyme (ACE) inhibitors may be effecting in causing regression (Paoletti et al, 2002). Hemodialysis patients may be more prone to side effects of certain drugs than patients with earlier stages of CKD. The presence of and propensity to these side effects may be easily overlooked. For example, minoxidil may potentiate or be confused with uremic pericardial effusion (Levin et al, 2010). A 2009 systematic review and meta-analysis of eight randomised controlled trials (three with and five without hypertensive patients) that enrolled 1679 dialysis patients found that lowering blood pressure with antihypertensive therapy was associated with decreased risks of cardiovascular events (RR of 0.71, 95% CI 0.55-0.99), all cause mortality (RR 0.80, 0.66-0.96) and cardiovascular mortality (0.71, 0.50-0.99) (Heerspink et al, 2009). Although there was significant variation in attained blood pressure, the overall mean decrease in systolic and diastolic blood pressure with active therapy was 4 to 5 mmHg and 2 to 3 mmHg, respectively. There were no studies that compared the efficacy of different antihypertensive agents. Additional limitations included the low number of patients, lack of information concerning volume control, and marked variations in blood pressure reduction (Tomson, 2009). Despite these limitations, it generally appears that renin-angiotensin-system blockers, beta blockers, and calcium-chanell blockers provide similar efficacy in dialysis patients. Recommendations on antihypertensive drugs are usually based on their efficacy in blood pressure reduction, interdialytic and intradialytic pharmacokinetics, side-effect profile, independent cardioprotective effects and non-cardiovascular effects of the specific class, as well as on the comorbidities of the patient. Calcium-chanell blockers are both effective and well tolerated in dialysis patients, even in those who are volume expanded (London et al, 1990). The only randomized prospective study found, that amlodipine, compared with placebo, improved overall mortality among hypertensive dialysis patients (Tepel et al, 2008). Calcium-channel blockers are particularly useful in patients with left ventricular hypertrophy and diastolic dysfunction. Calcium-channel blockers do not require supplementary postdialysis dosing. ACE inhibitors are well tolerated and are particularly effective in patients with heart failure due to systolic dysfunction and in many patients after myocardial infarction. The 2006 K/DOQI guidelines also suggest that ACE inhibitors and/or angiotensin II receptor blockers (ARB) are preferred in dialysis patients with significant residual renal function (K/DOQI, 2006). These agents may help preserve native kidney function. ACE inhibitors and ARB are associated with a decrease in left ventricular mass among hemodialysis patients (Canella et al, 1997, Tai et al, 2010). ARB and ACE inhibitors have similar issues in terms of adverse effects, including hyperkalemia and possible dampened erythropoiesis (Hörl & Hörl, 2004). Beta blockers are particularly indicated in patients who have had a recent myocardial infarction. As in nonuremic subjects, ESRD patients who have heart failure due to systolic dysfunction may also benefit from therapy with a beta blockers. Such therapy should be initiated at very low doses to minimize the risk of hemodynamic deterioration. In addition, beta blockers should be used cautiously in patients also taking a calcium-channel blocker, since there are often additive negative chronotropic and inotropic actions.

7. Summary

Hypertension is common in hemodialysis patients with major implications for survival. Accurate measure of blood pressure is an essential precursor for management. Pre- and post-dialysis blood pressure measurement may not reflect the average blood pressure experienced by the patient. Most management decisions for the diagnosis and treatment of hypertension are made using blood pressure measurements made in the dialysis center. However, ABPM and home blood pressure recordings may be of superior prognostic value. They are generally superior to the dialysis center blood pressure measurements in predicting long-term prognosis. In addition, ABPM and home blood pressure recordings significantly and strongly predict cardiovascular events. The reference standard for diagnosing hypertension among hemodialysis patients is 44-48 hour interdialytic ABPM. Hypervolemia that is not clinically obvious is the most common treatable cause of hypertension among patients with ESRD; thus, volume control should be the initial therapy to treat hypertension in most hemodialysis patients. Reducing dietary and dialysate sodium is an often overlooked strategy to improve blood pressure control. The treatment should be guided by blood pressure obtained outside the dialysis center. In general, all antihypertensive drugs can be used in the hemodialysis population with doses determined by dialyzability and hemodynamic instability. Renin-angiotensin-aldosterone system inhibitors have been shown to improve cardiovascular morbidity and mortality and are recommended as the initial pharmacologic therapy for hypertensive hemodialysis patients.

8. References

Agarwal, R, Bouldin, JM, Light, RP, Garg, A (2011 Feb 17). Inferior vena cava diameter and left atrial diameter volume but not dry weight. *Clin J Am Soc Nephrol;* (Epub ahead of print)

Agarwal R (2010). Blood pressure and mortality among hemodialysis pateints. *Hypertension,* Vol 55, pp. 762-768.

Agarwal, R, Sinha, AD (2009). Cardiovascular protection with antihypertensive drugs in dialysis patients: systematic review and meta-analysis. *Hypertension,* Vol. 53, pp. 860-866.

Agarwal, R, Peixoto, AJ, Santos, SF, et al (2009a). Out-of-office blood pressure monitoring in chronic kidney disease. *Blood Press Monit,* Vol. 14, pp. 2-11.

Agarwal, R, Satyan, S, Alborzi, P, et al (2009b). Home blood pressure measurements for managing hypertension in hemodialysis patients. *Am J Nephrol,* Vol. 30, pp. 126-134.

Agarwal R, Andersen MJ, Light RP (2007). Location not quantity of blood pressure measurements predicts mortality in hemodialyis patients. *Am J Nephrol,* Vol. 28, pp. 210-217.

Agarwal, R, Peixoto, AJ, Santos, SF, et al (2006a). Pre- and postdialysis blood pressure are imprecise estimates of interdialytic ambulatory blood pressure. *Clin J Am Soc Nephrol,* Vol. 1, pp. 389-398.

Agarwal, R, Andersen, MJ, Bishu, K, Saha, C (2006b). Home blood pressure monitoring improves the diagnosis of hypertension in hemodialysis patients. *Kidney Int,* Vol. 69, pp. 900-906.

Agarwal, R, Brim, NJ, Mahenthiran, J, et al (2006c). Out-of-hemodialysis-unit blood pressure is a superior determinant of left ventricular hypertrophy. *Hypertension,* Vol. 47, pp. 62-68.

Agarwal, R (2005). Hypertension and survival in chronic hemodialysis patients - Past lessons and future opportunities. *Kidney Int,* Vol. 67, pp. 1-13.

Agarwal, R (2003). Systolic hypertension in hemodialysis patients. *Semin Dial,* Vol 16, No.3, pp. 208-213.

Agarwal, R, Nissenson, AR, Batlle, D, et al (2003). Prevalence, treatment, and control of hypertension in chronic hemodialysis patients in the United States. *Am J Med,* Vol. 115, pp. 291-297.

Agarwal, R (2002). Assessment of blood pressure in hemodialysis patients. *Semin Dial,* Vol. 15, pp. 299-304.

Agarwal, R, Lewis, RR, Davis, JL, Becker, B (2001). Lisinopril therapy for hemodialysis hypertension - hemodynamic and endocrine responses. *Am J Kidney D*is, Vol. 38, pp. 1245-50.

Agarwal, R, Lewis, RR (2001). Prediction of hypertension in chronic hemodialysis patients. *Kidney Int,* Vol. 60, pp. 1982-1989.

Amar J, Vernier I, Rossignol E, et al (2000). Nocturnal blood pressure and 24-hour pulse pressure are potent indicators of mortality in hemodialysis patients. *Kidney Int*, Vol. 57, pp. 2485-2491.

Aucella, F, Maas, R, Vigilante, M, et al (2009). Methylarginines and mortality in patients with end stage renal disease: a prospective cohort study. *Atherosclerosis*, Vol. 207, No. 2, pp. 541-545.

Augustyniak, RA, Tuncel, M, Zhang, W, et al (2002). Sympathetic overactivity as a cause of hypertension in chronic renal failure. *J Hyperten,* Vol.20, No.1, pp. 3-9.

Bellinghieri, G, Santoro, D, Mazzaglia, G, Savica, V (1999). Hypertension in dialysis patients. *Miner Electrolyte Metab*, Vol. 25, pp. 84-89.

Birchem, JA, Fraley, MA, Senkottaiyan, N, Alpert, MA (2005). Influence of hypertension on cardiovascular outcomes in hemodialysis patients. *Semin Dial*, Vol. 18, pp. 391–5.

Bobrie, G, Chatellier, G, Genes, N, et al (2004). Cardiovascular prognosis of »masked hypertension« detected by blood presure self-measuremnt in elderly treated hypertensive patients. *JAMA*, Vol. 291, pp. 1342-1349.

Bode-Boger, SM, Boger, RH, Kuhn, M, et al (1996). Recombinant human erythropoietin enhances vasoconstrictor tone via endothelin-1 and constrictor prostanoids. *Kidney Int*, Vol. 50, No. 4, pp. 1255-1261.

Brunet, P, Saingra Y, Leonetti, F, et al (1996). Tolerance of hemodialysis: a randomized cross-over trial of 5-h versus 4-h treatment time. *Nephrol Dial Transplant*, Vol. 11, Suppl. 8, pp. 46-51.

Burke, GL, Evans, GW, Riley, WA, et al (1995). Arterial wall thickness is associated with prevalent cardiovascular disease in middle-aged adults. The Atherosclerosis Risk in Communities (ARIC) Study. *Stroke*, Vol. 26, pp. 386-91.

Canella, G, Paoletti, E, Ravera, G, et al (2000). Inadequate diagnosis and therapy of arterial hypertension as causes of left ventricular hypertrophy in uremic dialysis patients. *Kidney Int*, Vol. 58, pp. 260-268.

Canella, G, Paoletti, E, Delfino, R, et al (1997). Prolonged therapy with ACE inhibitors induced a regression of left ventricular hypertrophy of dialyzed uremic patients independently from hypotensive effects. *Am J Kidney Dis*, Vol. 30, pp. 659-664.

Chan, CT (2009). Cardiovascular effects of home intensive hemodialysis. *Adv Chronic Kidney Dis*, Vol. 16, pp. 173-178.

Charra, B, Calemard, E, Ruffet, M, et al (1992). Survival as an index of adequacy of dialysis. *Kidney Int*, Vol. 41, No.5, pp. 1286-1291.

Charra, B, Laurent, G, Chazot, C, et al (1996). Clinical assessment of dry weight. *Nephrol Dial Transplant*, Vol. 11, Suppl 2, pp. 16-19.

Charra, B, Bergstrom, J, Scribner, BH (1998). Blood pressure control in dialysis patients: importance of lag phenomen. *Am J Kidney Dis*, Vol. 32, pp. 720-724

Chazot, C, Charra, B, Vo, VC, et al (1999). The Janus-faced aspect of ´dry weight´. *Nephrol Dial Transplant*, Vol. 14, pp. 121-124.

Chazot, C, Charra, B, Laurent, C, et al (1995). Interdialysis blood pressure control by long hemodialysis sessions. *Nephrol Dial Transplant*, Vol. 10, No. 6, pp. 831-837.

Cheriex, EC, Leunissen, KML, Janssen, JHA, Mooy, JMV, van Hooff, P (1989). Echography of the inferior vena cava is a simple and reliable tool for estimation of »dry weight« in haemodialysis patients. *Nephrol Dial Transplant*, Vol. 4, pp. 563-568.

Chobanian, AV, Bakris, GL, Black, HR, et al (2003). The Seventh Report of the Joint National Committee on Prevention, Detection, Evaluation, and Treatment of High Blood Pressure: the JNC 7 report. *JAMA*, Vol. 289, pp. 2560-2572.

Coomer RW, Schulman G, Breyer JA, Shyr Y (1997). Ambulatory blood pressure monitoring in dialysis patients and estimation of mean interdialytic blood pressure. *Am J Kidney Dis*, Vol. 29, pp. 678-684.

Conlon PJ, Walshe JJ, Heinle SK, Minda S, Krucoff M, Schwab SJ (1996). Predialysis systolic blood pressure correlates strongly with mean 24-hour systolic blood pressure and left ventricular mass in stable hemodialysis patients. *J Am Soc Nephrol*, Vol. 7, pp. 2658-2663.

Converse, RL, Jacobsen, TN, Toto, RD, et al (1992). Sympathetic overactivity in patients with chronic renal failure. *N Engl J Med*, Vol. 327, pp. 1912-1918.

Covic, A, Goldsmith, DJ, Venning, MC, Akrill, P (1999). Long-hours home hemodialysis-the best renal replacement therapy methods? *QJM*, Vol. 92, No. 5, pp. 251-260.

Culleton, BF, Hemmelgarn BR (2003). Is chronic kidney disease a cardiovascular disease risk factor? *Semin Dial*, Vol. 16: 95–100.

De Paula, FM, Peixoto, AJ, Pinto, LV, et al (2004). Clinical consequences of an individualized dialysate sodium prescription in hemodialysis patients. *Kidney Int*, Vol. 66, pp. 1232-1238.

Ekart, R, Hojs, R, Krajnc I (2001). Unkomplizierte Nierenzysten und arterielle Hypertonie. *Wien Klin Wochenschr*, Vol. 113, Suppl 3, pp. 43-46.

Ekart, R, Hojs, R, Hojs-Fabjan, T, Pečovnik Balon, B (2005). Predictive value of carotid intima media thickness in hemodialysis patients. *Artif Organs*, Vol. 29, pp. 615-619.

Ekart, R, Hojs, R (2006). Acquired cystic kidney disease and arterial hypertension in hemodialysis patients. *Wien Klin Wochensch*, Vol. 118, Suppl 2, pp. 17-22.

Ekart, R, Hojs, R, , Pečovnik Balon, B, Bevc, S, Dvoršak, B (2009). Blood pressure measurements and carotid intima media thickness in hemodialysis patients. *Therap Apher Dial*; Vol. 13 , pp. 288-293.

Eschbach, JW, Kelly, MR, Haley, NR, et al (1989). Treatment of anemia of progressive renal failure with recombinant human erythropoietin. *N Engl J Med*, Vol. 321, pp. 158-63.

Farmer, CKT, Donohoe, P, Dallyn, PE, et al (2000). Low-sodium hemodialysis without fluid removal improves blood pressure control in chronic hemodialysis patients. *Nephrology*, Vol. 5, pp. 237-241.

Farmer, CK, Goldsmith, DJ, Cox, J, et al (1997). An investigation of the effect of advancing uremia, renal replacement therapy and renal transplantation on blood pressure diurnal varaibility. *Nephrol Dial Transplant*, Vol. 12, pp. 2301-2307.

Foley, RN, Parfrey, PS, Harnett, JD, Kent, GM, Murray, DC, Barre, PE (1996). Impact of hypertension on cardiomyopathy, morbidity and mortality in end-stage renal disease. *Kidney Int*, Vol. 49, pp. 1379-1385.

Foley, RN, Parfrey, PS, Sarnak, M (1998). The clinical epidemiology of cardiovascular disease in chronic renal disease. *Am J Kidney Dis*, Vol. 32, S112-S115.

Foley, RN, Herzog, CA, Collins, AJ (2002). Blood pressure and long-term mortality in United States hemodialysis patients: USRDS Waves 3 and 4 study. *Kidney Int*, Vol. 62, pp. 1784-1790.

Foley, RN, Agarwal, R (2007). Hypertension is harmful to dialysis patients and should be controlled. *Semin Dial*, Vol. 20, pp. 518-22.

Fujiwara, N, Osanai, T, Kamada, T, et al (2000). Study on the relationship between plasma nitrite and nitrate level and salt sensitivity in human hypertension: modulation of nitric oxide synthesis by salt intake. *Circulation*, Vol. 101, pp. 856-861.

Furchgott, RF (1996). The discovery of endothelium-derived relaxing factor and its importance of the identification of nitric oxide. *JAMA*, Vol. 276, pp. 1186-1188.

Guerin, AP, Pannier, B, Marchais, SJ, London, GM (2006). Cardiovascular disease in the dialysis population: prognostic significance of arterial disorders. *Curr Opin Nephrol Hypertens*, Vol. 15, pp. 105-115.

Hand, MF, Haynes, WG, Johnstone, HA, et al (1995). Erythropoietin enhances vascular responsiveness to norepinephrine in renal failure. *Kidney Int*, Vol. 48, pp. 806-813.

Heerspink, HJ, Ninomiya, T, Zoungas, S, et al (2009). Effect of lowering blood pressure on cardiovascular events and mortality in patients on dialysis. A systematic review and meta-analysis of randomised controlled trials. *Lancet*, Vol. 373, 1009-1015.

Henrich, WL, Katz, FH, Molinoff, PB, Schrier, RW (1977). Competitive effects of hypokalemia and volume depletion on plasma renin activity, aldosterone and catecholamine concentrations in hemodialysis patients. *Kidney In*, Vol. 12, pp. 279-284.

Henrich, WL, Mailloux, LU (2010). Hypertension in dialysis patients, In: *www.uptodate.com*

Herzog, CA, Mangrum, JM, Passman, R (2008). Sudden cardiac death and dialysis patients. *Semin Dial*, Vol. 21, pp. 300-307.

Hopkins K, Bakris GL (2009a). Assessing blood pressure control in dialysis patients: finally a step forward. *Hypertension*, Vol. 53, pp. 448-449.

Hopkins, K, Bakris, GL (2009b). Hypertension goals in advanced-stage kidney disease. *Clin J Am Soc Nephrol*, Vol. 4, S92-S94.

Hörl, WH (2010). Hypertension in end-stage renal disease: different measures and their prognostic significance. *Nephrol Dial Transplant*, Vol. 25, pp. 3161-3166.

Hörl, MP, Hörl, WH (2004). Drug therapy for hypertension in hemodialysis patients. *Semin Dial*, Vol. 17, pp. 288-294.

Ishikawa I (1991). Uremic acquired renal cystic disease. Natural history and complications. *Nephron*, Vol. 58, pp. 257-267.

Ishimitsu, T, Tsukada, H, Ogawa, Y, et al (1993). Genetic predisposition to hypertension facilitates blood pressure elevation in hemodialysis patients treated with erythropoietin. *Am J Med*, Vol. 94, pp. 401-406.

Kalantar-Zadeh K, Kilpatrick RD, McAllister CJ, et al (2005). Reverse epidemiology of hypertension and cardiovascular death in the hemodialysis population: the 58th annual fall conference and scientific sessions. *Hypertension*, Vol. 45, pp. 811-815.

Karnik, JA, Young, BS, Lew, NL, et al (2001). Cardiac arrest and sudden death in dialysis units. *Kidney Int*, Vol. 60, pp. 350-357.

Kato, A, Takita, T, Maruyama, Y, Kumagai, H, Hishida A (2003). Impact of carotid atherosclerosis on long-term mortality in chronic hemodialysis patiens. *Kidney Int*, Vol. 64, pp. 1472-1477.

Katzarski KS, Nisell J, Randmaa I, Danielsson A, Freyschuss U, Bergström J (1997). A critical evaluation of ultrasound measurement of inferior vena cava diameter in assessing dry weight in normotensive and hypertensive hemodialysis patients. *Am J Kidney Dis*, Vol. 30, pp. 459-465.

Katzarski, KS, Charra, B, Luik, AJ, et al (1999). Fluid state and blood pressure control in patients treated with long and short haemodialysis. *Nephrol Dial Transplant*, Vol. 14, pp. 369-375.

Kayikcioglu, M, Tumuklu, M, Özkahya, M, et al (2009). The benefit of salt restriction in the treatment of end-stage renal disease by hemodialysis. *Nephrol Dial Transplant*, Vol. 24, pp. 956-962.

Klassen, PS, Lowrie, EG, Reddan, DN, et al (2002). Association between pulse pressure and mortality in patients undergoing maintenance hemodialysis. *JAMA*, Vol. 287, pp. 1548-1555.

K/DOQI Clinical Practice Guidelines and Clinical Practice Recommendations (2006). Updates Hemodialysis adequacy Peritoneal Dialysis adequacy Vascular Access. *Am J Kidney Dis*, Vol. 48, Suppl. 1, S2-S90.

K/DOQI Workgroup (2005). K/DOQI clinical practice guidelines for cardiovascular disease in dialysis patients. *Am J Kindey Dis,* Vol. 45, No. 4, Suppl 3, pp. S1-S153.

Koppensteiner, R, Stockenhuber, F, Jahn, C, et al (1990). Changes in determinants of blood rheology during treatment with hemodialysis and recombinant human erythropoietin. *BMJ*, Vol. 300, pp. 1626-1627.

Kornerup, HJ, Schmitz, O, Danielsen, H, et al (1984). Significance of the renin-angiotensin system for blood pressure regulation in end-stage renal disease. *Contrib Nephrol*, Vol. 41, pp. 123-127.

Laurent, G, Charra, B (1998). The results of an 8h thrice weekly hemodialysis schedule. *Nephrol Dial Transplant*, Vol. 13, Suppl. 6, pp. 125-131.

Levin, NW, Kotanko, P, Eckardt, KU, et al (2010). Blood pressure in chronic kidney disease stage 5D-report from a Kidney Disease: Improving Global Outcomes controversies conference. *Kidney Int*, Vol. 77, pp. 273-284.

Lebel, M, Kingma, I, Grose, JH, Langlois, S (1995). Effect of recombinant human erythropoietin therapy on ambulatory blood pressure in normotensive and in untreated borderline hypertensive hemodialysis patients. *Am J Hypertens*, Vol. 8, pp. 545-551.

Lindner, A, Charra, B, Sherrard, DJ, Scribner, BH (1974). Accelerated atherosclerosis in prolonged maintenance hemodialysis. *N Engl J Med*, Vol. 290, 697-701.

Li, Z, Lacson, Jr E, Lowrie, EG, et al (2006). The epidemiology of systolic blood pressure and death risk in hemodialysis patients. *Am J Kidney Dis*, Vol. 48, pp. 606-615.

Lins, RL, Elseviers, M, Rogiers, P, et al (1997). Importance of volume factors in dialysis related hypertension. *Clin Nephrol*, Vol. 48, pp. 29-33.

Liu M, Takahashi H, Morita Y, Maruyama S, Mizuno M, Yuzawa Y, et al (2003). Non-dipping is a potent predictor of cardiovascular mortality and is associated with autonomic dysfunction in hemodialysis patients. *Nephrol Dial Transplant*, Vol. 18, pp. 563-569.

Locatelli, F, Marcelli, D, Conte, F, et al (2001). Survival and development of cardiovascular disease by modality of treatment in patients with end-stage renal disease. *J Am Soc Nephrol*, Vol 12, pp. 2411-2417.

Locatelli, F, Covic, A, Chazot, A, et al (2004). Hypertension and cardiovascular risk assessment in dialysis patients. *Nephrol Dial Transplant*, Vol. 19, No. 5, pp. 1058-1068.

London, GM, Marchais, SJ, Guerin, AP, et al (1990). Salt and water retention and calcium blockade in uremia. *Circulation*, Vol. 82, pp. 105-113.

Luther, JM, Golper, TA (2008). Blood pressure targets in hemodialysis patients. *Kidney Int*, Vol. 73, No. 6, pp. 667-668.

Mailloux, LU, Haley, WE (1998). Hypertension in the ESRD patient; Pathophysiology, Therapy, Outcomes, and Future Directions. *Am J Kidney Dis*, Vol. 32, No. 5, pp. 705-719.

Mailoux, LU (2000). The overlooked role of salt restriction in dialysis patients (editorial). *Semin Dial*, Vol. 13, Nr. 3, pp. 150-151.

Mallamaci, F, Tripepi, G, Maas, R, et al (2004). Analysis of the relationship between norepinephrine and assymetric dimethyl arginine levels among patients with end-stage renal disease. *J Am Soc Nephrol*, Vol. 15, pp. 435-441.

Manlucu, J, Gallo, K, Heidenheim, PA, Lindsay, RM (2010). Lowering postdialysis plasma sodium (conductivity) to increase sodium removal in volume-expanded hemodialysis patients: a pilot study using a biofeedback software system. *Am J Kidney Dis*, Vol. 56, pp. 69-76.

Martin, LC, Franco, RJS, Gavras, I, Matsubara, BB, Okoshi, K, Zanati, SG, et al (2006). Is 44-hour better than 24-hour ambulatory blood pressure monitoring in hemodialysis? *Kidney Blood Press Res*, Vol. 29, pp. 273-279.

McGregor, DO, Buttimore, AL, Nicholls, MG, Lynn, KL (1999). Ambulatory blood pressure monitoring in patients receiving long, slow home hemodialysis. *Nephrol Dial Transplant*, Vol. 14, No.11, pp. 2676-2679.

Mezzeti, A, Pierdomenico, SD, Constantini, F, et al (1997). White-coat resistant hypertension. *Am J Hypertens*, Vol. 10, No. 11, pp. 1302-1307.

Mitra, S, Chandna, SM, Farrington K (1999). What is hypertension in chronic hemodialysis? The role of interdialytic blood pressure monitoring. *Nephrol Dial Transplant 1999*, Vol. 14, pp. 2915-2921.

Moriya H, Oka M, Maesato K, et al (2008). Weekly averaged blood pressure is more important than a single-point blood pressure measurement in the risk stratification of dialysis patients. *Clin J Am Soc Nephrol*, Vol. 3, pp. 416-422.

Myers, MG, Meglis, G, Polemidiotis, G (1997). The impact of physician vs automated blood pressure readings on office induced hypertension. *J Hum Hypertens*, Vol. 11, No. 8, 41-493.

Okada, K, Abe, M, Hagi, C, et al (2005). Prolonged protective effect of short daily hemodialysis against dialysis- induced hypotension. *Kidney Blood Press Res*, Vol. 28, pp. 68-76.

Paoletti, E, Cassottana, P, Bellino, D, et al (2002). Left ventricular geometry and adverse cardiovascular events in chronic hemodialysis patients on prolonged therapy with ACE inhibitors. *Am J Kidney Dis*, Vol. 40, pp. 728-736.

Pedersen, JF, Emamian, SA, Nielsen, MB (1993). Simple renal cyst: relations to age and arterial blood pressure. *Br J Radiol*, Vol. 66, pp. 581-584.

Pedersen, JF, Emamian, SA, Nielsen, MB (1997). Significant association between simple renal cysts and arterial blood pressure. *Br J Radiol*, Vol. 79, pp. 688-692.

Peixoto, AJ, Gowda, N, Parikh, CR, Santos, SF (2010). Long-term stability of serum sodium in hemodialysis patients. *Blood Purif*, Vol.29, pp. 264-267.

Peixoto, AJ, Santos, SF (2010). Blood pressure management in hemodialysis: what have we learned ? *Curr Opin Nephrol Hypertens*, Vol 19, pp. 561-566.

Peixoto, AJ, Santos, SF, Mendes, RB, et al (2000). Reproducibility of ambulatory blood pressure monitoring in hemodialysis patients. *Am J Kidney Dis*, Vol. 36, pp. 983-900.

Port, FK, Hulbert-Shearon, TE, Wolfe, RA, et al (1999). Predialysis blood pressure and mortality risk in a national sample of maintenance hemodialysis patients. *Am J Kidney Dis*, Vol. 33, No. 3, pp. 507-517.

Preston, RA, Epstein, M (1997). Ischemic renal disease: an emerging cause of chronic renal failure and end-stage renal disease. *J Hypertens*, Vol. 15, pp. 1365-1377.

Rahman M, Griffin V, Heyka R, Hoit B (2005). Diurnal variation of blood pressure; reproducibility and association with left ventricular hypertrophy in hemodialysis patients. *Blood Press Monit*, Vol. 10, pp. 25-32.

Raine, AE, Bedford, L, Simpson, AW, et al (1993). Hyperparathyroidism, platelet intracellular free calcium and hypertension in chronic renal failure. *Kidney Int*, Vol. 43, pp. 700-705.

Rosansky, SJ, Menachery, SJ, Wagner, CM, Jackson, K (1995). Circadian blood pressure variation versus renal function. *Am J Kidney Dis*, Vol. 26, pp. 716-721.

Salem, MM, Bower, J (1996). Hypertension in the hemodialysis population: any relation to one-year survival? *Am J Kidney Dis*, Vol. 28, pp. 737-740.

Sankaranarayanan, N, Santos, SF, Peixoto, AJ (2004). Blood pressure measurement in dialysis patients. *Adv Chronic Kidney Dis*, Vol 11, pp. 134-142.

Santos, SF, Peixoto, AJ (2008). Revisiting the dialysate sodium prescription as a tool for better blood pressure and interdialytic weight gain management in hemodialysis patients. *J Am Soc Nephrol*, Vol. 3, pp. 522-530.

Santos, SF, Mendes, RB, Santos, CA, et al (2003). Profile of interdialytic blood pressure in hemodialysis patients. *Am J Nephrol*, Vol. 23, pp. 96-105.

Schmid, H, Hartmann, B, Schiffl, H (2009). Adherence to prescribed oral medication in adult patients undergoing chronic hemodialysis: a critical review of literature. *Eur J Med Res*, Vol. 14, pp. 185-190.

Stefanidis, I, Wurth, P, Mertens, PR, et al (2004). Plasma endothelin-1 in hemodialysis treatment - the influence of hypertension. *J Cardiovasc Pharmacol*, Vol. 44, Suppl 1, S43-S48.

Tai, DJ, Lim, TW, James, MT, et al (2010). Cardiovascular effects of Angiotensin converting enzyme inhibition or Angiotensin receptor blockade in hemodialysis: a meta-analysis. *Clin J Am Soc Nephrol*, Vol. 5, pp. 623-630.

Tattersall, J, Martin-Malo, A, Pedrini , L, et al (2007). European best practice guidelines on hemodialysis. *Nephrol Dial Transplant*, Vol. 22, Suppl 2, ii5-ii22.

Tepel, M, Hopfenmueller, W, Scholze, A, et al (2008). Effect of amlodipine on cardiovascular events in hypertensive hemodialysis patients. *Nephrol Dial Transplant*, Vol. 23, pp. 3605-3612.

Thein, H, Haloob, I, Marshall, MR (2007). Associations of a facility level decrease in dialysate sodium concentration with blood pressure and interdialytic weight gain. *Nephrol Dial Transplant*, Vol. 22, pp. 2630-2639.

Thompson, AM, Pickering, TG (2006). The role of ambulatory blood pressure monitoring in chronic and end-stage renal disease. *Kidney Int*, Vol. 70, pp. 1000-1007.

Tomson, CR (2009). Blood pressure and outcome in patients on dialysis. *Lancet*, Vol. 373, pp. 981-982.

Tripepi G, Fagugli RM, Dattolo P, et al (2005). Prognostic value of 24-hour ambulatory blood pressure monitoring and of night/day ratio in nondiabetic, cardiovascular events-free hemodialysis patients. *Kidney Int*, Vol. 68, pp. 1294-1302.

Vallance, P, Leone, A, Calver, A, et al (1992). Accumulation of an endogenous inhibitor of nitric oxide synthesis in chronic renal failure. *Lancet*, Vol. 339, pp. 572-575.

Walsh, M, Culleton, B, Tonelli, M, Manns, B (2005). A systematic review of the effect of nocturnal hemodialysis on blood pressure, left ventricular hypertrophy, anemia, mineral metabolism, and health-related quality of life. *Kidney Int*, Vol. 67, pp. 1500-1508.

Zager, PG, Nikolic, J, Brown, RH, et al (1998). "U" curve association of blood pressure and mortality in hemodialysis patients. *Kidney Int*, Vol. 54, pp. 561-569.

Zoccali, C (2003). Arterial pressure components and cardiovascular risk in end-stage renal disease. *Nephrol Dial Transplant*, Vol. 18, pp. 249-252.

Zoccali, C, Mallamaci, F, Mass, R, et al (2002). Left ventricular hypertrophy, cardiac remodeling and assimetric dimethyl arginine (ADMA) in hemodialysis patients. *Kidney Int*, Vol. 62, pp. 339-345.

Zoccali, C, Mallamaci, F, Tripepi, G, et al (1999). Prediction of left ventricular geometry by clinic, pre-dialysis and 24-h ambulatory BP monitoring in hemodialysis patients: CREED investigators. *J Hypertens*, Vol. 17, pp. 1751-1758.

Zoccali, C, Benedetto, FA, Tripepi, G, et al (1998). Noctural hypoxemia, night-day arterial pressure changes and left ventricular geometry in dialysis patients. *Kidney Int*, Vol. 53, pp. 1078-1084.

5

Antidiabetic Therapy in Type 2 Diabetic Patients on Hemodialysis

Georg Biesenbach and Erich Pohanka
2nd Department of Medicine, Section Nephrology, General Hospital Linz, Austria

1. Introduction

Diabetic nephropathy is the most common cause for end-stage renal disease (ESRD). Chronic renal failure is associated with miscellahous alterations in carbohydrate and insulin metabolism.. Moreover, several specific therapies employed in renal insufficiency also influence pharmacological therapy of diabetes in uraemic patients.. In patients with altered renal function, therapeutic possibilities are limited due to the accumulatin of some oral agents and/or their metabolites at the reduced glomerular filtration rate (GFR). The connection between kidney and insulin metabolism is well known for many years (Horton et al, 1968). For insulin metabolism the kidneys are one of its target organs. Chronic renal failure is associated to multiple alterations in the carbohydrate and insulin metabolism that should be taken into account when treating diabetic patients with altered renal function (DeFronzo et al, 1973). Specific therapeutic needs (oral agents or insulin) will be determined based on the degree of insulin resistance or insulin deficiency of patients with renal insufficiency (Rabkin e al,1984). A good metabolic control is not only important in the early phase of diabetic nephropathy but also in diabetic patients with ESRD. It was shown in several studies, that metabolic control under antidiabetic therapy is a predictor for prognosis of patents with renal replacement therapy (Morokia et al, 2001). A good glycemic control can reduce the progression of atherosclerosis (Oomichi et al, 2006) and improve the survival in patients treated with hemodialysis (Kovesdy et al, 2008). Though, in a recent study it was suggested that aggressive glycemic control cannot be routinely recommended for all diabetic hemodialysis patients on the basis of reducing mortality risk (Williams et al, 2010). The majority of uremic type 2-diabetic patients need insulin, however, a smaller part of these diabetic patients can also be treated with oral antidiabetic agents.
The problem of the topic of this study is the fact, that there are only few data in the literature concerning antidiabetic therapy in type 2 diabetic patients with ESRD (Biesenbach et al, 2010). This paper offers a review of the relevant findings related to insulin therapy in diabetic patients with ESRD. Additionally, we review the relevant aspects related to oral antidiabetic therapy in diabetic patients with impaired renal function.

2. Insulin metabolism and insulin therapy

The insulin metabolism is changed in uremic patients. In insulin-treated diabetic patients suffering from renal insufficiency the insulin requirement is reduced in renal insufficiency.

Additionally, hemodialysis influences insulin metabolism and the glycemic control under antidiabetic therapy. In this overview the insulin metabolism in uremic patients and the insulin therapy as well as oral antidiabetic therapy will be discussed.

2.1 Insulin metabolism in uremic patients

Insulin is a polypeptide hormone (51-amino acids), the molecular weight of approximately 6000 Da, The Half-life (t1/2) of insulin is short (3–5 min). Under fasting conditions the insulin secretion rate is 0.5–1 unit/h. After meal insulin secretion shows a 3–10 fold increase (Polonsky et al 1986). In healthy subjects insulin is secreted into the portal system, insulin passes through the liver, where about 75% is metabolized, with the remaining 25% metabolized by the kidneys. About 60% of the insulin in the arterial bed is filtered by the glomerulus, and 40% is actively secreted into the nephric tubules. Most of the insulin in the tubules is metabolized into amino acids, and only 1% of insulin is secreted intact (Mak et al,´1992). As parameter for endogenous insulin secretion C-peptide can be used. Unlike insulin, C-peptide is not metabolized during its first pass through the liver and, approximately 70% of its plasma clearance is performed in the kidney (Block et al, 1972)

For diabetic patients receiving exogenous insulin, renal metabolism plays a more significant role since there is no first-pass metabolism in the liver. As renal function starts to decline, insulin clearance does not change appreciably, due to compensatory peritubular insulin uptake. But once the GFR drops below 20-30mL/min, the kidneys clear significantly less insulin, an effect causally determined by a decrease in the hepatic metabolism of insulin that occurs in uremia. Despite an increase in insulin resistance caused by renal failure, the net effect is a reduced requirement for exogenous insulin in ESRD as the result of periodic improvement in uremia, acidosis, and phosphate handling (Shrishrimal et al, 2009).

Thus, in the presence of impaired renal function, the type 1 as well as type 2 diabetic patients require less insulin, mainly due to prolonged insulin clearance (Biesenbach et al, 2003). For these reasons the American College of Physicians recommends to decrease insulin doses by 25% of initial insulin dose when GFR is 50-10 ml/min and by 50% when GFR is less than 10 ml/min (Aronoff et al 1999). Other factors that contribute to decreasing exogenous insulin requirements in CRF diabetic patients are the reduction of renal gluconeogenesis, uraemia-induced anorexia and weight loss (Charpentier, et al, 2000)

In ESRD, both uremia and dialysis can complicate glycemic control by affecting the secretion, clearance, and peripheral tissue sensitivity of insulin. Several factors, including uremic toxins, may increase insulin resistance in ESRD, leading to a blunted ability to suppress hepatic gluconeogenesis and regulate peripheral glucose utilization. In type 2 diabetes without kidney disease, insulin resistance leads to increased insulin secretion. This does not occur in ESRD because of concomitant metabolic acidosis and vitamin D deficiency (Shrishlrimal et al, 2009).Impairment of renal function is associated with insulin resistance, this resistance can be improved by start of hemodialysis (Rabkin et al, 1984) Hemodialysis alters insulin secretion,insulin clearance, and resistance.

In an own study the mean decrease of required insulin dose dependent on time was slightly lower in type 1 diabetes with 2,8 IU/year versus 3.8 IU/year in type 2 diabetes (NS). The decline in insulin requirement increased significantly when GFR decreased below 30 ml/min.

The reduction of insulin requirement at the beginning of decline of renal function may be explained by study associated improvement of glycemic control.

We also measured C-peptide at the beginning and the end of renal function impairment, the mean difference was not significant with 2.2 versus 2.7 ng /ml, Thus, we assumed that residual insulin secretion has no significant impact on the reduction in insulin requirement dependent on GFR Insulin therapy in patients on hemodialysis is associated with hyperinsulinemia and a higher incidence of hypoglycaemia compared to patients without dialysis (Loipl et al, 2005). In rare cases insulin substitution can be stopped in type 2 diabetic patients with already low insulin requirement already in the pre-dialysis phase.

2.2 Practical managing of insulin therapy in patients on hemodialysis

Most type 2 diabetic patients with ESRD need insulin therapy. In patients with renal insufficiency it may be considered that intensive insulin therapy can help to improve glycaemic control more than conservative insulin therapy. There is lack of relevant pharmacokinetic studies for the various types of insulin in patients with different degrees of renal insufficiency (Snyder & Berns, 2004): Due to the absence of comparative studies there are no therapeutic guidelines that define insulin adjustments based on GFR (Bilous et al, 2004). In hemodialysis patients with type 2 diabetes insulin requirements is usually reduced in probable relationship with an improvement in insulin resistance associated with the dialytic procedure (Schmidtz et al, 1984). Additionally, a reduced insulin clearance may contribute to the decrease in requirement of insulin. On the basis of evidence, it can be recommend a basis-bolus insulin regime with the long-acting insulin glargine (Lantus®) or detemir (Levemir®) for basal requirements, along with a rapid-acting insulin analogue such as lispro (Humalog®), insulin aspart (NovoLog®. Novorapid®) or insulin glulisine (Apidra®) before meals. Duration of action of insulin glargine is significantly longer than that of human NPH insulin (IProtaphan®, Basal®), Humulin®) with a less pronounced peak of action (Iglesias et al, 2008). In the literature the Tmax averages were 8.6 hours for insulin glargine compared to 5.4 hours for NPH insulin. Lower FPG (fasting plasma glucose) levels with fewer episodes of hypoglycemia are achieved with insulin glargine compared to NPH insulin. Insulin glargine is metabolized at the carboxyl terminal of the B chain to two metabolites) with activity similar to that of human insulin (Ersoy et al, 2006). Few studies were published comparing analogue insulin and regular insulin (Aisenpreis et al, 1999). Both, short acting as well as long acting insulin analogues have advantages in comparison to regular insulin. During the last years in most centers the NPH insulin was replaced by the long acting insulin analogues glargine or detemir. Meanwhile, several studies have described the use of insulin analogues in ESRD (O'Mara et al, 2010). Nevertheless, clinical efficacy and safety profile of insulin analogues are not clearly defined in chronic renal failure. Since of potentially carcinogenic and proliferative effects have not yet been disproved. Most studies with analogues to date have excluded diabetic patients with advanced diabetic complications. Therfore, there is little information regarding the use of these analogues in renal insufficiency. The main advantage of the short-acting insulin analogue is the shorter absorption, the most important advantage of the long-acting insulin analogues is the lower risk of hypoglycemia, thus improving glycemic control and improving quality of life (Jehle et al, 1999). In insulin-treated type 2 diabetic patients with low insulin requirement (<20 IU/day) a conventional insulin regime may such also be used, such as daily 1-2 injections of a long acting insulin or a pre-mixed insulin-combination (NPH-insulin and normal insulin or short-acting insulin analogues). When GFR decreases to10-50 mL/min, the total dose of both, regular insulin or insulin analogue should be reduced by 25%. In patients with ESRD, the insulin dose should be reduced by 50%.

However, there are great interindividual differences in the decrease of insulin requirement (Biesenbach et al, 2003)
The insulin requirement in hemodialysis patíents in dialysis is very different. In an own study we investigated the insulin requirement during the first dialysis year in insulin-treated type 2 diabetic patients dependent on rest diuresis. Patients were divided into two groups according to their diuresis. Group 1, of patients with preserved near-normal urine production (>1 l/day) during the first dialysis year (n = 12), and group 2, of patients with significant reduction of urine excretion (<0.5 l/day) within 3 months after start of dialysis (n = 12). All patients were dialysed three times per week (total dialysis time 12 h weekly). The HbA1c- were similar in both groups and did not significantly change during the first year. Insulin requirement in the patients with normal diuresis decreased from 24 IU/day at the start of dialysis to 14 ± 8 IU/day 1 year later (41% reduction, P < 0.05). In the group with reduced diuresis, the required insulin dose remained the same with 28 ± 12 and 26 ± 8 IU/day, respectively (7% reduction). We concluded that in insulin-treated diabetic patients the insulin requirement can be different due to differences in the residual renal function. During the first year hemodialysis the insulin requirement can further drop in patients with decreasing diuresis (Biesenbach et al, 2008). However, the evidencce of this study limited due to the small patient groups.
The targets of therapy in patients with ESRD are similar as in subjects with normal GFR; The targets are a hemoglobin A1c value between 6% and 7%, a fasting blood glucose level less than 140 mg/dL, and a postprandial glucose level less than 200 mg/dL. The individual targets of therapy may be changed depending on the higher risk for hypoglycemia in patients on hemodialysis (Uzu et al, 2008)

3. Oral antidiabetic drug therapy

Type 2 diabetic patients with ESRD need in the majority insulin therapy, however, some patients are treated by oral anti-diabetic drugs or diet alone. In type 2 diabetes and terminal renal failure several drugs can be used. Nevertheless, Most oral antidiabetic drugs are not recommended under hemodialysis therapy.

3.1 Old oral antdiabetic drugs

Three "old" agents have been approved for patients with renal insufficiency.
Sulfonylurea (SU) drugs can be used in diabetic patients with ESRD (Charpentier et al, 2009): Gliquidone (Glurenorm®) can be used with normal dose, gliclazide (Diamicron®) and glimepiride (Amaryl®) in reduced dose (50%). Under hemodialysis SU drugs should rather be avoided due to the higher risk of hypoglycaemia. Glibenclamid (Euglucon®)is absolutely contraindicated in renal insufficiency due to severe hypoglyceimia (Krepinsky et al, 2000).

Alpha-glucosidase inhibitors

Both, the alpha-glucosidase inhibitor acarbose (Glucobay®) and especially miglitol (Diastabol®) are contraindicated in ESRD (Yale 2005)

Biguanides

Metformin (Glucophage®, Diabetex®, Metformin®) is a biguanide that reduces hepatic gluconeogenesis and glucose output. It is contraindicated in patients with renal disease (s-creatinine >1.1 mg/dl in women and >1.4 mg/dl in men) and also in congestive heart failure due to the risks of lactic acidosis. However, in some studies the authors suggestsed that the use of metformin in patients who are over the age of 80 years, have congestive heart failure or have renal insufficiency leads to a benefit that far outweighs the potential harm. (McCormack et al, 2005)

3.2 New antidiabetic drugs

In this group three "new"agents are included: insulin secretizers (glinide), insulin sensitizers (glitazone) and the new group of GLP 1 agonists and DDP inhibitors (gliptine) (Mohideen et al, 2005)

Meglitinides

The are two glinides,: repaglinide (Novonorm®; Prandin®) and nateglinide (Starlix®) are insulin secretagogues, both can be used in renal failure, but not recommended for patients on hemodialysis (Nagai et al, 2003)

Thiazolidinedione (glitazone)

Pioglitazone (Actos®) do not need dosing adjustment. Main adverse effect of this agents is edema, therefore it is contraindicated in heart failure, especially when combined with insulin therapy. Since the end of 2010 only pioglitazone is available. Rosiglitazone (Avandia®) was removed due to an increased cardiovascular risk (Thompson-Culkin et al, 2002)

Incretine (GLP-1 Analogues and Gliptins)

Glucagon-like peptide-1 (GLP-1) stimulates glucose-dependent insulin release from pancreatic beta cells and inhibits inappropriate postprandial glucagon release. It also slows gastric emptying and reduces food intake. Dipeptidyl peptidase IV (DPP-IV) is an active ubiquitous enzyme that deactivates a variety of bioactive peptides, including GLP-1. **Exenatide** (Byetta®) is a naturally occurring GLP-1 analogue that is resistant to degradation by DPP-IV and has a longer half-life. Given subcutaneously, no dose adjustment is required if the glomerular filtration rate (GFR) is greater than 30 mL/min, The drug's label has been updated to note that the drug should not be used in patients with severe renal impairment;
Exenatide is absolutely contraindicated in patients on hemodialysis (Kuehn, 2011) **Sitagliptin** (Januvia®) was the first oral DPP-IV inhibitor, the usual dose of sitagliptin is 100 mg once daily, with reduction to 50 mg for patients with a GFR of 30 to 50 mL/min, and 25 mg for patients with a GFR < 30 mL/min (Bergman et al, 2007). Further vildagliptin (Galvus®), normal dose 2x50 mg daily, a dose reduction is recommended for patients with moderate to severe renal impairment (Thuren et al, 2008).

4. Fluctuation of blood glucose and monitoring of glycemic control

Several factors can negatively influence glycaemic control in diabetic patients. These include poor food intake, insufficient exercise, uraemia-induced anorexia, insulin metabolism disorders, especially insulin resistance and reduced insulin clearance, and inadequate drug therapy. IIn diabetic patients with ESRD additional factors can cause blood glucose (BG) fluctuations.

4.1 Fluctuations of blood glucose under hemodialysis

High fluctuations of blood glucose (BG) are characteristically in insulin-dependent diabetic patients on hemodialysis. Several factors contribute to these wide fluctuations in BG-levels and increase the risk of hypoglycemic events. Hemodialysis may cause hypoglycemia due to a decrease of plasma glucose and immunoreactive insulin. Patients undergoing hemodialysis may become hypoglycemic and not be aware of it. There is no hormonal imbalance causing the hypoglycemia and the hormonal response to the hypoglycemia is blunted. Patients with an initial plasma glucose of 5.5 mmol/l (100 mg/dl) or less who are hemodialyzed and who do not eat during dialysis may be particularly at risk, especially if they are on insulin or taking glucose-lowering medication. These should be dialyzed with a dialysis fluid containing at least 5.5 mmol/l (100 mg/dl) glucose. (Jackson et al, 2000). In patients with poor metabolic control, hyperglycemia appears immediately post-hemodialysis; this was attributed partly to the hemodialysis-induced decrease in the plasma immunoreactive insulin levels. In summary, hemodialysis causes hypoglycemia during dialysis and hyperglycemia post-dialysis by absolute or relative plasma immunoreactive insulin deficiency (Shrishrimal, 2009). The dextrose concentration in the dialysate can affect glucose control in both ways. Dialysates with lower dextrose concentrations may be associated with hypoglycemia, dialysates with higher dextrose can lead to hyperglycemia. Most dialysis centers are using dialysate with 100mg/dl glucose concentration Furthermore, there it was reported that hypoglycemia is usual at the day following hemodialysis, the authors recommended a reduction of the basal insulin dose at these days. Recent study has demonstrated a significant 25% reduction in basal insulin requirements the day after dialysis compared to the day before. No significant change in bolus insulin was oserved, and overall the reduction of total insulin requirements was −15% (Sobngwi et al, 2010)

Insulin in peritoneal dialysis

The fluctuations of blood glucose, hyperinsulinemia and the rare formation of insulin antibodies under subcutaneous insulin (sc) injection can be prevented by peritoneal dialysis PD). Investigations of insulin in patients treated with PD indicate that the intraperitoneal (ip) administration on of insulin leads to more even glucose levels, but that when dialysis fluids with glucose concentrations higher than 13.6 g/L are used, the absorption of glucose from the abdominal cavity is greater in PD with ip insulin treatment than it is with sc administration (Quellhorst, 2002)

The raised glucose absorption from the abdominal cavity in ip insulin administration must be regarded as a disadvantage. Investigations of insulin in PD showed, that after a dwell time of 30 min, the absorption of insulin from the abdominal cavity in the patients with diabetes was much higher than in the patients without diabetes. In several studies the authors compared both routes of insulin administration. they observed a better fall of HbA1c after switching from sc to ip administration (Grodstein et al, 1981)

4.2 Monitoring of glycemic control

It is well known that hemoglobin A(1c) is no exact parameter for glycemic control in uremic diabetic patients (Joy et al , 2002). Especially, the hemoglobin A(1c) level can be falsely high in ESRD, but it is still a reasonable measure of glycemic control in this population. The cause of the falsely evated level in diabetic patients with ESRD is the elevated blood urea nitrogen, which causes formation of carbamylated hemoglobin, which is indistinguishable from glycosylated hemoglobin. Other factors such as the shorter red life span of red blood cells, iron deficiency, recent transfusion, and use of erythropoietin-stimulating agents may also cause underestimation of glucose control. In a recent study it was reported that glycated albumin is a better glycemic indicator than glycated hemoglobon values in hemodialysis patientswith diabetes (Inaba, eet al, 2007) However, in the clinical practise glycated hemoglobin was not replaced by glycated albumin or fructosamine

5. Metabolic control and vascular diseases dependent on antidiabetic therapy

There are only few data in the literature concerning metabolic control under different - antidiabetic therapy. In a recent study we investigated metabolic control and vascular diseases in 64 type 2 diabetic patients under chronic hemodialysis therapy. 42 patients (65%) received insulin therapy (n=42) versus 12 patients oral antidiabetic drug therapy (19%). 10 patients were treated with diet alone (16%). Observation period was the first year of hemodialysis (Biesenbach et al, 2010). The baseline data are summarized in table 1, The

	Oral SU	Insulin	Diet alone
Number (n)	12	42	10
Age (years)	63±16	62±11	62±11
Female (n/%)	6 (50%)	24 (57%)	5 (50%)
Body weight	78±21	79±18	76±16
Diabetes duration (years)	13±4	16±5**	6±3**
C-Peptide (ng/ml)	2.2±1.1	1.8±0.9*	2.4±1.1*
Hypertension (n)	10 (87%)	38 (90%)	8 (80%)
Antihypertensive drugs (n/%)	2,3 (0- 4)	2,1 (0-4)	2.0 (0-3)
Statine (n/%)	4 (33%)	14 (33%)	4 (40%)
Smoker (n/%)	4 (33%)	12 (28%)	3 (33%)

*p<0.05, **p<0.01

Table 1. Baseline data before the start of hemodialysis in patients with sulfonylurea (SU) or insulin therapy and/or diet alone

5.1 Metabolic control dependent on antidiabetic therapy

HbA1c values were similar in each groups at the start of HD as well as after one year. Hypoglycemia occurred more frequently in the insulin-treated patients, however the difference was not significant. The triglycerides were significantly lower in the insulin-treated patients (138+28 versus 176+46 mg/dl, (p<0.05). The body weight was similar in each group, during 12 months a slightly weight loss (1-2%) could be observed in the group with oral antidiabetic and insulin therapy. The metabolic control in the three patient groups is presented in table 2 and 3 as well as table 4.

The C-peptide at the start of HD was lower in the insulin treated patients with 1.8±0.9 ng/ml versus 2.2±1.1 and 2.4±1.1 ng/ml in the other groups (p<0.05). During the first 12 months after the start of hemodialysis in the patient group with SU therapy two patients became insulin dependent, on the other group insulin therapy could be stopped in two cases, a reduction of insulin dose was necessary in 2 patients (48%).

	At start of HD	after 12 months	changes
HbA1c (%)	7.6±1.3	7.7±1.2	+ 1%
Hypo (n/patient/month)	0.6	0.9	+50%
Body weight (kg)	78±21	76±18	-2%
Cholesterol (mg/dl)	168±44	156±33	-7%
Triglycerides (mg/dl)	188+48	176±46	-6%
SU gliclazid/glimerpirid (n)	6/6	4/4	
SU changed to insulin (n)	0	2	16%
SU changed to diet alone (n)	0	2	16%

Table 2. Metabolic control at the start and after 12 months hemodialyis in patients with sulfonylurea (SU) as oral antidiabetic therapy.

	At start of HD	after 1 year	changes (%)
HbA1c (%)	7.9±1.1	7.7±0.8	-2%
Hypoglycemia (n/patient/month)	0.6	1.1	+83%
Body weight (kg)	79±18	78±17	-1%
Cholesterol (mg/dl)	154±42	144±36	-6%
Triglycerides (mg/dl)	144±38	138±28	-4%
Insulin dose (U/patient/day)	28±6*	22±5*	-21%
Insulin changed to SU (n)	0	1	8%
Insulin changed to diet alone (n)	0	1	8%

*$p<0.05$

Table 3. Metabolic control at the start and after 12 months hemodialysis in patients with insulin therapy.

	At the start of HD	after 1 year	changes (%)
HbA1c (%)	7.4±0.8	7.1±0.6	-4%
Hypoglycemia (n/patient/month)	0,4	0,6	+50%
Body weight (kg)	76±16	76±12	0%
Cholesterol (mg/dl)	182±38	178±33	-3%
Triglycerides (mg/dl)	164±32	160±33	-3%
Diet alone changed to insulin	0	0	0%
Diet alone changed to antidiabetic drug	0	1	10%

Table 4. Metabolic control at the start and after12 months hemodialysis in patients with diabetes diet alone.

5.2 The prevalence of vascular diseases depended on antidiabetic therapy

The prevalence of vascular diseases was only slightly higher in the insulin-treated patients (NS). The prevalence of coronary artery disease was 45% in the CAD group versus 33% and 30% in the other two groups. This may be caused by a significantly higher diabetes duration. The prevalences are also shown in figure 1 The similar prevalence of macroangiopathy at the start of dialysis is not surprisingly, in each patient groupthe vascular risk factors were similar. The renal disease in type 2 diabetic patients at ESRD is in the majority a diabetic nephropathy (70-80%) The other diabetic patients mostly suffer from a vascular nephropathy (15-25%). It may be assumed that patients with vascular disease need more often only diet alone. In an earlier study we reported, that during the last 3 years before start of dialysis, progression of diabetic and vascular nephropathy with fall in GFR, were similar, and the prevalence of vascular diseases too (Biesenbach et al, 2006). Surprisingly, there is no relevant study in the literature concerning differences in the antidiabetic therapy between patients with diabetic and vascular nephropathy. In a recent study comparing the outcome of patients with diabetic and vascular nephropathy, we reported that insulin was used in 67% of the patients with diabetic nephropathy versus in only 25% of those with vascular nephropathy (Stieglmayr et al, 2010)

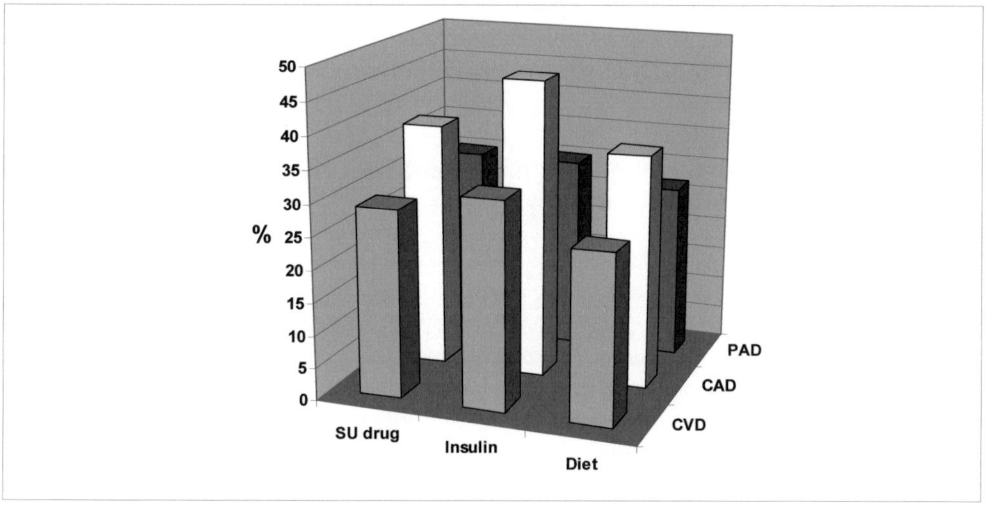

Fig. 1. Prevalence of cerebrovascular disease (CVD), coronary artery disease (CAD) and peripheral artery disease (PAD) dependent on anti-diabetic therapy with diet alone, Insulin or sulfonylurea (SU) drug.

6. Conclusions

Antidiabetic therapy in patients with ESRD can be difficult, both, the administration of oral antidiabetic drugs as well as the insulin injction. To obtain a good glycemic control in chronic renal insufficiency multiple factors intrinsic to diabetes, renal insufficiency and therapy has to be taken into account. Insulin resistance and and hyperinsulinaemia can impair the capacity of antidiabetic therapy. The requirement of insulin decreases in renal insufficiency due to reduced insulin clearance. Intensive insulin therapy is the adequate method for improving glycaemic control in ESRD. The most common side effect of insulin is hypoglycemia. In the few studies reported until now, the use of insulin analogues in uremic patients has been associated with potential advantages and benefits with regard to glycaemic control, yet without any significant elevation in hypoglycaemic event frequency. Intensified insuin therapy, the basis bolus regime, shoud be prefered, in type 2 diabetes wth low insulin requirement a conventional insulin therapy can also be used.

7. Summary – important factors of antidiabetic therapy in ESRD

- Wide fluctations in blood glucose levels are characteristically in diabetic patients on hemodialysis
- Most of the diabetic patients with ESRD need insulin- therapy, only a small group of these patients can be treated with oral antidiabetic drugs
- Several oral antidiabetic drugs like glinide, glitazone and gliptine as well as some SU agents can be used in patients with renal insufficiency, in patients on hemodialysis in most cases a drug dose reduction by 50% is necessary in most cases.
- Most diabetes drugs are excreted at least in part by the kidney, so that patients in ESRD are at greater risk of hypoglycemia
- Impairment of renal functon is associated with reduced insulin clearance , therfore, insulin doses should be lowered in patients with low GFR.
- In patients with insulin therapy hypoglycaemia occurs more frequently during dialysis and hyperglycemia after dialysis due to insulin deficiency-
- The hemoglobin A1c level can be falsely high in ESRD, but there is no alternative, it is still a reasonable measure of glycemic control
- The prevalence of vascular diseases is not significantly different in the the patients with insulin versus oral antidiabetic therapy

8. References

Aisenpreis U, Pfu¨ tzner A, Giehl M, Keller F, Jehle PM. *Pharmacokinetics and pharmacodynamics of insulin lispro compared with regular insulin in haemodialysis patients with diabetes mellitus.* Nephrol Dial Transplant 14 (Suppl. 4): 5–6, 1999

Aronoff GR, Berns JS, Brier ME et al. eds. *Drug Prescribing in Renal Failure. Dosing Guideline for Adults,* 4th edn. Philadelphia: American College of Physicians, 1999.

Bergman AJ, Cote J, Yi B et al. *Effect of renal insufficincy on the pharmacokinetics of sitagliptin, a dipeptidyl peptidase-inhibitor* Diabetes Care 30: 1862-1864, 2007

Biesenbach G, Bodlaj G, Ebner S, Biesenbach P, Pieringer H *Metabolic control and vascular diseases under oral antidiabetic drug versus insulin therapy and/or diet alone during the first year of hemodialysis in type 2 diabetic patients with ESRD* Int Urol Nephrol 20: 642-645 2010.

Biesenbach G, Raml A, Schmekal B, Eichbauer-Sturm G. .*Decreased insulin requirement in relation to GFR in nephropathic Type 1 and insulin-treated Type 2* diabetic patients. Diabet Med. 8:642-45, 2003

Biesenbach G, Bodlaj G, Pieringer H, SedlakM. Influence of residual diuresis on insulin requirement in insulin-treated type 2 diabetic patients during the first year of hemodialysis. Nephrol Dial Transplant. 23(1):422-423, 2008

Biesenbach G, Schmekal B, Pieringer H, Janko O *Rate of decline of GFR and progression of vascular disease in type 2 diabetic patients with diabetic or vascular nephropathy during the last three years before startimg dialysis therapy*. Kidney Blood Press Res. 29(5):267-672.,2006

Block M, Mako M, Steiner D, Rubenstein A. *Circulating -peptide immunoreactivity studies in normal and diabetic patients*. Diabetes 21: 1013–1024, 1972

Bridget M. Kuehn. *Exenatide and kidney function*. YAMA 302: 2466, 2010

Charpentier G, Riveline JP, Varroud-Vial M. *Management of drugs affecting blood glucose in diabetic patients with renal failure.* Diabetes Metab 26: 73–85. 2002

DeFronzo RA, Andres R, Edgar P, Walker WG. *Carbohydrate metabolism in uremia. A review.* Medicine 52: 469–481. 1973

Ersoy A, Ersoy C, Altinay T. *Insulin analogue usage in a haemodisis patient with type 2 diabetes mellitus.* Nephrol Dial Transplant. 21(2):553-554, 2006

Grodstein GP, Blumenkrantz MJ, Kopple JD; Moran JK, Coburn JW: *Glucose absorption during continuous ambulatory peritoneal dialysis.* Kidney Int 19: 564, 1981

Horton ES, Johnson C, Lebovitz HE. Carbohydrate metabolism in uremia. Ann Intern Med 1968; 68: 63–74. 1968

Jehle PM, Aisenpreis U, Bundschu D, Keller F. Advantages *of insulin lispro (short-acting) in terminal kidney failure*. Fortschr Med 20: 41–42. 1999

Iglesias P and Diez J *Insulin therapy in renal disease* Diabetes, Obesity and Metabolism, 10, 811–823, 2006

Inaba M, Okuno S, Kumeda Y, et al. (2007) Osaka CKD Expert Research Group. *Glycated albumin is a better glycemic indicator than glycated hemoglobin values in hemodialysis patients with diabetes: effect of anemia and erythropoietin injection.* J Am Soc Nephrol 18:896- 903, 2007

Jackson MA, Holland MR, Nicholas J, Lodwick R, Forster D, Macdonald IA (2000). *Hemodialysis-induced hypoglycemia in diabetic Patients* Clin Nephrol. 54:30-34, 2000

Joy MS, Cefali WT, Hogan SL, Nachman PH *Long-term glycemic control measurements in diabetic patients receiving hemodialysis.* Am J Kidney Dis 2002; 39:297–307, 2002

Kovesdy Kovesdy C, Sharma K, Kalantar-Zadeh. *Glycemic control in diabetic CKD patients: where do we stand?* Am J Kidney Dis 52: 6766-777, 2008

Jackson MA, Holland MR, Nicholas J, Lodwick R, Forster D, Macdonald IA (2000). *Hemodialysis-induced hypoglycemia in diabetic Patients* Clin Nephrol. 54:30-34, 2000

Loipl J, Schmekal B, Biesenbach G *Long-term impact of chronic hemodialysis on glycemic control and serum lipids in insulin-treated type 2-diabetic patients.* Ren Fail. 27(3):305-308, 2005

Mak RH, DeFronzo RA *Glucose and insulin metabolism in uremia.* Nephron 61:377-382, 2002

McCormack , Johns H, Hildesdey H Metformin's contraindications should be contraindicated *Canadian Med Ass J 173: 1503, 2005*

Mohadee P, Bornemann M.Sugihara J, G, Arakaki R T*he metabolic effects of triglitazone in patients with diabetes and end stage renal disease.* Endokrine 38.181-186, 2005

Morioka T, Emoto M, Tabata T et al *Glycemic control is a predictor for survival of diabetic patients on hemodialsis.* Am J KidneyDis 24: 909-913, 2001

Nagat T, Imamura M, Lizuka K, Mori M. *Hypoglycemia due to nateglinide admnistration in diabetic patients with chronic renal failure.* Disbetes Res Clin Pract 59:191-194, 2003

O'Mara NB. *Agents for the treatment of diabetes mellitus.* Semin Dial.23:475-479, 2010

O0michi T, Emoto M, Tabata T et al *Impact of glycemic control on survival of diabetic patientson chronic regular hemodialysis.* Diabetes Care 29: 1496-1500, 2006

Polonsky KS, Licinio-Paixao J, Given BD et al. Use of biosynthetic human C-peptide in the measurement of insulin secretion rates in normal volunteers and type I diabetic patients. J Clin Invest 77: 98–105. 1986

Quellhorst. *Insulin therapy during peritoneal dialysis: pros and cons of various forms of administration.* . J Am Soc Nephrol. 13 Suppl 1:S92-6. 2002

Rabkin R, Ryann MP, Duckwords WC. *The renal metabolism of insdulin.* Diabetologia 27; 351-357, 1984

Shrishrimal, P Hart, F Michota *Managing diabetes in hemodialysis patients: Observations and recommendations* Cleveland Clinic Journal of Medicine . 76 11; 649-655, 2009

Schmidtz O, Alberti KG, Orskov H. *Insulin resistance in uraemic insulin-dependent diabetics. Effect of dialysis therapy as assessed by the artificial endocrine pancreas.* Acta Endocrinol 105: 371–378, 1984

Snyder RW, Berns JS *Use of insulin and oral hyüoglycemic medications in atients with diabetes and advanced kidney.* Semin Dial 7:365-370, 2004

Stieglmayr S, Khayyat AH, Bodlaj G, Pieringer H, Biesenbach G. *Comparable outcomes in type 2 diabetic patients with diabetic or vascular nephropathy treated by hemodialysis.* Nephron Clin Pract 114 (2) 104-107, 2010

Thompson-Culkin K, Zussman B, Miller AK Freed MI et al *Pharmacokinetics of rosiglitazone in patients with end-stage renal disease.* J Int Med Res 30: 391-399, 2002

Uzu T, Hatta T, Deji N, Izumiya T et al. *Target for glycemic control in type 2 diabetic atients on hemodialysis: effects of amemia and erythropoietin injection on HbA(1c).* Ther Apher Dial 13: 89-94, 2009

Williams ME *Insulin Management of a Diabetic Patient on Hemodialysis* Seminar Dialysis 5(1); 69-73, 2007

Yale J-F *Oral Antihyperglycemic Agents and Renal Disease: New agents, New Concepts* J Am Soc Nephrol 16: S7–S10, 2005

6

Treatment Protocol for Controlling Bone Metabolism Parameters in Hemodialysis Patients

Pablo Molina, Pilar Sánchez-Pérez, Ana Peris,
José L. Górriz and Luis M. Pallardó
*Department of Nephrology, Hospital Universitario Dr Peset &
Division of Nephrology, Hospital Francesc de Borja, Valencia
Spain*

1. Introduction

Abnormal mineral metabolism and severe secondary hyperparathyroidism play a key role in the pathophysiology of skeletal and extraskeletal calcification and are associated with increased morbidity and mortality among hemodialysis (HD) patients (Block GA et al., 1998, 2004; Ganesh et al., 2001; London GM et al., 2003). As a result of these findings, the National Kidney Foundation introduced guidelines in 2003 on controlling parathyroid hormone (PTH), calcium (Ca), phosphorous (P) and calcium-phosphorous ion product (CaxP) in these patients (National Kidney Foundation-Kidney Disease Outcomes and Quality Initiative, 2003). However, in spite of the publication of the K/DOQI guidelines, most HD patients remained outside the recommended targets (Al Aly et al., 2004; Arenas et al., 2006; Lorenzo et al., 2006; Maduell et al., 2005). Historically, Ca-containing phosphate binders and vitamin D have provided the main strategies for reducing P and PTH levels (Slatopolsky et al., 1986). However, the overuse of Ca-containing phosphate binders and active vitamin D can result in hypercalcemia, high CaxP level and Ca overload, which may accelerate vascular disease and hasten death. These side effects potentially require temporary cessation of vitamin D and a reduction in Ca-containing binder administration. This cycle results in a temporary worsening of secondary hyperparathyroidism, allowing bone disease progression (Block et al., 1998, 2000; Johnson et al., 2002; Moe et al., 2003). Hence, new treatment strategies are required (Jindal et al., 2006; Moe et al., 2009;).

Since 2006, two new drugs, paricalcitol and cinacalcet, have been available in daily clinical practice for secondary hyperparathyroidism treatment. Paricalcitol is a vitamin D metabolite that has some advantages over calcitriol, the standard form of vitamin D used worldwide. Paricalcitol suppresses PTH faster than calcitriol (Sprague et al., 2001), and may have a lesser Ca and P intestinal absorption capacity, with smaller increases in Ca and P serum (Llach et al., 2001). Patients who receive paricalcitol may also have a significant survival advantage over those who receive calcitriol (Teng et al., 2003). Despite these advantages, the occurrence of hypercalcemia and high CaxP, when high doses of paricalcitol are used, is not unusual (Goodman, 2001; Martin & Gonzalez, 2001).

Cinacalcet, the first calcimimetic available, has provided a new approach for severe secondary hyperparathyroidism. It increases the sensitivity of the Ca-sensing receptor on the parathyroid cell surface to extracellular Ca ions, thereby inhibiting the release of PTH. All clinical trials concluded that cinacalcet is effective in reducing PTH while simultaneously lowering Ca, P and CaxP levels in HD patients (Block et al, 2004; Goodman et al., 2002; Lindberg et al., 2005; Quarles et al., 2003). All these effects could facilitate achievement of the K/DOQI recommended targets (Block et al., 2008; Messa et al, 2008; Moe et al., 2005).

Given the difficulty of achieving K/DOQI targets, and the absence of treatment algorithms that take into account both drug treatment (conventional drugs like phosphate binders, and new drugs like paricalcitol and cinacalcet) and HD features, such as the length of dialysis session or the dialysate Ca concentration recommended, our HD Unit has, since 2006, implemented a new treatment protocol for controlling bone metabolism parameters. The aim of our study was to evaluate the long-term effect of applying this protocol on achieving K/DOQI targets.

2. Materials and methods

2.1 Study design

This is a single-centre, intervention study. HD patients were eligible for inclusion if they were adults (age ≥18 years) and if they had attended our HD unit for at least 3 months from Jan 2006 to April 2008. Patients who had been on HD therapy for less than 3 months, or who presented excessively suppressed parathyroid hormone (PTH <10 pg/mL) secondary to previous parathyroidectomy, were excluded. Starting in April 2006, the new protocol treatment was applied to 52 of the 57 patients attending our unit over this two year period. Five patients were excluded (in every case because of a stay in our HD unit of less than 3 months).

2.2 Interventions

This intervention study consisted of three stages: an assessment stage 3 months before applying the protocol (base period), and the 12 and 24 month effectiveness assessment phases. During the base period (January-March 2006), calcitriol was the only drug available for hyperparathyroidism treatment, and a bath containing 2.5 mEq/L of Ca was preferentially used, as K/DOQI guidelines recommended. Since April 2006, treatment for control bone metabolism parameters, including cinacalcet administration, has been adjusted according to our new protocol. All patients treated with calcitriol, were changed to paricalcitol. Dialysate Ca content was determined individually, based on the protocol. In all three stages, Ca acetate was the only Ca-containing phosphate binder used, in order to limit the total dosage of elemental Ca provided. The preferred non-Ca phosphate binder used was sevelamer, up to a maximum dose of 4800 mg per day. Only if P remained >5.5 mg/dL, in spite of full doses of Ca acetate and sevelamer, was treatment with aluminium hydroxide considered. In line with K-DOQI guidelines, we tried to maintain serum Ca levels within the normal range for our laboratory (8.4-10.2 mg/dL), and preferably towards the lower end (8.4-9.5 mg/dL); P below 5.5 mg/dL; CaxP below 55 mg^2/dL^2; and PTH levels between 150 and 300 pg/mL. The protocol consisted in three treatment algorithms, depending on the PTH level. When parathyroid hormone level was less than 150 pg/mL (Figure 1), depending on Ca levels, the dose of cinacalcet or paricalcitol was reduced gradually, until a minimum dose (oral cinacalcet, 30 mg three times per week; intravenous paricalcitol, 2.5 µg once per week) was reached. If PTH levels continued to be oversuppressed, we considered a reduction in dialysate Ca concentration from 3.0 to 2.5 mEq/L or a reduction in the dose of Ca acetate, in order to stimulate the PTH secretion.

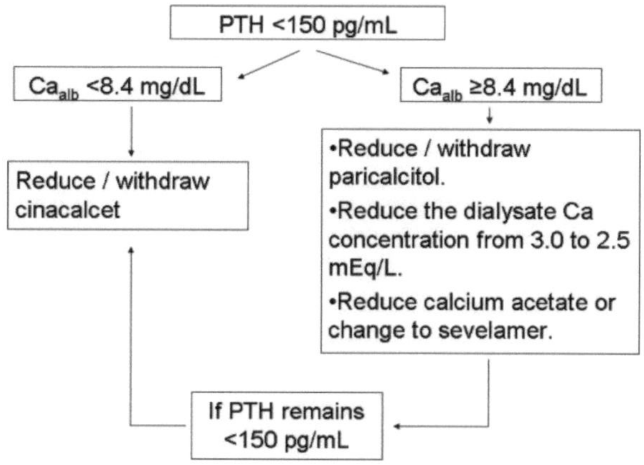

Fig. 1. Algorithm treatment when parathyroid hormone level was less than 150 pg/mL.

When parathyroid hormone level was within the target range (Figure 2), osteodystrophy treatment was modified according to Ca and P levels. If Ca levels ≥9.5 mg/dL and P levels were within the range, the doses of paricalcitol or Ca acetate were reduced. A reduction in dialysate calcium concentration to 2.5 mEq/L was also considered. If P levels were >5.5 mg/dL and Ca levels were within the range, we increased the dose of phosphate binders and we considered lengthening the time of dialysis session. If both Ca and P levels were too high, Ca acetate was replaced by non-Ca phosphate binders and paricalcitol dosage was reduced or replaced by cinacalcet. In this case, we also considered a reduction in dialysate Ca concentration to 2.5 mEq/L and an increase in the length or frequency of dialysis session.

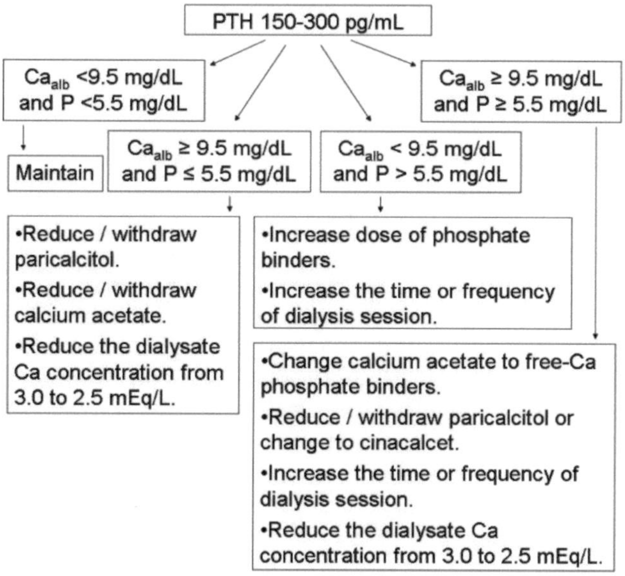

Fig. 2. Algorithm treatment when parathyroid hormone level was within the target range.

When parathyroid hormone was over 300 pg/mL (Figure 3), and Ca <9.5 mg/dL, dialysate Ca concentration were raised from 2.5 to 3.0 mEq/L, and we increased paricalcitol or cinacalcet, depending on whether the P and CaxP levels were normal or too high, respectively. Increases in the length of dialysis session and in the Ca acetate dosage were also considered. When Ca levels were between 9.5 to 10.2 mg/dL and CaxP <55 mg^2/dL^2, cinacalcet was preferentially used. If PTH remained too high, in spite of full doses of cinacalcet, we considered changing Ca acetate to sevelamer and increasing dialysate Ca concentration or adding low doses of paricalcitol, carefully monitoring CaxP levels. When Ca levels were too high or within the high-normal range and CaxP >55 mg^2/dL^2, paricalcitol was reduced or withdrawn and the cinacalcet dosage was increased. We also considered increasing the length or frequency of dialysis session and the dosage of non-Ca phosphate binders, and reducing the dialysate Ca concentration.

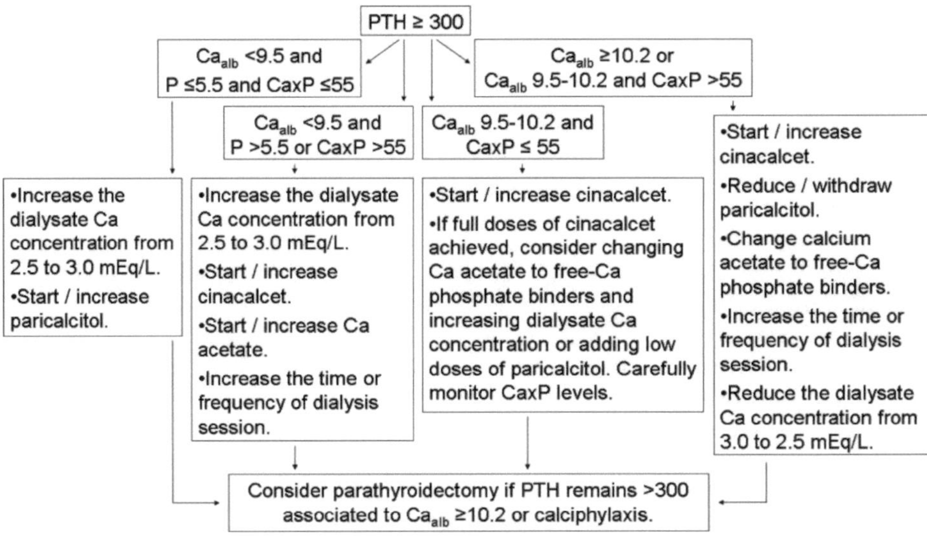

Fig. 3. Algorithm treatment when parathyroid hormone was over 300 pg/mL.

2.3 Laboratory tests

All blood samples were collected at the start of the dialysis session following the longest interdialysis period. The samples were analyzed for serum Ca, P and intact PTH. All K-DOQI parameters were measured at least monthly. In total, 863 blood samples were analyzed (median: 16.9 samples per patient). Total serum Ca and P were measured by colorimetric assay (Roche Diagnostics GmbH, Mannheim, Germany), the reference value for serum calcium being 8.6–10.4 mg/dL and for phosphate 3.5–5.5 mg/dL. The serum levels of total Ca were adjusted for circulating albumin levels (reference values: 3.4-4.8 g/dL). Albumin levels were assessed by Albumin BCG Method (Roche Diagnostics GmbH, Mannheim, Germany). PTH levels were assessed by an electrochemiluminescence immunoassay (Elecsys, Roche Diagnostics GmbH, Mannheim, Germany). The reference range for healthy adults is 15–65 pg/mL.

2.4 Renal replacement therapy

Patients received standard HD or post-dilution hemodiafiltration (HDF) treatment, lasting between 3h and 4h30m, three times per week.Dialysis prescription was monitored to maintain Kt/V>1.2- Polysulphone or AN69st membrane dialysers were used. Blood flow was at least 300mL/min and dialysate flow 750 mL/min. Dialysate composition was Ca 2.5 or 3.0, Na 139 or 140, K 1.5 or 1.9, bicarbonate 34, 37 or 40.8, mEq/L. Infusate composition for patients on HDF was Na 145, Cl 85, bicarbonate 60 mmol/L, with an infusion flow of 2 L/hour. The dialysis equipment employed was Bellco® or Hospal®.

2.5 Statistics

Student's unpaired *t*-test was used to compare the three phase means of all PTH, Ca, P and CaxP values. The proportion of patients within K/DOQI target ranges over the 2 years following the implemention of the protocol was used to evaluate effectiveness. Percentages were compared using the chi-square test. We analyzed potential factors involved in the evolution of bone metabolism parameters, such as phosphate binder dosage, the cinacalcet and paricalcitol used, and the features of HD employed. Results are expressed as mean and standard deviation. A multivariate analysis of the factors associated with the achievement of all four K/DOQI target ranges during the last year were assessed using logistic regression analysis. A value of $p<0.05$ was considered statistically significant.

3. Results

3.1 Patients

Fifty-two patients were studied, twenty-nine men and twenty-three women, 66.7±17.7 years old (range, 25 to 86 years) with a mean time on HD therapy of 71±84 months (range, 4 to 318 months). The etiology of renal failure was hypertensive nephrosclerosis (n=12), diabetic nephropathy (n=10), glomerulonephritis (n=9), interstitial nephritis (n=8), polycystic kidney disease (n=2), Alport's syndrome (n=1), and undetermined (n=10). The demographics of the patients studied at each stage of the study are summarized in Table 1. Mean observation time was 16.7±9.4 months.

	Baseline	1 year	2 years
Number of patients dialysed	30	36	43
Number of prevalent patients	25	28	30
Number of incident patients	5	8	13
Mean age of patients (years)	67.7 ± 16.9 (25 - 84)	67.2 ± 17.3 (25 - 85)	66.6 ± 16.4 (31 - 86)
Mean time on HD (months)	113 ± 89 (12 - 294)	94 ± 89 (6 - 306)	70 ± 86 (3 - 318)
Mean serum albumin (g/dL)	3.8 ± 0.3 (3.5 - 4.6)	3.8 ± 0.3 (2.8 - 4.6)	3.7 ± 0.4 (2.5 - 4.6)
% of diabetic patients	20%(6)	17%(6)	26%(11)

Table 1. Demographic characteristics of patient population at each stage of the study.

3.2 Evolution of biochemical parameters

Changes in the adjusted Ca (Ca_{Alb}), P, CaxP, and PTH levels before and after implementing the protocol are shown in Table 2. Ca_{Alb}, CaxP and PTH levels decreased significantly throughout the study, with a mean decrease of 3.5% (p=0.016), 8.2% (p=0.023) and 39.4% (p=0.002), respectively. Although there was a reduction in P levels, the difference did not reach statistical significance (p=0.075).

	Baseline	1 year	2 years	p
Ca_{Alb} (mg/dL)	9.46 ± 0.57 (8.26 - 10.45)	9.20 ± 0.529 (7.54 – 10.24)	9.13 ± 0.56 (7.35 – 10.40)	0.016
P (mg/dL)	4.97 ± 1.09 (3.29 - 7.91)	4.62 ± 0.94 (3.02 - 6.7)	4.56 ± 0.84 (3.05 - 6.79)	0.075
CaxP (mg^2/dL^2)	47.36 ± 11.33 (29.97 - 79.81)	42.58 ± 9.03 (27.10 - 63.26)	41.65 ± 8.27 (26.91 - 65.52)	0.023
PTH (pg/mL)	343 ± 209 (11 - 864)	239 ± 126 (36 - 678)	208 ± 107 (42 - 704)	0.002

Table 2. Evolution of Biochemical Parameters.

Mean corrected calcium, serum phosphorus, ion calcium-phosphorus product, and intact parathyroid hormone levels at each stage of the study were compared using Student's unpaired t-test.

3.3 Achievement of K/DOQI target levels

The percentages of patients achieving the K/DOQI targets are summarized in Figure 4. In the base period, the proportion of patients achieving P, CaxP and PTH targets were 67%, 73% and 13% respectively. An improvement in the achievement of these three targets was observed, reaching 84%, 93% and 72% of patients, respectively. This improvement was significant in CaxP and PTH levels ($p=0.024$ and $p<0.001$, respectively). The increase in the percentage of patients achieving P target did not reach statistical significance ($p=0.074$). The proportion of patients achieving Ca_{Alb} levels remained above 90% throughout the study ($p=0.644$). Overall, the rate of patients with all four K-DOQI parameters within target ranges improved significantly from 10.0 at baseline, to 33.3% ($p=0.023$) and to 60.5% ($p<0.001$) during the first and second year after implementing the protocol, respectively (Figure 5).

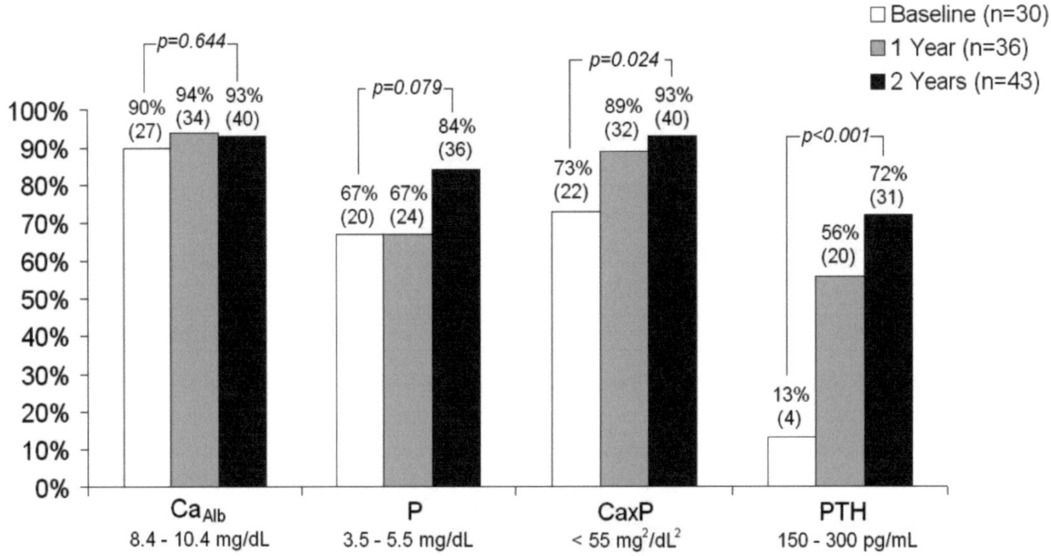

Fig. 4. Percentage (%) of patients achieving each K/DOQI target by time period.

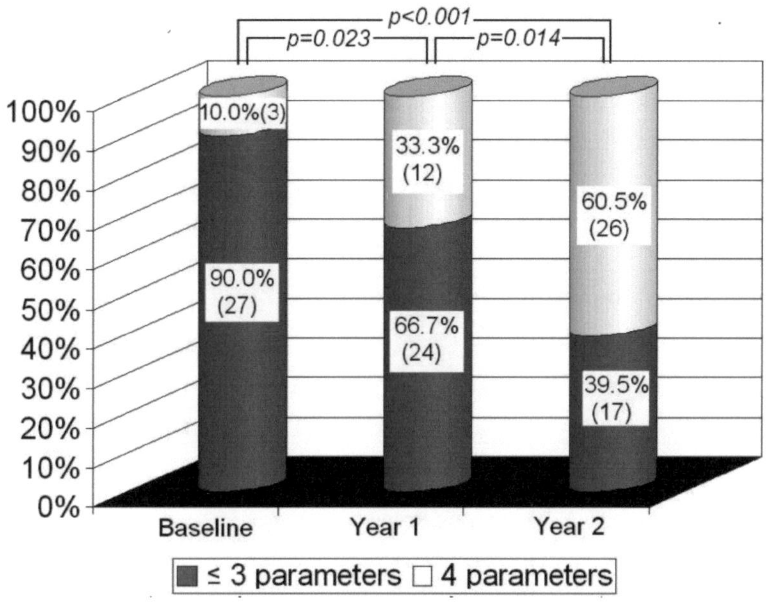

Fig. 5. Percentage (%) of patients achieving all four K/DOQI targets by time period.

3.4 Medication use

Treatment of osteodystrophy over time is shown in Table 3. As the protocol stated, all patients treated with calcitriol were changed to paricalcitol, which was administered to approximately a third of the patients throughout the study. Cinacalcet was the other drug available for HPT, and was administered to 22% and 26% of patients during the first and second year after implementing the protocol, respectively. Two drugs were administered in combination to 5 (12%) and 6 (14%) patients in each assessment stage. Ca acetate was the only calcium-based phosphate binder used, and the proportion of patients receiving this drug remained unchanged (70% of patients, approximately). The mean total dosage of elemental calcium provided by calcium acetate increased from 451±151 to 562±275 mg/day without statistical significance (p=0.079). The proportion of patients under treatment with aluminium hydroxide at the start of the study was significantly reduced from 20% (n=6) to 5% (n=2) (p=0.047). Its dose remained unchanged throughout the study.

Mean total dosage of calcium acetate is expressed as elemental calcium provided by calcium acetate. Mean doses were compared using Student's unpaired *t*-test. Percentages were compared using the chi-square test. Abbreviations: n: number of patients; n.a.: not applicable. †Mean dose of aluminium hydroxide cannot be computed because the standard deviations of both groups were 0.

3.5 Renal replacement therapy

Changes in HD features over time are shown in Table 4. After implementing the protocol, a 3.0 mEq/L dialysate Ca concentration became the most widely used (7% vs. 72%; p=0.001), and a significant increase in the proportion of patients under convective therapy was detected (30% vs. 67%; p=0.034). The length of dialysis session and the HD dose remained unchanged.

	Baseline (n=30)	1 year (n=36)	2 years (n=43)	*p*
Rocaltrol n, (%) patients on treatment mean dose (μg/week)	13 (43%) 1.44 ± 0.21 (0.75 - 1.50)	-	-	n.a. n.a.
Paricalcitol n, (%) patients on treatment mean dose (μg/week)	-	16 (44%) 9.93 ± 5.19 (2.50 - 22.50)	14 (33%) 9.38 ± 4.87 (5.00 – 20.00)	n.a. n.a.
Cinacalcet n, (%) patients on treatment mean dose (mg/day)	-	8 (22%) 35.7 ± 17.8 (15 - 60)	11 (26%) 45.0 ± 34.6 (15 - 120)	n.a. n.a.
Calcium acetate n, (%) patients on treatment mean dose (mg/day)	20 (67%) 451 ± 151 (254 - 762)	28 (78%) 553 ± 242 (127 - 1143)	28 (65%) 562 ± 275 (127 - 1143)	0.547 0.079
Sevelamer n, (%) patients on treatment mean dose (mg/day)	20 (67%) 4760 ± 1916 (2400 - 7200)	22 (61%) 4255 ± 1645 (2400 - 7200)	26 (61%) 4062 ± 1662 (800 - 7200)	0.386 0.179
Aluminium hydroxide n, (%) patients on treatment mean dose (mg/day)	6 (20%) 699 ± 0 (699 - 699)	2 (6%) 699 ± 0 (699 - 699)	2 (5%) 699 ± 0 (699 - 699)	0.047 †

Table 3. Treatment of osteodystrophy at each stage of the study.

	Baseline (n=30)	1 year (n=36)	2 years (n=43)	*p*
Dialysate Ca concentration, n (%) Patients with Ca 2.5 Patients with Ca 3.0	28 (93%) 2 (7%)	6 (17%) 30 (83%)	12 (28%) 31 (72%)	0.001
Dialysis type, n (%) Hemodialysis Hemodiafiltration	21 (70%) 9 (30%)	11 (31%) 26 (69%)	14 (33%) 29 (67%)	0.034
Length of dialysis session (hours/week)	11.2 ± 1.3 (9.0 – 13.5)	11.4 ± 1.3 (9.0 – 13.5)	11.6 ± 1.3 (9.0 – 13.5)	0.481
Kt/V	1.39 ± 0.24 (0.90 – 1.84)	1.50 ± 0.20 (1.10-1.91)	1.42 ± 0.22 (1.01-1.90)	0.439

Table 4. HD features at each stage of the study.

Student's unpaired *t*-test was used to compare means of length of dialysis session and Kt/V values. Percentages were compared using the chi-square test. Abbreviations: n: number of patients; URR: urea reduction ratio.

3.6 Factors associated with achieving K/DOQI targets

Data on each group of patients within and outside all four K/DOQI target ranges during the last year were compared (Table 5). The use of cinacalcet (39% vs. 6%; p=0.017) and the use of a 3.0 mEq/L dialysate Ca concentration (85% vs. 53%; p=0.028) were significantly more frequent in the group of patients who achieved all K/DOQI targets than in the group

	≤ 3 K/DOQI targets achieved (n=17)	All 4 K/DOQI targets achieved (n=26)	*p*
Gender, n (%) Female Male	9 (53%) 8 (47%)	10 (39%) 16 (61%)	0.267
Age (years)	67.98 ± 15.88	65.62 ± 17.03	0.650
Mean time on HD (months)	50.21 ± 55.56	82.17 ± 100.22	0.756
Diabetes mellitus, n (%)	6 (35%)	5 (19%)	0.493
Mean serum albumin (g/dL)	3.69 ± 0.41	3.76 ± 0.36	0.575
Mean 25 OH vit D (ng/mL)	11.9 ± 4.5	12.4 ± 4.5	0.770
Dialysate Ca concentration, n (%) Patients with Ca 2.5 Patients with Ca 3.0	8 (47%) 9 (53%)	4 (15%) 22 (85%)	0.028
Dialysis type, n (%) Hemodialysis Hemodiafiltration	7 (41%) 10 (59%)	7 (27%) 19 (73%)	0.259
Length of dialysis session (hours/week)	11.4 ± 1.4	11.5 ± 1.2	0.434
Kt/V	1.37 ± 0.22	1.46 ± 0.21	0.178
Residual diuresis†, n (%)	3 (18%)	7 (27%)	0.375
Paricalcitol n, (%) patients on treatment mean dose (µg/week)	4 (24%) 8.13 ± 4.73	10 (39%) 9.79 ± 5.05	0.247 0.573
Cinacalcet n, (%) patients on treatment mean dose (mg/day)	1 (6%) 30	10 (39%) 46.7 ± 36.6	0.017 0.909
Calcium acetate n, (%) patients on treatment mean dose (mg/day)	11 (65%) 577 ± 323	17 (65%) 553 ± 250	0.608 0.434
Sevelamer n, (%) patients on treatment mean dose (mg/day)	10 (39%) 4000 ± 1131	16 (62%) 4100 ± 1957	0.554 0.870
Aluminium hydroxide n, (%) patients on treatment	2 (12%)	0 (0%)	0.151

Table 5. Characteristics of the patients who achieved all K/DOQI target ranges during the second year period and those who did not. Mean total dosage of calcium acetate is expressed as elemental calcium provided by calcium acetate. Student's unpaired *t*-test was used to compare means. Percentages were compared using the chi-square test. Abbreviation: n, number of patients; 25 OH vit D, 25-Hydroxyvitamin D; URR, urea reduction ratio. † Residual diuresis is defined as diuresis >1000 mL/24h and residual KtV ≥0.4.

outside ranges. Although there was a higher proportion of patients under paricalcitol treatment (39% vs. 24%) and convective therapy (73% vs. 59%) in the group achieving all targets, the differences did not reach statistical significance (p=0.247 and p=0.259, respectively). There were no differences in the use of phosphate binders or the dialysis dose. A multivariate analysis found that the use of a 3.0 mEq/L dialysate Ca concentration (OR 5.756; 1.102-30.077; p=0.038) and treatment with cinacalcet (OR 12.684; 1.115-144.352; p=0.041) were the factors associated with achieving all K/DOQI targets.

4. Discussion

In spite of applying the K/DOQI Clinical Practice Guidelines for Bone Metabolism and Disease, achievement of K/DOQI targets reminds difficult. In 2006, coinciding with the availability in daily clinical practice of paricalcitol and cinacalcet, our HD Unit implemented a new treatment protocol for controlling the bone metabolism parameters better. As Figures 1, 2 and 3 show, this protocol consisted of three practical treatment algorithms, based on the use of cinacalcet and paricalcitol and the individualization of the dialysate Ca concentration employed, as the main strategies for hyperparathyroidism control, and of dialysis adequacy and combined therapy with sevelamer and Ca acetate for controlling Ca and P levels. Although other algorithms for controlling bone metabolism parameters have been developed (Cannata & Drueke, 2000; Messa et al, 2008; Torregrosa et al., 2011), this, we believe, is the first one to take into account both the drug treatment and HD features, such as the length of dialysis session or the dialysate Ca concentration recommended.

Application of this new treatment protocol was effective and resulted in significant reductions in mean Ca_{Alb}, CaxP and PTH levels (Table 2), with a higher proportion of patients achieving the recommended goals. Noteworthy is the 60.5% of patients with all four K-DOQI parameters within target ranges in the second year after implementing the protocol (Figure 5). This improvement in K/DOQI targets maintained over time could have a direct impact in the survival of patients, given that the simultaneous control of all bone and mineral metabolisms have been showed to be associated with improved survival (Danese et al., 2008).

Implementation of the protocol entailed the administration of paricalcitol and cinacalcet, a preferential use of convective therapies, and the most widely used dialysate Ca concentration of 3.0 mEq/L (Tables 4 and 5). However, it is not easy to assess which of the measures carried out, following implementation of the protocol, has the greatest effect on improving the K/DOQI targets observed, given the multiple factors involved in PTH secretion and in Ca and P levels. We, therefore, compared the characteristics of the patients who achieved all K/DOQI target ranges during the second year of study and those who did not (Table 5). Although there was higher HD dose and a higher proportion of patients under paricalcitol treatment and convective therapy in the group within all the targets, a multivariate analysis showed that the use of a 3.0 mEq/L dialysate Ca concentration and the treatment with cinacalcet were the only two factors significantly associated with achievement of all K/DOQI targets.

These findings are consistent with the literature. Cinacalcet, the first calcimimetic available in daily clinical practice, has proven effective for lowering PTH, Ca, P and CaxP levels in HD patients (Block et al, 2004; Goodman et al., 2002; Lindberg et al., 2005; Quarles et al., 2003). This ability to lower PTH, while limiting the risks of hyperphosphatemia or hypercalcemia, has improved the achievement of the proposed treatment goals (Block et al., 2008; Messa et al., 2008; Moe et al., 2005), allowing it to be used synergistically in combination with vitamin D sterols (Chertow et al., 2006; Messa et al., 2008). Our protocol took this favourable and complementary effect of combined treatment into account: 60% of the patients who were on paricalcitol treatment and achieved all K/DOQI goals during the second year of study, also received treatment with cinacalcet. In conclusion, we cannot explain the great improvement in K/DOQI goals achieved throughout the study without the use of cinacalcet, either alone or in association with paricalcitol. It's to note the absence of significant association between the use of paricalcitol and achievement of control of all K/DOQI targets. We think it might be related to the fact that 43% of the patients were previously treated with calcitriol. Hence it's difficult to detect any advantages in improving bone metabolism parameters with the use of paricalcitol. Despite these results, we still recommend the preferential use of paricalcitol over calcitriol, given the benefits observed in other studies with the selective vitamin D receptor activation (Llach et al., 2001; Sprague et al.,2001; Teng et al., 2003).

Greater use of a 3.0 mEq/L dialysate Ca concentration was the other factor significantly associated with achieving all K/DOQI targets (85% of patients within all targets). Although optimal dialysate Ca concentration for HD patients has been set at 2.5 mEq/L according to K-DOQI guidelines, this recommendation is opinion-based and could negatively affect secondary hyperparathyroidism (Argilés et al., 1998; Fernández, et al., 1995). Several studies have reported better control of secondary hyperparathyroidism, without risk of severe hypercalcemia, after raising the dialysate Ca concentration from 2.5 to 3.0 mEq/L (Argilés, 1995; Malberti & Raviani, 2004; Molina et al., 2008). A Ca concentration of 3.0 mEq/L has, therefore, been suggested as the first choice for the majority of patients on HD (Cannata & Drueke, 2000; Torregrosa et al, 2011; Touissant et al., 2006). In any case, the best approach would be to individualize the prescription of dialysate Ca concentration, as the K-DOQI guidelines noted.

Noteworthy is the absence of significant changes observed in the use of phosphate binders, with the exception of aluminium hydroxide, the use of which was significantly reduced, as evidence of better control of bone metabolism parameters. Although the proportion of patients receiving Ca acetate remained unchanged, the mean total dosage of elemental Ca provided showed a tendency to increase (451±151 vs 562±275 mg/day; p=0.079). The lack of statistical significance could be due to the limited number of patients. This raise in Ca provided by Ca-containing phosphate binders has been previously reported in another study with cinacalcet therapy (Block et al., 2008), where excessively high doses of Ca provided by binders were necessary in order to avoid hypocalcemia. In our study, however, the mean total dosage of elemental Ca provided remained below the maximum dose recommended by K/DOQI guidelines. We speculate that the relatively small average dose of cinacalcet used (45.0±34.6 mg/day), the preferential use of a dialysate Ca concentration of 3.0 mEq/L and the administration of paricalcitol could explain the absence of the need for excessively high doses of Ca acetate. Finally, we should emphasize the desirability of only using Ca acetate, as the Ca-

containing phosphate binder, in order to limit the total dosage of elemental Ca provided.
The current study has several limitations. This was an intervention study without a control group. It would have been interesting to study additional markers of bone metabolism such as bone mass, skeletal fracture rates, cardiovascular calcification or arterial function, given that they could provide more valuable information on the overall assessment of renal bone disease than K-DOQI core measurement standard biomarkers. Other limitations of our study were the limited number of patients, which is common in a single-centre study. However, this was compensated for by the long follow-up period and the relatively high number of blood samples analyzed.

5. Conclusion

Two years after its implementation, the proposed treatment protocol for control bone metabolism parameters has greatly increased the achievement of K/DOQI treatment targets in most of the HD patients. The protocol entailed the administration of cinacalcet, the replacement of calcitriol by paricalcitol, and the incorporation of individual dialysate Ca concentration prescriptions into the algorithm, with a preferential use of a dialysate Ca concentration of 3.0 mEq/L.

6. Acknowledgment

The authors express their gratitude to George Mattingley, Jacqueline Clarke, Sam Landete and Arantxa Caño for their collaboration in translating this text. The authors also thank Francisco Maduell, MD, for his assistance in the development of the manuscript.

7. References

Al Aly Z, González EA, Martin KJ & Gellens ME. (2004). Achieving K/DOQI Laboratory Target Values for Bone and Mineral Metabolism: An Uphill Battle. *Am J Nephrol*, Vol.24, No.4, (August 2004), pp. 422-426. ISSN 0250-8095

Arenas MD, Alvarez U de F, Gil MT, Soriano A, Egea JJ, Millán I, Amoedo ML, Muray S & Carretón MA. (2006). Application of NKF-K/DOQI Clinical Practice Guidelines for Bone Metabolism and Disease: changes of clinical practices and their effects on outcomes and quality standards in three haemodialysis units. *Nephrol Dial Transplant*, Vol.21, No.6, (June 2006), pp. 1663-1668. ISSN 0931-0509

Argilés A. (1995). Points to remember when selecting dialysate calcium concentration. *Nephrol Dial Transplant*, Vol.10, No.4, (April 1995), pp. 451-454. ISSN 0931-0509

Argilés A, Mourad G. (1998). How do we have to use the calcium in the dialysate to optimize the management of secondary hyperparathyroidism? *Nephrol Dial Transplant*, Vol.13, Suppl.3, (April 1998), pp. S62-S64. ISSN 0931-0509

Block GA, Hulbert-Shearon TE, Levin NW & Port FK. (1998). Association of serum phosphorus and calcium x phosphate product with mortality risk in chronic hemodialysis patients: A national study. *Am J Kidney Dis*, Vol.31, No.4, (April 1998), pp. 607-617. ISSN 0272-6386

Block GA, Port FK. (2000). Re-evaluation of risks associated with hyperphosphatemia and hyperparathyroidism in dialysis patients: Recommendations for a change in management. *Am J Kidney Dis*, Vol.35, No.6, (June 2000), pp. 1226-1237. ISSN 0272-6386

Block GA, Martin KJ, de Francisco ALM, Turner SA, Avram MM, Suranyi MG, Hercz G, Cunningham J, Abu-Alfa AK, Messa P, Coyne DW, Locatelli F, Cohen RM, Evenepoel P, Moe SM, Fournier A, Braun J, McCary LC, Zani VJ, Olson KA, Drüeke TB & Goodman WG. (2004). Cinacalcet for secondary hyperparathyroidism in patients receiving hemodialysis. *N Engl J Med*, Vol.350, No.5, (April 2004), pp. 1516-1525. ISSN 0028-4793

Block GA, Klassen PS, Lazarus JM, Ofsthun N, Lowrie EG & Chertow GM. (2004). Mineral metabolism, mortality, and morbidity in maintenance hemodialysis. *J Am Soc Nephrol*, Vol.15, No.8, (August 2004), pp. 2208-2218. ISSN 1046-6673

Block GA, Zeig S, Sugihara J, Chertow GM, Chi EM, Turner SA & Bushinsky DA. (2008). Combined therapy with cinacalcet and low dose of vitamin D sterols in patients with moderate to severe secondary hyperparathyroidism. *Nephrol Dial Transplant*, Vol.23, No.7, (July 2008), pp. 2311-2138. ISSN 0931-0509

Cannata JB & Drueke TB. (2000). Clinical algorithms on renal osteodystrophy. *Nephrol Dial Transplant*, Vol.15, Suppl.5, (October 2000), pp. S39-S57. ISSN 0931-0509

Chertow GM, Blumenthal S, Turner S, Roppolo M, Stern L, Chi EM & Reed J. (2006). Cinacalcet hydrochloride (Sensipar) in hemodialysis patients on active vitamin D derivates with controlled PTH and elevated calcium x phosphate. *Clin J Am Soc Nephrol*, Vol.1, No.2, (March 2006), pp. 305-312. ISSN 1555-9041

Danese MD, Belozeroff V, Smirnakis K & Rothman KJ. (2008). Consistent control of mineral and bone disorder in incident hemodialysis patients. *Clin J Am Soc Nephrol*, Vol.3, No.5, (September 2008), pp. 1423-1429. ISSN 1555-9041

Fernández E, Borràs M, Pals B & Montoliu J. (1995). Low-Calcium Dialysate Stimulates Parathormone Secretion and its Long-Term Use Worsens Secondary Hyperparathyroidism. *J Am Soc Nephrol*, Vol.6, No.1, (July 1995), pp. 132-135. ISSN 1046-6673

Ganesh SK, Stack AG, Levin NW, Hulbert -Shearon T & Port FK. (2001). Association of elevated serum PO4, CaxPO4 product, and parathyroid hormone with cardiac mortality risk in chronic hemodialysis patients. *J Am Soc Nephrol*, Vol.12, No.10, (October 2001), pp. 2131-2138. ISSN 1046-6673

Goodman WG. (2001). Recent developments in the management of secondary hyperparathyroidism. *Kidney Int*, Vol.59, No.3, (March 2001), pp. 1187-1201. ISSN 0085-2538

Goodman WG, Hladik GA, Turner SA, Blaisdell PW, Goodkin DA, Liu W, Barri YM, Cohen RM & Coburn JW. (2002). The calcimimetic agent AMG 073 lowers plasma parathyroid hormone levels in hemodialysis patients with secondary hyperparathyroidism. *J Am Soc Nephrol*, Vol.13, No.4, (April 2002), pp. 1017-1024. ISSN 1046-6673

Jindal K, Chan CT, Deziel C, Hirsch D, Soroka SD, Tonelli M & Culleton BF. (2006). Clinical Practice Guidelines for the Canadian Society of Nephrology: Mineral Metabolism. *J Am Soc Nephrol,* Vol.17, No.3, Suppl.1, (March 2006), pp. S1-S27. ISSN 1046-6673

Johnson CA, McCarthy J, Bailie GR, Deane J & Smith S. (2002). Analysis of renal bone disease treatment in dialysis patients. *Am J Kidney Dis,* Vol.39, No.6, (June 2002), pp. 1270-1277. ISSN 0272-6386

Lindberg JS, Culleton B, Wong G, Borah MF, Clark RV, Shapiro WB, Roger SD, Husserl FE, Klassen PS, Guo MD, Albizem MB & Coburn JW. (2005). Cinacalcet HCl, an oral calcimimetic agent for the treatment of secondary hyperparthyoridism in hemodialysis and peritoneal dialysis: A randomized double-blind, multicenter study. *J Am Soc Nephrol,* Vol.16, No.6, (March 2005), pp. 800-807. ISSN 1046-6673

Llach F& Yudd M. (2001). Paricalcitol in dialysis patients with calcitriol-resistant secondary hyperparathyroidism. *Am J Kidney Dis,* Vol.38, No.5 (Suppl 5), (November 2001), pp. S45-S50. ISSN 0272-6386

London GM, Guerin AP, Marchais SJ, Metivier F, Pannier B & Adda H (2003). Arterial media calcification in end-stage renal disease: Impact on all-cause and cardiovascular mortality. *Nephrol Dial Transplant,* Vol.18, No.9, (September 2003), pp. 1731-1740. ISSN 0931-0509

Lorenzo V, Martín-Malo A, Pérez-García R, Torregrosa JV, Vega N, de Francisco AL & Cases A. (2006). Prevalence, clinical correlates and therapy cost of mineral abnormalities among haemodialysis patients: a cross-sectional multicentre study. *Nephrol Dial Transplant,* Vol.21, No.2, (February 2006), pp. 459-465. ISSN 0931-0509

Maduell F, Górriz JL, Pallardó LM, Pons R & Santiago C. (2005). Assessment of phosphorus and calcium metabolism and its clinical management in hemodialysis patients in the community of Valencia. *J Nephrol,* Vol.18, No.6, (December 2005), pp. 739-748. ISSN 1121-8428

Malberti F & Ravani P. (2004). The choice of the dialysate calcium concentration in the management of patients on haemodialysis and heamodiafiltration. *Nephrol Dial Transplant,* Vol.18, Suppl.7, (August 2004), pp. S37-S40. ISSN 0931-0509

Martin KJ & Gonzalez EA. (2001). Vitamin D analogues for the management of secondary hyperparathyroidism. *Am J Kidney Dis,* Vol.38, No.5 (Suppl 5), (November 2001), pp. S34-S40. ISSN 0272-6386

Messa P, Macário F, Yaqoob M, Bouman K, Braun J, von Albertini B, Brink H, Maduell F, Graf H, Frazão JM, Bos WJ, Torregrosa V, Saha H, Reichel H, Wilkie M, Zani VJ, Molemans B, Carter D & Locatelli F. (2008). The OPTIMA study: assessing a new cinacalcet (Sensipar/Mimpara) treatment algorithm for secondary hyperparathyroidism. *Clin J Am Soc Nephrol,* Vol.3, No.1, (January 2008), pp. 36-45. ISSN 1555-9041

Moe S & Drueke TB. (2003). Management of secondary hyperparathyroidism: The importance and the callenge of controlling parathyroid hormone levels without elevating calcium, phosphorous and calcium-phosphorous product. *Am J Nephrol*, Vol.23, No.6, (November 2003), pp. 369-379. ISSN 0250-8095

Moe SM, Chertow GM & Coburn JW. (2005). Achieving NKF-K/DOQI bone metabolism and treatment goals with cinacalcet HCl. *Kidney Int*, Vol.67, No.2, (February 2005), pp. 760-771. ISSN 0085-2538

Moe SM, Drüeke TB, Block GA, Cannata-Andía JB, Elder GJ, Fukagawa M, Jorgetti V, Ketteler M, Langman CB, Levin A, MacLeod AM, McCann L, McCullough PA, Ott SM, Wang AY, Weisinger JR, Wheeler DC, Persson R, Earley A, Moorthi R & Uhlig K. (2009). KDIGO clinical practice guideline for the diagnosis, evaluation, prevention, and treatment of Chronic Kidney Disease-Mineral and Bone Disorder (CKD-MBD).Kidney Disease: Improving Global Outcomes (KDIGO) CKD-MBD Work Group. *Kidney Int*, Vol.76, Suppl.113, (August 2009), pp. S1-S130. ISSN 0085-2538

Molina P, Sánchez P, Garrigós E & Peris A. (2008). Marked improvement in bone metabolism parameters after raising the dialysate calcium concentration from 2.5 to 3 mEq/L in non-hypercalcemic hemodialysis patients. *Hemodial Int*, Vol.12, No.1, (January 2008), pp. 73-79. ISSN 1492-7535

National Kidney Foundation-Kidney Disease Outcomes and Quality Initiative. (2003). K/DOQI Clinical Practice Guidelines for Bone Metabolism and Disease in Chronic Kidney Disease. *Am J Kidney Dis*, Vol.42, Suppl.3, (October 2003), pp. S1-S201. ISSN 0272-6386

Quarles LD, Sherrard DJ, Adler S, Rosansky SJ, McCary LC, Liu W, Turner SA & Bushinsky DA. (2003). The calcimimetic AMG 073 as a potential treatment for secondary hyperparathyroidism of end–stage renal disease. *J Am Soc Nephrol*, Vol.14, No.3, (March 2003), pp. 575-583. ISSN 1046-6673

Slatopolsky E, Weerts C, Lopez-Hilker S, Norwood K, Zink M, Windus D & Delmez J. (1986). Calcium carbonate as a phosphate binder in patients with chronic renal failure undergoing dialysis. *N Eng J Med*, Vol.315, No.3, (July 1986), pp. 157-161. ISSN 0028-4793

Sprague SM, Lerma E, McCormmick D, Abraham M & Battle D. (2001). Suppression of parathyroid hormone secretion in hemodialysis patients: comparison of paricalcitol with calcitriol. *Am J Kidney Dis*, Vol.38, No.5 (Suppl 5), (November 2001), pp. S51-S56. ISSN 0272-6386

Teng M, Wolf M, Lowrie E, Ofsthun N, Lazarus JM & Thadhani R. (2003). Survival of patients undergoing hemodialysis with paricalctiol or calcitriol therapy. *N Engl J Med*, Vol.349, No.5, (July 2003), pp. 446-456. ISSN 0028-4793

Torregrosa JV, Bover J, Cannata J, Lorenzo V, de Francisco ALM, Martínez I, Rodríguez M, Arenas L, González E, Caravaca F, Martín-Malo A, Fernández E & Torres A. (2011). Spanish Society of Nephrology recommendations for controlling mineral and bone disorders in chronic kidney disease patients (S.E.N.-M.B.D.) *Nefrologia*, Vol.31, Suppl.1, (March 2011), pp. S3-S32. ISSN 0211-6995

Toussaint N, Cooney P & Kerr PG. (2006). Review of dialysate calcium concentration in hemodialysis. *Hemodial Int*, Vol.10, No.4, (October 2006), pp. 326-337. ISSN 1492-7535

7

Dialysis Disequilibrium Syndrome: A Neurological Manifestation of Haemodialysis

Thomas Flannery
Queen's University Belfast/Belfast Health & Social Care Trust
Northern Ireland

1. Introduction

Renal insufficiency has many protean effects on the central nervous system. Early symptoms such as fatigue, clumsiness, and impaired concentration may progress to hallucinations, agitation, disorientation and coma if the renal insufficiency is untreated. The pathophysiology of these changes, due to uraemic encephalopathy are thought to be mediated by impaired neurotransmission (Burn & Bates, 1998). Dialysis of patients with end-stage renal disease (ESRD) helps to minimize the effects of uraemic encephalopathy. However, dialysis of uraemic patients may in itself, also have deleterious effects on the nervous system. One of the potential neurologic sequelae of this treatment modality is dialysis disequilibrium syndrome. First described in 1962, the dialysis disequilibrium syndrome (DDS) is a central nervous system disorder that remains an important clinical problem in dialysis patients. It is characterized by neurologic symptoms of varying severity that are thought to be due primarily to cerebral oedema. Classically, DDS arises in individuals starting haemodialysis due to chronic renal failure and is associated, in particular, with "aggressive" (high solute removal) dialysis (Port et al., 1973).

2. Incidence

Dialysis disequilibrium syndrome has been reported most frequently after rapid haemodialysis and in certain high-risk groups (Arieff, 1989). However, this syndrome is likely to be under-reported given the often mild nature of DDS-type symptoms. First-time haemodialysis patients are at greatest risk, particularly if the blood urea nitrogen (BUN) levels are markedly elevated (above 175 mg/dL or 60 mmol/L). In addition, patients with a sudden change in their dialysis regime, in particular, cases with increased dialysis flow rates are susceptible. Children and elderly patients may remain at increased risk, in particular those with a sudden change in their haemodialysis regime (Flannery et al, 2008). Patients with pre-existing neurologic disease, such as head injury, stroke or malignant hypertension, are also at greater risk for developing DDS (Peterson, 1964; Yoshida et al., 1987).

3. Pathogenesis

Although DDS has been recognized for more than forty years, the pathogenesis of DDS remains debated and incompletely understood. However, what is established and central to the diagnosis of DDS is a raised intracranial pressure. While many theories have been proposed, it is likely that the mechanism(s) underlying the intracranial hypertension are multifactorial.

3.1 "The reverse urea effect"

Haemodialysis rapidly removes small solutes such as urea, particularly in patients who have marked uraemia. Urea is generally considered an "ineffective" osmole, because of its ability to permeate cell membranes. However, this ability to cross the cell membrane may take several hours to reach completion. This "lag period" may be particularly relevant in the brain where the blood-brain barrier may contribute to a plasma-brain urea concentration gradient. As a result, urea transiently acts as an effective osmole, promoting water movement into the brain. In addition, the reduction in BUN lowers the plasma osmolality, thereby creating a transient osmotic gradient that promotes water movement into the cells. In the brain, this water shift across the blood-brain-barrier produces cerebral oedema and a variable degree of acute neurological dysfunction depending on the severity and speed of BUN reduction (Silver et al., 1996). The extracellular volume depletion associated with aggressive dialysis and consequent cerebral hypoperfusion may exacerbate the patient's clinical status. Absolute increases in brain water content have been demonstrated in a rat model of uraemia undergoing rapid haemodialysis that was accounted for by an increase in the ratio of brain to plasma urea (Silver et al., 1992; Silver, 1995). Downregulation of central nervous system urea transporters have also been proposed as a mechanism contributing to the delay in urea clearance from the brain, although there has been little additional evidence to confirm this theory (Hu et al., 2000).

3.2 Intracerebral acidosis

A number of reports suggest that the "reverse urea effect" cannot solely account for the development of cerebral oedema in DDS since urea movement out of the brain is sufficiently rapid to prevent a large osmotic gradient developing between the brain and extracellular fluid (Arieff et al, 1973). The rate of removal of urea from brain closely parallels its rate of removal from plasma, but the clearance of urea from the cerebrospinal fluid (CSF) is delayed (Arieff, 1989). Studies in dialysis patients have shown that there is often a substantial rise in the P_{CO2} of lumbar CSF, with a concomitant fall in its pH during haemodialysis (Arieff et al., 1973; Fraser & Arieff, 1988). Studies in uraemic dogs treated with rapid haemodialysis have shown that, despite a rise in the pH of arterial blood, the pH of the CSF fell. It has been found in animal models that the decrement in the pH of the CSF is associated with a concomitant decline in the pH of the brain, and this finding is probably a factor in the pathogenesis of the DDS (Areiff et al., 1976). This decrease in cerebral intracellular pH, resulting in the displacement of bound sodium and potassium by the excess hydrogen ions can increase intracellular osmolality and promote water movement into the brain.

An additional contributing factor to the intracerebral acidosis mechanism is the idiogenic osmole principle proposed by Arieff (1973). The increased osmolality of the extracellular fluid in uraemia may induce an adaptive accumulation of intracellular organic osmolytes to limit cerebral cell dehydration (Arieff et al., 1973). During haemodialysis, retention of these organic osmolytes contributes to a paradoxical reduction in intracellular pH resulting in increased brain osmolality and cerebral oedema (Arieff et al., 1976; Trachtman et al., 1993).

These brain organic osmolytes may include glutamine, glutamate, taurine, and myoinositol. However, an increase in brain organic osmolytes has not been confirmed in all studies. A fall in the pH of CSF may contribute to a depression of the sensorium, and intracellular acidosis of brain cells could result in a rise of brain intracellular osmolality. Such an increase of osmolality could lead to cytotoxic oedema. The resulting cerebral oedema may be related to a decrease in intracellular pH of the cerbral cortex, probably as a consequence of an increase in intracellular organic acids.

3.3 Dialysis disequilibrium syndrome-induced interstitial oedema

The advent of magnetic resonance imaging (MRI), in particular diffusion-weighted imaging (DWI), has increased physicians' ability to evaluate brain water content. The apparent diffusion coefficient (ADC) measured by DWI, is sensitive in detecting dynamic changes in tissue water. This technique is useful in identifying neurological disorders where there is a derangement in the brain water dynamics e.g. stroke (Warach et al., 1995) and has recently been proposed as a useful investigation in patients with suspected DDS (Chen et al., 2007). In this study, the authors found that haemodialysis increased the ADC values of brain water, especially in white matter, indicating that interstitial oedema rather than cytotoxic oedema is more important in the pathogenesis of DDS-related brain oedema.

Foci of bright areas of white matter were found in all patients on T2-weighted images. The ADC values in white and gray matter in ESRD patients before and after haemodialysis, were significantly greater than those of the healthy controls ($p<0.005$). Regarding the impact of haemodialysis, the ADC of frontal lobe white matter increased significantly after haemodialysis ($p=0.036$). The authors concluded that because ADC is an indicator of interstitial as opposed to cytotoxic oedema, that DDS is a manifestation of an increase in interstitial fluid compartment, especially after first haemodialysis. Other contributing factors may include uraemic toxin-associated dysfunction of the blood-brain barrier in patients with ESRD before their first haemodialysis (Jeppsson et al., 1982). Hypertension is also prevalent in patients with ESRD at the initiation of long-term dialysis therapy, which may accelerate atherosclerosis and cause damage to cerebral vasculature in patients with ESRD, leading to the increase of the ADC (Goksan, et al., 2004).

4. Evaluation of patients with suspected DDS

Dialysis disequilibrium syndrome should be a diagnosis of exclusion in haemodialysis patients who develop new-onset neurological symptoms. Important differential diagnoses include uraemic encephalopathy, subdural haematoma, metabolic disturbances (hyponatraemia, hypoglycaemia), and drug-induced encephalopathy. Indeed, drug accumulation resulting in neurotoxicity may be a problem with drugs that are normally excreted by the kidney. Even in complex cases however, a detailed clinical evaluation coupled with relevant investigations will usually help to make the diagnosis of DDS.

4.1 Symptoms and signs

The classical DDS refers to acute symptoms developing during or immediately after haemodialysis. Early findings include headache, nausea, disorientation, restlessness, blurred vision, and asterixis. These and other vague symptoms such as muscle cramps, anorexia, and dizziness developing near the end of a dialysis treatment are also part of this syndrome.

Papilloedema has also been reported to be associated with DDS and this can be a useful clinical sign in confirming the presence of raised intracranial pressure (Im et al., 2007). More severely affected patients may develop confusion, seizures, coma, and even death, although with greater awareness of DDS, these extreme cases are now very rare.

4.2 Radiographic evaluation

With the greater availability of computed tomography (CT) and magnetic resonance imaging (MRI) scanners, haemodialysis patients with new-onset neurological symptoms can readily undergo brain imaging to exclude a structural cause of their symptoms. Furthermore, with the technical advances in MR imaging, patients with suspected DDS can be imaged for brain water content using DWI sequences (Walters et al., 2001). As mentioned previously, an increase in ADC values have been reported in patients undergoing first-time haemodialysis in keeping with the associated increase in interstitial fluid water content (Chen et al., 2007). However, it is important to bear in mind that longstanding silent cerebral white matter lesions are present in up to one third of patients with chronic renal disease (Martinez-Vea et al., 2006). These lesions may be related to vascular risk factors, particularly hypertension, and reflect ischaemic brain damage caused by generalized vascular damage (Chen et al., 2007).

4.3 Electroencephalography

It appears that modern methods of dialysis have altered the clinical features of the DDS. Most of the seizures, coma and deaths related to DDS were reported before 1970, whereas the symptoms frequently reported since then are generally mild, consisting of headache, nausea, fatigue, weakness and muscle cramping ((Harris & Townsend, 1989). As a consequence, although the use of electroencephalography (EEG) has decreased significantly in the investigation and monitoring of DDS patients, it may occasionally be required in the evaluation of some patients.

The EEG recording typically consists of bilateral bursts of high-voltage rhythmic delta waves and occasional spike and wave patterns on a high-voltage dysrhythmic background (Kennedy, 1970). In addition to the initial diagnostic applications, EEG has been used to monitor the effects of changing the dialysis fluid constituents (e.g. acetate versus bicarbonate). Neyer et al (1983) observed EEG changes more frequently in the acetate dialysis group compared with the bicarbonate group. Although values for serum urea, osmolarity and sodium was similar in both groups, correction in metabolic acidosis varied. After acetate haemodialysis, a negative base excess and fall in PaCO2 was observed while in the bicarbonate group, the $PaCO_2$ rose and the base excess was positive. This report indicated the importance of the biochemical composition in haemodialysis fluid and in general, bicarbonate-based dialysate fluid has substituted acetate-based solutions. With the improvements in brain imaging, and less frequent severe cases of DDS, EEG has become less frequently used investigation for DDS-suspected cases.

4.4 Intracranial pressure monitoring

Although brain imaging has improved with more advanced MR sequences, the detection of DDS in patients with a coexistent disorder of the central nervous system can be problematic. In such cases DDS may be a contributing factor to the clinical features and may contribute to an elevation of intracranial pressure. In such cases, in particular neurosurgical patients (e.g.

head trauma, intracranial haemorrhage, suspected shunt malfunction) intracranial pressure (ICP) monitoring can be a useful diagnostic and monitoring adjunct. The intracranial pressure of patients suspected of DDS, has been shown to rise almost immediately after the initiation of haemodialysis (Yoshida et al., 1987) and reach maximal values approximately two hours later (Fig. 1). Maximal recordings greater than 50 mmHg are possible (Flannery et al., 2008) indicating that increased ICP during haemodialysis may be extreme and potentially harmful.

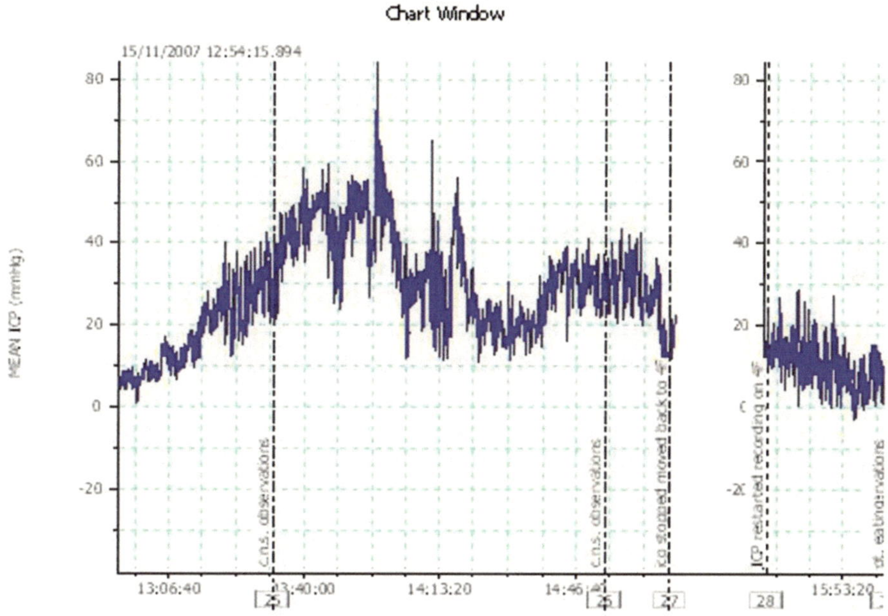

Fig. 1. A typical ICP recording obtained before, during, and at the end of Haemodialysis. (taken with permission from "Dialysis disequilibrium syndrome: a consideration in patients with hydrocephalus", Journal of Neurosurgery Paediatrics 2008; 2: 143-145).The ICP recording can be seen to rise shortly after commencement of dialysis (less than one hour) and return to normal fairly soon after dialysis was completed.

5. Treatment of DDS

The management of DDS can be categorized into preventive and therapeutic measures.

5.1 Prevention of DDS

Prevention is the mainstay of therapy in the DDS, particularly in first-time haemodialysis patients who are at greatest risk. Consequently, the mode of dialysis is important in reducing the likelihood of DDS. In general, DDS is seen less frequently with non-haemodialysis modalities such as continuous ambulatory peritoneal dialysis (Bertrand et al., 1983; Dettori et al., 1982). Unfortunately, in some cases these alternative modes of dialysis may not be suitable e.g. peritoneal adhesions, patient intolerance, etc. Where haemodialysis is the only suitable option, a number of precautions can be taken to facilitate a gradual reduction in BUN and minimize the risk of DDS. These include intermittent haemodialysis using less efficient dialyzers with a smaller surface area and by reducing the duration and blood flow rate of dialysis (Bagshaw et al., 2004). It is also important to ensure that chronic dialysis patients do not undergo a sudden change in their dialysis regime perhaps implemented by a change in personal circumstances e.g. moving to a new dialysis unit (Flannery et al., 2008).

5.2 Treatment of DDS symptoms

Aside from measures to optimise dialysis parameters and minimizing the risk of DDS, the primary objective of DDS treatment is the reduction of raised intracranial pressure. Symptoms of DDS, in particular the milder symptoms, are generally self-limited and usually dissipate within several hours. However, the initial reports of DDS often contained cases of severe morbidity and even mortality. It is from these early reports that much of our knowledge of management of DDS symptoms arises (Port et al, 1973; Arieff et al, 1978; Harris & Townsend, 1989).

Early studies indicated that DDS was successfully treated by the addition of either hyperosmotic or hyperoncotic solute (glucose, glycerol, albumin, urea, fructose, sodium chloride, mannitol) to the dialysate or by the substitution of sodium bicarbonate for sodium lactate (or acetate) in the dialysate (Port et al., 1973; Pagel et al., 1982; Rodrigo et al., 1977; Arieff et al., 1973; Fraser & Arieff, 1988). The purpose of such manoeuvres was to minimize rapid alterations in the plasma osmolality or bicarbonate during dialysis. In uraemic animals undergoing rapid haemodialysis, the addition of glycerol or mannitol to the dialysate prevented many of the manifestations of experimental DDS. Studies on uraemic patients undergoing haemodialysis with glycerol or mannitol added to the dialysate suggest that these agents lessen the symptoms that may be associated with DDS. The substitution of bicarbonate for acetate or lactate in the dialysate appears to diminish cardiovascular instability and may prove useful in decreasing the symptoms of DDS in some patients (Arieff, 1989).

Intravenous mannitol may be given to elevate the plasma osmolality if ICP is increased and is a safe and effective clinical method for preventing ICP increase (Kennedy, 1970; Rodrigo et al., 1977). In the event of persistently elevated ICP in spite of medical measures, Yoshida et al report ventricular drainage as a relatively safe and effective surgical method of preventing irreversible brain herniation and death. The authors also proposed that a ventricular catheter allows for serial CSF sampling to monitor osmolality and urea concentration in complex cases to optimise dialysis parameters (Yoshida et al., 1987).

Although seizures are much less frequently observed compared with earlier reports, it may be necessary in some cases to administer prophylactic anti-epileptic medication to high-risk cases. A typical regimen might be a loading dose of 1000 mg Phenytoin followed by 300 mg daily until uraemia has been controlled. Severe DDS with seizures can also be rapidly reversed by raising the plasma osmolality with either hypertonic saline or mannitol. However, caution needs to be exercised in the selection of appropriate anti-epileptic medication as some are primarily excreted by the renal route.

6. Other neurological sequelae of haemodialysis

Dialysis disequilibrium syndrome is essentially a diagnosis of exclusion and dialysis patients presenting with neurological symptoms should be evaluated to exclude another pathological process. These disorders may require additional modes of treatment.

6.1 Subdural haematoma

Subdural haematomas have been reported in 1.0 to 3.3% of patients undergoing haemodialysis. Contributory factors are coagulation problems associated with the uraemic state, and the use of anticoagulants for dialysis (Rashkin & Fishman, 1976). There is often no preceding history of trauma. The clinical manifestations are variable and can resemble those of DDS. Up to 20% of subdural haematomas are bilateral and may cause gait disturbance predisposing patients to falls and head trauma. Cases with associated mass effect may require neurosurgical intervention following the reversal of anti-coagulant medication.

6.2 Wernicke's encephalopathy

Although thiamine is a water-soluble vitamin, and might be therefore expected to cross the dialysis membrane with ease, there have been only a few reports of Wernicke's encephalopathy in patients undergoing longterm dialysis (Burn & Bates, 1998). The deficiency state is likely to develop due to a combination of factors including chronic malnourishment due to anorexia, a genetic predisposition and the use of glucose containing intravenous fluids. It should also be noted that classic features of Wernicke's encephalopathy e.g. opthalmoplegia, may be absent in dialysis patients (Jagadha et al., 1987).

6.3 Dialysis dementia

Dialysis dementia was first documented by Alfrey et al (1972), and typically the disorder is progressive unless treated. Dialysis dementia may be part of a multisystem disorder which includes vitamin D resistant osteomalacia, proximal myopathy, and iron deficient microcytic, hypochromic anaemia (Burn & Bates, 1998). A mixed dysarthria and dysphasia with dysgraphia has been reported as one of the earliest signs of dialysis dementia in up to 95% of cases. The patient may initially have a stuttering, hesitant speech, which only occurs during and immediately after dialysis. Initially the patient may also be more apathetic and become depressed. As the disorder progresses, language function becomes more severely and persistently involved (Burn & Bates, 1989).

Convulsions develop in up to 60% in the later stages, and psychosis with hallucinations and paranoid delusions may be prominent. Frank dementia becomes obvious in over 95% of patients with patients becoming immobile and mute in the preterminal stages (Chokroverty et al., 1976).

7. Conclusions

Although severe DDS is less common than initial reports due to improvements in modes of dialysis, milder forms of DDS may go unnoticed by the clinician. It is important to be aware of this diagnosis, particularly in high-risk groups, with the aim of prevention and early detection to limit the potentially more serious consequences of DDS.

8. Acknowledgement

The author is grateful to the editorial office of the Journal of Neurosurgery for permission to use Fig. 1.

9. References

Alfrey, A.C., LeGendre, G.R., & Kaehny, W.D. (1976). The dialysis encephalopathy syndrome: possible aluminium intoxication. *N Eng J Med*, Vol.294, No.4, (January 1976), pp. 184-188, ISSN 0028-4793

Arieff, A., Massry, S., Barrientos, A., & Kleeman C. (1973). Brain water and electrolyte metabolism in uraemia: effects of slow and rapid haemodialysis. *Kidney Internat*, Vol.4, No.3, (September 1973), pp. 177-187, ISSN 0085-2538

Arieff, A., Guisado, R., Massry, S.G., & Lazarowitz, V. (1976). Central nervous system pH in uraemia and the effects of haemodialysis. *J Clin Invest*, Vol.58, No.2, (August 1976), pp. 306-311, ISSN 0021-9738

Arieff, A.I, Lazarowitz, V.C., & Guisado, R. (1978). Experimental dialysis disequilibrium syndrome: prevention with glycerol. *Kidney Int*, Vol.14, No.3, (September 1978), pp. 270-278, ISSN 0085-2538

Arieff, A.I. (1989). More on the Dialysis disequilibrium syndrome. *Western J Med*, Vol.151, No.1, (July 1989), pp. 74-76, ISSN 0093-0415

Arieff, A.I. (1994). Dialysis disequilibrium syndrome: current concepts on pathogenesis and prevention. *Kidney Int*, Vol.45, pp. 629-635, ISSN 0085-2538

Bagshaw, S.M., Peets, A.D., Hameed, M., Boiteau, P.J.E., Laupland, K.B., & Doig, CJ. (2004). Dialysis disequilibrium syndrome: brain death following haemodialysis for metabolic acidosis and acute renal failure – a case report. BMC Nephrology, Vol.5, No.9, (August 2004), pp. 1-5, ISSN 1471-2369

Bertrand, Y.M., Hermant, A., Mahieu, P., & Roels, J. (1983). Intracranial pressure changes in patients with head trauma during haemodialysis. *Intensive Care Med,* Vol.9, (November 1983), pp. 321–323, ISSN 0342-4642

Chen, C.L., Lai, P.H., Chou, K.J., Lee, P.T., Chung, H.M., & Fang, H.C. (2007). A preliminary report of brain oedema in patients with uraemia at first haemodialysis: evaluation by diffusion-weighted imaging. *Am J Neuroradiol* Vol.28, No.1, (January 2007), pp. 68-71, ISSN 0195-6108

Chokroverty, S., Bruetman, M.E., Berger, V., & Reyes, M.G. (1976). Progressive dialytic encephalopathy. *J Neurol Neurosurg Psychiatry*, Vol. 39, No. 5, (May 1976), pp. 411-419, ISSN 1468-330X

Dettori, P., La Greca, G., Biasioli, S., Chiaramonte, S., Fabris, A., Feriani, M., Pinna, V., Pisani, E., & Ronco, C. (1982). Changes of cerebral density in dialyzed patients. *Neuroradiology*, Vol.23, No.2, (April 1982), pp. 95-99, ISSN 0028-3940

Flannery, T., Shoakazemi, A., McLaughlin, B., Woodman, A., & Cooke, S. (2008). Dialysis disequilibrium syndrome: a consideration in patients with hydrocephalus. *J Neurosurg Paed,* Vol.2, No.1, (August 2008), pp. 143-145, ISSN 1933-0707

Fraser, C.L., & Arieff, A.I. (1988). Nervous system complications in uraemia. *Ann Intern Med,* Vol.109, No.2, (July 1988), pp. 143-153, ISSN 0003-4819

Goksan, B., Karaali-Savrun, F., Ertan, S., & Savrun, M. (2004). Haemodialysis-related headache. *Cephalgia*, Vol.24, No.4, (April 2004), pp. 284-287, ISSN 1468-2982

Harris, C.P. & Townsend, J.J. (1989). Dialysis disequilibrium syndrome [Clinicopathologic Conference]. West J Med, Vol.151, No.1, (July 1989), 52-55, ISSN 0093-0415

Hu, M.C., Bankir, L., Michelet, S., Rousselet, G., & Trinh-Trang-Tan, M.M. (2000). Massive reduction of urea transporters in remnant kidney and brain in uraemic rats. *Kidney Internat,* Vol.58, No.3, (September 2000), pp. 1202-1210, ISSN 0085-2538

Im, L., Atabay, C., & Eller, A.W. (2007). Papilloedema associated with dialysis disequilibrium syndrome. *Semin Opthalmol*, Vol.22, No.3, (July-September 2007), 133-135, ISSN 0882-0538

Jagadha, V., Deck, J.H., Halliday, W.C., & Smyth, H.S. (1987). Wernicke's encephalopathy in patients on peritoneal dialysis or haemodialysis. *Ann Neurol*, Vol.21, No.1, (January 1987), pp. 78-84, ISSN 0364-5134

Jeppsson, B., Freund, H.R., Gimmon, Z., James, J.H., von Meyenfeldt, M.F., & Fischer, J.E. (1982). Blood-brain barrier derangement in uraemic encephalopathy. *Surgery*, Vol.92, No.1, (July 1982), pp. 30-35, ISSN 0039-6060

Kennedy, A.C. (1970). Dialysis Disequilibrium syndrome. *Electroencephalogr Clin Neurophysiol*, Vol.29, No.2, (August 1970), pp. 206-219, ISSN 0013-4694

Martinez-Vea, A., Salvado, E., Bardaji, A., Gutierrez, C., Ramos, A., Garcia, C., Compete, T., Peralta, C., Broch, M., Pastor, R., Angelet, P., Marcas, L., Sauri, A., & Oliver, J.A. (2006). Silent cerebral white matter lesions and their relationship with vascular risk factors in middle-aged predialysis patients with CKD. *Am J Kidney Dis*, Vol.47, No.2, (February 2006), pp. 241-250, ISSN 0272-6386

Neyer, U., Woss, E., Haller, R., & Kross, R. (1983). Headache and EEG changes caused by acetate and bicarbonate dialysis. *Acta Med Austriaca*, Vol.10, No.1, (January 1983), pp. 15-23, ISSN 1563-2571

Pagel, M.D., Ahmad, S., Vizzo, J.E., & Scribner, B.H.. (1982). Acetate and bicarbonate fluctuations and acetate intolerance during dialysis. *Kidney Int*, Vol.21, No.3, (March 1982), pp. 513-518, ISSN 0085-2538

Peterson, H., & Swanson, A.G. (1964). Acute encephalopathy occurring during haemodialysis. The reverse urea effect. *Arch Intern Med*, Vol.113, (June 1964), pp. 877-880, ISSN 0003-9926

Port, F.K., Johnson, W.J., & Klass, D.W. (1973). Prevention of dialysis disequilibrium syndrome by use of high sodium concentration in the dialysate. *Kidney Int*, Vol.3, No.5, (May 1973), pp. 327-333, ISSN 0085-2538

Rashkin, N.H., & Fishman, R.A. (1976). Neurologic disorders in renal failure (Part II). *N Engl J Med*, Vol.294, No.4, (January 1976), pp. 204-210, ISSN 0028-4793

Rodrigo, F., Shideman, J., McHugh, R., Buselmeier, T., & Kjellstrand, C. (1977). Osmolality changes during haemodialysis. Natural history, clinical correlations, and influence of dialysate glucose and intravenous mannitol. *Ann Intern Med*, Vol.86, No.5, (May 1977), pp. 554-561, ISSN 0003-4819

Silver, S.M., DeSimone, J.A. Jr., Smith, D.A., & Sterns, R.H. (1992). Dialysis disequilibrium syndrome (DDS) in the rat: role of the "reverse urea effect". *Kidney Internat*, Vol.42, No.1, (July 1992), pp. 161-166, ISSN 0085-2538

Silver, S.M. (1995). Cerebral oedema after rapid dialysis is not caused by an increase in brain organic osmolytes. *J Am Soc Nephrol*, Vol.6, No.6, (December 1995), pp. 1600-1606, ISSN 1046-6673

Silver, S.M., Stearns, R.H., & Halperin, M.L. (1996). Brain swelling after dialysis: old urea or new osmoles? *Am J Kidney Dis*, Vol.28, No.1, (July 1996), pp. 1–13, ISSN 0272-6386

Trachtmann, H., Futterweit, S., Tonidanel, W., & Gullans, S. (1993). The role of organic osmolytes in the cerebral cell volume regulatory response to acute and chronic renal failure. *J Am Soc Nephrol*, Vol.3, No.12, (June 1993), pp. 1913-1919, ISSN 1046-6673

Walters R., Fox N., Crum W., Taube D., & Thomas D. (2001). Haemodialysis and cerebral oedema. *Nephron,* Vol.87, No.2, (February 2001), pp. 143-147, ISSN 0028-2766

Warach, S., Gaa, J., Siewert, B., Wielopolski, P., & Edelman, P.R. (1995). Acute human stroke studied by whole brain echo planar diffusion-weighted magnetic resonance imaging. *Ann Neurol*, Vol.37, No.2, (February 1995), pp. 231-241, ISSN 0364-5134

Yoshida, S., Tajika, T., Yamasaki, N., Tanikawa, T., Kitamura, K., Kudo, K., Lyden, P. (1987). Dialysis dysequilibrium syndrome in neurosurgical patients. *Neurosurgery*, Vol.20, No.5, (May 1987), pp. 716–721, ISSN 0148-396X

8

Cardiovascular Disease in End Stage Renal Disease Patients

Lukas Haragsim and Baroon Rai
University of Oklahoma,
United States of America

1. Introduction

Cardiovascular disease is the primary cause of preventable death in industrialized countries (1). It is on a steady rise in many other countries where it had not been traditionally recognized as a major disease burden. There has been a lot of attempts to define the risk factors associated with cardiovascular disease. Similar efforts have been made in defining the treatment and the secondary prevention of cardiovascular diseases.
End Stage Renal Disease (ESRD) patients form a vulnerable sub-group of general population. In 2007, the adjusted annual mortality of dialysis patients in the United States was 19 % (USRDS 2008 Annual Data Report) (2). Cardiovascular and infection related complications are the major cause of morbidity and mortality in this group (3). ESRD patients have a high prevalence of cardiovascular risk factors leading to a phenomenally high cardiovascular morbidity and mortality. In fact it remains the single most important cause of death in ESRD patients. In 2005-2007 it accounted for 45 % of all deaths in ESRD patients (4). Cardiac arrest was responsible for almost half of these deaths (5). This apparently disproportionate burden of cardiovascular disease in ESRD patients is likely due to the many traditional risk factors that both these diseases share. In addition, we are learning more about other non-conventional risk factors unique to ESRD patients that promote and accelerate the atherosclerotic process that underlies most cardiovascular diseases.
In this chapter we will discuss the significant risk factors of cardiovascular diseases in ESRD patients. We will also discuss the treatment and intervention aspects of cardiovascular disease, especially in reference to hemodialysis patients.

2. Risk factors

2.1 Diabetes

Prevalence of diabetes in ESRD patients is about 50% (6). Both macrovascular and microvascular benefits of good glycemic control have been established for both type 1 and type 2 diabetes. Various prospective trials have tried to define a range of glycemic control (target hemoglobin A1c) with maximal cardiovascular and mortality benefit. It appears, at least in general population, that the benefits of better glycemic control follow a J shaped curve with worse outcomes for hemoglobin A1c both above and below the optimal range. Two large randomized trials failed to show any benefit in the reduction of major macrovascular disease in type 2 diabetic patients with intensive glycemic control.

In the ADVANCE (Action in Diabetes and Vascular Disease: Preterax and Diamicron Modified Release Controlled Evaluation) trial, there was no difference between the incidence of major cardiovascular event, cardiovascular mortality or all cause mortality between the intensive control group with median HbA1c 6.5 % and the standard group with median HbA1c 7.3%. Interestingly benefit was seen in the combined incidence of macrovascular and microvascular complications (HR 0.9, CI 0.82-0.98, P=0.01). (7) This was attributed to the reduction of nephropathy, a microvascular complication, in the intensive group.

In the ACCORD trial, which was another large prospective randomized study, 10,251 patients with a median HbA1c of 8.1 % was assigned to receive intensive therapy (target of 6% and below) or standard therapy (target of 7-7.9%). The primary outcome of interest was a composite of nonfatal MI, nonfatal stroke or death from cardiovascular cause. Though there was no significant difference in the primary outcome, the intensive-therapy group had an increased rate of death; the differences in mortality appeared within 1 to 2 years and persisted during the follow-up period. For ethical reasons, the intensive glycemic treatment was discontinued 17 months before the scheduled end of the study and the patients were switched to the standard glycemic regimen. (8)

Both of these studies did not include dialysis patients and it is not certain whether the conclusions can be directly applied to dialysis patients. Aggressive blood sugar control using multiple drug classes is not recommended. A target HbA1c of 7 % may be appropriate, more along the treatment line of the standard regimen in the ACCORD trial.

2.2 Hyperlipidemia

There is a wealth of data on the benefits of lowering of lipids especially with use of statins in both the primary and secondary prevention of cardiovascular disease. There have been multiple randomized studies which have shown reduced risk of cardiovascular events in patients with normal renal function and varying degrees of chronic kidney disease. Given these studies and other observational studies on dialysis patients, it was generally assumed hemodialysis patients would benefit from lipid lowering too. However, two recent randomized prospective trials (AURORA and 4D) studies did not conform to this notion. The studies failed to show any benefits in reaching the primary end points of cardiovascular death, non-fatal myocardial infarction and stroke in hemodialysis patients, with the use of statins and significant reduction in total and LDL cholesterol.

In the 4D(die deutsche diabetes dialyse) study; a multicenter randomized double-blind and prospective study, 1255 patients with type 2 diabetes who were on maintenance hemodialysis, were randomly assigned to receive either 20 mg of atorvastatin or placebo. The primary outcome measured was the composite of cardiovascular death, non-fatal myocardial infarction and stroke. After four weeks, atorvastatin successfully lowered LDL cholesterol (121 to 72 mg/dl) versus no change with the placebo (125 to 120 mg/dl). During a median follow-up of four years, 469 patients (37%) reached the primary end point; 226 assigned to atorvastatin and 243 assigned to placebo (RR, 0.92; 95% CI,0.77 to 1.1; *P=0.37*). Atorvastatin did not change the incidence of any single components of the primary end point with the exception of fatal stroke for which RR was 2.03, (95% CI,1.05 to 3.93; *P=0.04*). There was however a significant reduction in the combined cardiac events (RR,0.82;95% CI,0.81 to 1.55; *P=0.49*), but there was no reduction in the total mortality (RR,0.93; 95% CI,0.79 to 1.08; *P=0.33*). (9)

ESRD patients with diabetes have an average annual rate of incidence of myocardial infarction or death from coronary artery disease of about 8%, which is higher than any other cohorts included in prospective statin trials. Despite this high incidence and the significant lipid lowering effect with the atorvastatin, there was no reduction in the composite of cardiovascular death, non-fatal MI and non-fatal stroke in the 4D study. Though patients with LDL cholesterol over 190 mg/dl were excluded, subgroup analysis did not reveal any difference in the composite outcome for any level of LDL or for patients with prior history of coronary artery disease. Even more interesting was the increased occurrence of fatal stroke in the atorvastatin group compared to the placebo group (11). This is in contrast to the Collaborative Atorvastatin in Diabetes Study (CARDS) which reported that people with type 2 diabetes who received atorvastatin had a RR for stroke of 0.52 (95% CI, 0.31 to 0.89) compared with the placebo group (12).

The 4D study was the first large scale randomized study which did not show overall benefit from potent dose of statin and significant reduction in the LDL cholesterol, challenging the general assumption about the log-linear relation of level of LDL cholesterol and the risk of cardiovascular disease. The result is in accordance with observational data in patients on hemodialysis therapy that has not linked dyslipidemia with reduced survival; opposite trends have been noted in some. But 4D results are in contrast to an observational retrospective analysis of hemodialysis patients in the US Renal Data System (USRDS) Morbidity and Mortality Study, Wave 2, which indicated that the risk of cardiovascular death decreases by 36% in statin users compared with non-users (13). This finding demonstrates the difficulty associated with basing treatment decisions on uncontrolled observational studies.

Another study that had similar conclusions was the AURORA study (Rosuvastatin and Cardiovascular events in patients undergoing Hemodialysis). It was a well designed, large randomized prospective trial. It involved 2776 patients, 50 to 80 years of age on maintenance hemodialysis, who were randomly assigned to either rosuvastatin 10 mg daily or placebo. The combined primary end point was death from cardiovascular causes, nonfatal myocardial infarction or nonfatal stroke. Secondary end points included death from all causes and individual cardiac and vascular events. During a median follow-up period of 3.8 years, 396 patients in the rosuvastatin group and 408 patients in the placebo group reached the primary end point (9.2 and 9.5 events per 1000 patient-years, respectively; hazard ratio for the combined end point in the rosuvastatin group vs. the placebo group, 0.96; 95% CI, 0.84 to 1.11; *P=0.59*). Rosuvastatin had no effect on individual components of the primary end point. There was also no significant effect on all-cause mortality (13.5 vs. 14.0 events per 100 patient-years; hazard ratio, 0.96; 95% CI, 0.86 to 1.07; *P=0.51*). This study further corroborated the lack of benefit with statin therapy in ESRD patients shown earlier by the 4D study. However there was no significant effect of statin in the incidence of stroke as seen in 4D study, but there was a marginal increase in the incidence of hemorrhagic stroke in pts with diabetes who were being treated with rosuvastatin (12 events vs. 2, P=0.03). (14)

This lack of benefit may be due to the underlying difference in the pathogenesis and outcome of cardiovascular events in ESRD patients from that in non-dialysis population. (15) More than 50% of cardiac mortality in ESRD patients is due to arrhythmias and sudden cardiac death. The gradual build up of atherosclerotic burden that lipid lowering prevents, might not be as important in the prevention of cardiovascular mortality in this vulnerable population. Similarly the plethora of recognized and unrecognized risk factors for cardiovascular disease in ESRD likely undermines the effect of modification of single risk factor.

In the light of available evidence the National Kidney Foundation recommends against routinely initiating statins for dyslipidemia in ESRD patients (16). However, there is no consensus on continuing or withdrawing statin therapy in dialysis patients already being treated. Both these studies did not specifically address this question. Similarly diabetic patients with severe dyslipidemia with LDL-C>190 mg/dl (who were not included in these studies) may have some benefits of lipid lowering and should not be precluded from statin treatment. (17)

2.3 Hypertension

2.3.1 Prevalence and association with cardiovascular morbidity and mortality

A large number (50-80%) of dialysis patients have hypertension. The relationship between HTN and cardiovascular disease is a complicated one. ESRD patients have a host of co-morbid conditions and risk factors for cardiovascular disease which makes defining the role of one risk factor difficult. It is especially true for risk factor like HTN the effect of which in the progression of cardiovascular disease is slow, insidious and requires a prolonged period of time.

While severe uncontrolled HTN is clearly associated with increased left ventricular mass, LV stiffness and pulse velocity all linked to increased cardiovascular morbidity and mortality (18) (19); the optimal BP target, the preferred agent and the role of dry weight reduction have not been well established.

Udayaraj et al examined the association of BP and mortality among 2770 patients who were on PD in U.K between 1997 and 2004. They looked at the relationship of BP to all-cause mortality using time-stratified models. The median follow up was 3.7 years within which 1104 deaths were observed. In fully adjusted analyses, greater BP (SBP, DBP, MAP and PP) was associated with lower mortality for follow up less than a year but increased mortality for follow up more than six years. However in the subgroup of patients placed on the transplant waitlist (TWL) within six months of starting renal replacement therapy, higher BP was not associated with decreased mortality in the first year. Higher BP was associated with increased mortality at year four or five; earlier for those not enlisted in the transplant list. The TWL patients likely represented relatively healthy and homogenous population who did not need extensive investigation to assess fitness for transplantation. This relatively healthy sub-group likely benefit from better BP control (20).

Similarly Mazuchi et al studied the relationship of pre-dialysis systolic and diastolic BP to all-cause mortality in 450 hemodialysis patients who had survived at least two years on HD. The observation period was initiated at the beginning of the third year. Mortality was analyzed during the first two years of follow-up (years 3 and 4 of HD; early mortality) and after the second year of follow-up (>5 years of HD; late mortality). In the multivariate analysis which included, pre-dialysis BP, demographic features and co-morbid conditions as independent variables, SBP and DBP were significantly associated with death. The adjusted total mortalities were U shaped. When early mortality was analyzed, low BP (DBP<74.5 mm Hg) was significantly associated with mortality. When late mortality was analyzed, only high BP (SBP>160 mmHg) was significantly associated with mortality (21).

While these observational studies suggest this reverse association of HTN and cardiovascular events one should draw conclusions only after careful statistical analyses. Low BP could be a surrogate marker for severe co-morbid conditions like heart failure independently contributing to cardiovascular death; similarly competing risk factors, chronic inflammation, malnutrition and survival bias can confound the effects of BP in uncontrolled retrospective studies. (22)

2.3.2 Management of HTN

There is still a significant element of uncertainty in the management of HTN in dialysis patients. While lowering BP may have benefits in reducing the cardiovascular morbidity and mortality in dialysis patients, certain epidemiological studies have shown increased mortality in the short term with lower BP. It is also not clear what BP targets should be achieved.

There is a growing indication that home BP monitoring may have a better role in therapeutic decision making than the pre-dialysis BP that is often used. In a recent open-labeled randomized control trial by Silva et al. the patients who were treated on the basis of home BP achieved better BP control than those who were treated on the basis of pre-dialysis BP at 6 months. However, there was no difference noted in the LV mass index , a surrogate for cardiovascular outcome in between the two groups (23).

2.3.3 Role of antihypertensives

There are two recent meta-analyses published on the role of antihypertensives in HD patients. The authors specifically were interested in the question whether the published randomized studies supported the observation about the increase in mortality seen with lowering of BP in some epidemiological studies. Both meta-analyses concluded that use of antihypertensives was not associated with increased mortality and there were benefits in cardiovascular outcomes (24).

The first meta-analysis by Agrawal et al (Cardiovascular protection with antihypertensive drugs in dialysis patients, *Hypertension.* 2009; 53:860) included five published randomized studies and one unpublished randomized study. The authors found that there was an overall benefit of antihypertensive therapy compared with the control (or placebo) group; the combined hazard ratio for cardiovascular events was reduced by 31% using a fixed-effects model and by 38% using a random-effects model. The hypertensive group had a pooled hazard ratio of 0.49 (95% CI: 0.35 to 0.67) inferring a greater benefit than the normotensive group, the pooled hazard ratio being 0.86 (95% CI: 0.67 to 1.12). Heterogeneity between normotensive and hypertensive group was significant *(P=0.006).* Of note, there was no increase in the all-cause mortality (25).

A limitation of this meta-analysis, as admitted by the authors, was the presence of publication bias. Low precision studies with effect estimates that did not show benefit, were missing. The trial discussed in this review did not specifically target a lower BP and whether the outcome benefits observed in this meta-analysis were attributable to blood pressure lowering or some non-hemodynamic effects of these drugs is unclear.

The second meta-analysis by Heerspink et al included eight randomized control trials and provided data for 1679 patients and 495 cardiovascular events. Weighted mean systolic blood pressure was 4.5 mm Hg lower and diastolic blood pressure 2.3 mm Hg lower in actively treated patients than in the controls. Blood pressure lowering treatment was associated with lower risks of cardiovascular events (RR 0.71, 95% CI 0.55-0.92; p=0.009), all-cause mortality (RR 0.80, 0.66-0.96; p=0.014) and cardiovascular mortality (RR 0.71, 0.50-0.99; p=0.044) than control regimens. The effects seem to be consistent across a range of patient groups included in the studies (26).

2.3.4 Choice of antihypertensives

ACEI/ARBs Vs Other Anti-Hypertensive agents: In the non-ESRD population, angiotensin converting enzyme inhibitors (ACEIs) and angiotensin receptor blockers (ARBs) lead to reduction in LV mass, a validated surrogate endpoint for improved cardiovascular survival.

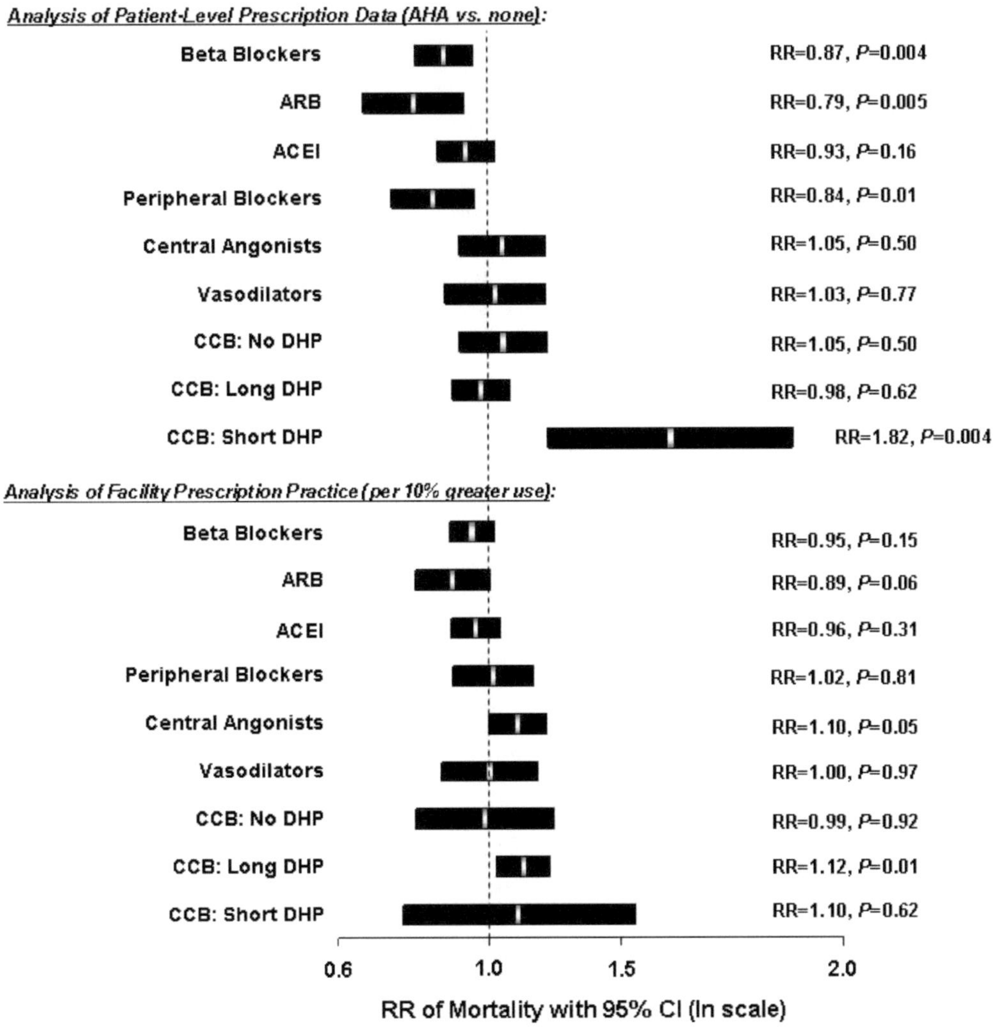

Fig. 1. Mortality Benefits with various Antihypertensive agents as seen in Dialysis Outcomes and Practice Pattern Study (DOPPS)
Prescription of antihypertensive agents to hemodialysis patients: time trends and associations with patient characteristics, country and survival in the DOPPS. Lopes AA, Young EW et al. Nephrol Dial Transplant 2009; 24(9):2809-16

LV hypertrophy is fairly common in ESRD patients and is probably multi-factorial contributed by chronic hypertension, volume overload, anemia and upregulation of renin-angiotensin system (27). Observational studies in dialysis patients have suggested blockade of RAS can lead to reduction in LV mass over and beyond the BP lowering effect (28). Though this LV mass reduction is known to translate as improved cardiovascular outcomes in general population, it remains to be proven whether such is the case in dialysis patients.
A recent meta-analysis by Tai DJ et al looked into the evidence for cardio-protective effects of ACEI/ARBs in dialysis patients. The primary outcome of interest was the composite of fatal and nonfatal CV events. The secondary outcomes were change in LV mass index,

change in systolic BP and change in LV ejection fraction. The authors pooled data from 8 randomized controlled trials which compared ACE/ARB to placebo or calcium channel blockers (22 out of 487 controls). There was no statistically significant reduction in the risk of fatal and non-fatal cardiovascular events (RR of 0.66, 95% CI 0.35-1.25; *P=0.2*), however there was a significant reduction in LV mass, with a weighted mean difference of 15.4 gm/m2 (95% CI 7.4-23.3;*P <0.001*) (29).

Dialysis Outcomes and Practice Pattern study (DOPPS) is a prospective observational study of practice patterns of prescription of antihypertensive agent associated with survival in twelve countries. The authors analyzed the usage of different class of antihypertensive among a total of 28, 513 hemodialysis patients enrolled in this study. There was a significant variation in the use of antihypertensive drug class in different countries. Facilities that treated 10% more patients with ARBs had, on average, 7% lower all-cause mortality, independent of patient characteristics and the prescription patterns of other antihypertensive medications (P=0.05). In the analysis of patient-level prescription data, the all-cause mortality was significantly (P < 0.05) lower for patients prescribed BBs, peripheral vasodilators and long-acting dihydropyridine CCBs and marginally significantly lower (P = 0.06) for patients prescribed ARBs. In contrast, the mortality risk was significantly higher for patients' prescribed short-acting dihydropyridine CCBs. Similar trends were observed for cardiovascular mortality. Beta-blockers (RR = 0.87, P = 0.004), ARBs (RR = 0.79, P = 0.005) and peripheral Vasodialtors (RR = 0.84, P = 0.01) were found to be significantly associated with lower risk of cardiovascular death in the analysis of patient level prescription. The risk of cardiovascular death was significantly higher for patients prescribed a short-acting dihydropyridine, a finding consistent with that for all-cause mortality (30).

2.3.5 BP control via lowering of dry weight

Challenging the dry weight to new targets has been an effective strategy to better control blood pressure in many chronic hemodialysis patients. PD patients with adequate volume control and daily or nocturnal hemodialysis patients typically have better BP control and require less antihypertensive treatment than conventional hemodialysis.

Kayikcioglu et al compared the benefit of non-pharmacologic therapy for control of LV mass among HD patients. In this cross-sectional study patients who were treated with salt and water restriction and dry weight reduction at one center were compared with patients who were primarily treated with antihypertensive treatment at another center. Despite similar systolic and diastolic BP, interdialytic weight gain and LV mass were lesser in the non-pharmacological group (31).

Similarly volume overloaded state has been linked to increased mortality in some observational studies. In a study cohort of 269 HD patients, volume overload defined as more than 15 % excess extracellular water (about 2.5 liters) as measured by body composition analyzer, was associated with increased mortality in a multivariate analysis (HR 2.1, *P=0.003*) (32).

However there is a subset of patients who develop significant intradialytic hypotension, cramps and lightheadedness or even paradoxical hypertension with more aggressive UF. In these patients reducing the dry weight would not be a favored approach as it would diminish compliance and even precipitate acute cardiovascular events. Identifying who would respond better to challenging dry weight and who would do better with antihypertensive agent alone would help the nephrologists in tailoring HD prescription to individual patient.

2.3.6 Relative plasma volume (RPV)

RPV can be a used as a marker of dry weight. It can be measured by continuously monitoring hematocrit during dialysis with commercially available equipment. Since it gives a real-time data on change in intravascular volume during hemodialysis it can be a valuable tool to adjust the rate and the amount of ultrafiltration. It would not only give a more objective assessment of dry weight but also the rate at which it can be achieved.

In a recent study by Sinha AD et al, 100 dialysis patients had their dry weight probed using continuous RPV monitoring during HD and were compared to 50 patients who served as time controls, over an 8 week period. RPV slopes were defined as flat when they were less than the median (1.33% per hour) at the baseline visit. The study found that flat RPV slopes suggest a volume-overloaded state for the following reasons: (1) probing dry weight in these patients led to steeper slopes; (2) those with flatter slopes at baseline had greater weight loss; (3) both baseline RPV slopes and the intensity of weight loss were found to be important for subsequent change in RPV slopes; and, most importantly, (4) RPV slopes predicted the subsequent reduction in interdialytic ambulatory systolic blood pressure. Those with the flattest slopes had the greatest decline in blood pressure on probing dry weight. Both baseline RPV slopes and the change in RPV slopes were important for subsequent changes in ambulatory blood pressure (33).

3. Hyperphosphatemia

Mineral bone disorder has been a focus of intense research in the last two decades and new evidence is unfolding linking this universal phenomenon in advanced CKD and ESRD to increased all cause and cardiovascular mortality. Most of the research has focused on increase in phosphorus as a risk factor for worse outcomes but there is increasing evidence that other mediators like calcium, PTH and vitamin D may contribute too.

An observational study by Ganesh SK et al. looked at the pooled data from two large random samples of prevalent hemodialysis patients in the early 1990s (n=12,833) and hyperphosphatemia was associated with increased risk of cardiac death. During a follow up period of 2 years after adjustments for patient demographics and non-cardiovascular co-morbid conditions, elevated phosphorus(>6.5mg/dl) was significantly associated with increased death from CAD (RR 1.41; $P < 0.0005$), sudden death (RR 1.2; $P < 0.01$), infection (RR 1.2; $P < 0.05$) and unknown causes (RR 1.25; $P < 0.05$) The RR of sudden death was also strongly associated with elevated Ca x PO4 product (RR 1.07 per 10 mg(2)/dl(2); $P < 0.005$) and serum parathyroid hormone levels greater than 495 pg/ml (RR 1.25; $P < 0.05$). (34)

In another observational study by Block et al, the authors looked at the relationship of serum calcium, phosphorus and PTH level with mortality and morbidity among 40,538 hemodialyis patients who had at least one measurement of calcium and phosphorus during the last 3 months of 1997. The sample was taken from Fresenius Medical Care North America Patient Statistical Profile system and the follow up time was 12-18 months. Several confounding variables were included in the analysis. Age, gender, race or ethnicity, diabetes and vintage (time since initiation of dialysis) were considered to represent "case mix". Multivariable adjustment included case mix plus body weight, URR (Urea Reduction Ratio), serum albumin, creatinine, predialysis BUN , bicarbonate, cholesterol, hemoglobin, ferritin and aluminium. After adjustment for case mix and laboratory variables, serum phosphorus concentrations > 5.0 mg/dl were associated with an increased relative risk of death.

(p< 0.001). Higher adjusted serum calcium concentrations were also associated with an increased risk of death, even when examined within narrow ranges of serum phosphorus. Moderate to severe hyperparathyroidism (PTH concentrations above _600 pg/ml) was associated with an increase in the relative risk of death, whereas more modest increases in PTH were not. (35)

Both these observational studies made adjustments for many confounding variables but given the complexity and interactions of multiple risk factors a definitive relationship between mineral metabolism disorder and cardiovascular or all-cause mortality in hemodialysis patients is difficult to establish. For example, hyperphosphatemia is often associated with non-compliant behavior and nutritional status (increased serum phosphate with higher dietary intake and with higher lean body mass) of the patient, both of which can affect patient morbidity and mortality.

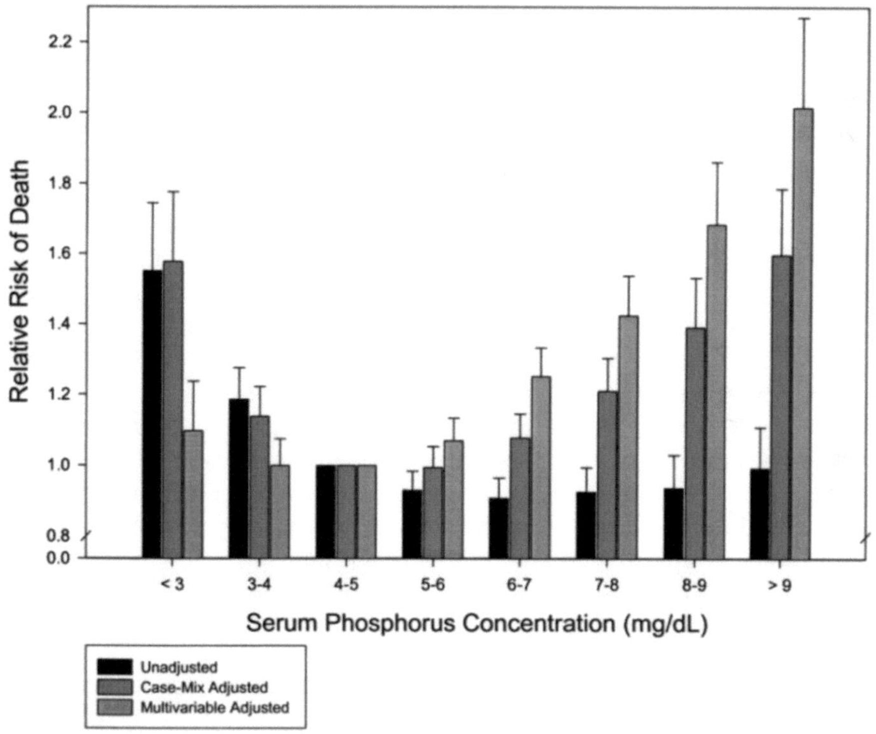

Fig. 2. Mortality Risks with Hyperphosphatemia in Hemodialysis patients.
Mineral Metabolism, Mortality, and Morbidity in Maintenance Hemodialysis. Block GA, Chertow GM et al. J Am Soc Nephrol 15: 2208–2218, 2004 (adopted)

3.1 Role in the pathogenesis of cardiovascular disease

Studies of various in vivo animal models and in vitro in tissues from patients, hyperphosphatemia have been shown to promote osteoblastic transformation of vascular smoothe muscles and matrix calcification in blood vessel wall. Similar process probably results in the vascular calcification seen in CKD and ESRD patients. However there is controversy as to whether vascular calcification itself is the cause for vascular dysfunction or whether it is an epiphenomenon to another common underlying process leading to vascular dysfunction.

Mc Cullough et al. in his recent paper proposed that vascular medial calcification seen in advanced CKD patients starts as intimal atherosclerotic lesion with cholesterol deposition. Based on pathological evidence and existing studies he believed Monckeberg sclerosis to be a manifestation of accelerated atherosclerosis in patients with CKD and a variant of advanced, calcified atherosclerosis with little inflammation and no clear evidence of independent, non-atherogenic process. High phosphate would promote osteoblastic transformation of vascular smooth muscle cells that already contained lipid deposits and enhanced deposition of calcium-hydroxyapatite crystals at the atherosclerotic plaque or in the lipid deposits in the vessel wall. In this model phosphate would promote medial calcification as part of an accelerated atherosclerotic process. (36)

In direct contrast, Drueke in his paper argued that medial calcification is a distinct disease entity unrelated to atherosclerosis. He believed medial calcification to be directly related to pathophysiological disturbance in mineral metabolism rather than to the conventional risk factors associated with atherosclerotic disease. He suggested that medial calcification can be induced experimentally in animals that are fairly resistant to atherosclerosis (such as wild type strains of rats and mice) by creating chronic renal failure and feeding vitamin D or its derivatives. Medial calcification can occur in the absence of intimal calcification in some experimental animal models. Whether this applies for humans is not known. Next, he cited a study by London et al, which showed using intravascular ultrasonography that hemodialysis patients with intimal atherosclerotic calcification have a higher risk of mortality than those with predominantly medial calcification. Based on these and other observations he concluded that medial calcification is different in origin and has different clinical implications than intimal calcification of atherosclerosis. (37)

Despite the controversy about the origin of medial calcification, there is a consensus on the role of hyperphosphatemia in promoting this accelerated calcification. Hyperphosphatemia leads to increased calcification and vascular stiffness. The resultant increase in aortic stiffness, aortic pulse wave velocity and left ventricular hypertrophy contributes to the high rate of cardiovascular morbidity and mortality in these patients.

4. Cardiovascular morbidity and mortality

Dialysis patients have a very high rate of mortality. In 2007, the adjusted annual mortality of dialysis patients in the United States was 19%. Bulk of this mortality is attributable to cardiovascular causes which contributes to about 40-45% of all deaths (38). Among cardiovascular causes, Sudden Cardiac Death (SCD) is the most common. It alone was responsible for 62 % of total cardiovascular deaths and 27 % of all cause deaths (39).

4.1 Sudden Cardiac Death (SCD)

4.1.1 Pathogenesis

We do not have a complete understanding of why SCD is such a disproportionate contributor to cardiovascular mortality in dialysis patients. The most common immediate cause for SCD is a ventricular tachyarrhythmia. In general population, these arrhythmias are often triggered by critical ischemia in a previously injured and often scarred myocardium. The wide prevalence of Left ventricular hypertrophy, anemia, the rapid fluid and electrolyte shifts during hemodialysis, endothelial dysfunction, myocardial interstitial fibrosis and low myocardial tolerance to ischemia possibly contribute to the high frequency of these arrhythmogenic events in dialysis patients (40).

Like in general population, obstructive coronary artery disease is likely a substrate for SCD in dialysis patients. It alone however is not a sufficient reason for the high incidence of SCD. This is supported by the observation that revascularization (both surgical and percutaneous) does not significantly reduce SCDs in the initial years. Data from USRDS Cardiovascular Special Studies Center show a rather unexpectedly high mortality after both CABG (2 year mortality of 43% for CABG using internal mammary graft) and PCI (2 year mortality of 48 % for bare metal stent) in the initial years. The annual mortality attributed to arrhythmias was 8.5% and 7 % for CABG and PCI respectively (41).

In general population, ventricular arrhythmia is the predominant fatal rhythm leading to SCD. Sustained monomorphic ventricular tachycardia and ventricular fibrillation are the most common ventricular arrhythmias in these terminal events. Myocardial scar or fibrotic tissue due to prior ischemic injuries and diminished LV function are the substrates while acute myocardial ischemia is the triggering event for these malignant arrhythmias (42). While this pathogenic mechanism is likely shared by hemodialysis patients there are probably additional mechanisms in play, like those mentioned earlier.

4.1.2 Incidence

The incidence of sudden cardiac death is not uniform over time. The risk increases with patient age and duration of dialysis. Data from USRDS study of all incident US dialysis patients (1995-1999), the rate of cardiac arrest progressively increased from 93 events per 1000 patients-years at 2 yrs after dialysis initiation to 164 events per 1000 patient-years 5 year after dialysis initiation (43). Interestingly, the rate of cardiac arrest in hemodialysis patients when compared to that of PD patients is significantly higher in the first 3 months (HR of 1.5), but rates are similar at 2 years and lower after 3 years (44). There is a temporal trend linking certain days of the week with more SCDs among dialysis patients than others. On Sunday preceding the dialysis on Monday (after a weekend without dialysis) the risk of SCD is three times the average risk. Mondays for patients who dialyze on Tuesdays hold similar risk. (45)

4.1.3 Prevention of SCD

4.1.3.1 B-Blockers

B-Blockers have been shown to be an effective drug for the primary prevention of SCD in non-dialysis patients and improve outcomes in patients with congestive heart failure. The USRDS Wave 3 and 4 studies showed decreased risk of death in patients who were on B-Blockers. Similarly in a randomized study in dialysis patients with dilated cardiomyopathy, there was a 68 % reduction in cardiovascular mortality ($P<0.0001$) and a trend towards reduction in the incidence of sudden death (HR 0.76, $P=0.12$) (46). There is however no randomized prospective study on the use of B-blockers for prevention of SCD in HD patients with preserved left ventricular function.

4.1.3.2 ACEI/ARBs

ACE inhibitors and ARBs have been shown to reverse ventricular hypertrophy, help with ventricular remodeling and have favorable effect on cardiovascular mortality over and beyond BP control in multiple prospective studies in non-dialysis patients. As previously discussed some observational studies have suggested survival benefits with the use of ACEI and ARBs compared to other antihypertensives. But there is no large prospective study on the benefits of ACE inhibitor or ARBs on cardiovascular mortality and in particular, on the incidence of SCDs in dialysis patients.

4.1.3.3 Implantable defibrillators

Role in primary prevention

There is a significant benefit in the primary prevention of Sudden Cardiac Death with the use of Implanted Cardioverter Defibrillator (ICD) in both ischemic and non-ischemic heart failure with low ejection fraction (EF<35%) (47) (48). The trials (MADIT1, MADIT 2, DEFINITE, MUST) that established this benefit however either excluded patients who were on dialysis or did not provide data on renal function of the subjects. While prospective randomized study on the benefits of ICDs in ESRD patients is lacking, the reduction in mortality seen with ICD use in non-dialysis patients is compellingly high (in the range of 30 % over a period of 20 months) and hence ICD should not be withheld on HD patients with low ejection fraction. However it is likely to be beneficial only if the patient is estimated to survive beyond a year and has a reasonable quality of life.

Impaired LV function with low ejection fraction (EF) increases the risk of SCD but many HD patients with relatively preserved LV function suffer SCDs. These patients clearly did not meet the requirement for ICD placement for SCD primary prevention. A retrospective study showed that 71 % of dialysis patients who died of sudden cardiac death had either normal left ventricular function or mild-moderate dysfunction (49). This reinforces the idea that there might not be one single predominant risk factor for sudden cardiac death in hemodialysis patients and interventions to reduce SCD have to be made at multiple levels.

Role in secondary prevention

Patients who survive sudden cardiac death or have had life-threatening ventricular arrhythmias are strongly recommended to have ICD implantation. ICD implantation has been found to be significantly superior to antiarrhythmic drug treatment and non-dialysis patients routinely get ICD implantation after such an event. However, ICD placement seems to be under-utilized in dialysis patients. In a retrospective study by Herzog et al, among ESRD patients who were hospitalized from 1996 to 2001 for cardiac arrest/ventricular fibrillation only 7.6 % of dialysis patients had ICD implantation. ICD implantation was independently associated with a 42% reduction in death risk [relative risk 0.58 (95% CI 0.5-0.66) (50).

Overall benefit and complications of ICD placement

In a meta-analysis by Sakhuja et. al, the authors investigated the mortality outcome of ICD placement in relation to renal function; particularly, the exposure of interest was dialysis. After initial screening, the study analyzed 6 retrospective cohort and 1 case-control studies (January 1999 to July 2008). Patients on dialysis had a 2.7 higher risk of mortality than patients not on dialysis despite the presence of ICDs. The authors suggested that despite the high risk of SCD in dialysis patients, there are other significant causes of death in dialysis patients that undermine the survival benefit offered by interventions aimed at reducing SCDs. Surprisingly, 4 out of 27 deaths in dialysis patients with documented cause were due to arrhythmias. This was attributed to inappropriately high defibrillation threshold for the ICD device (51). In another study, Wase et al found that >35% of dialysis patients had elevated defibrillation threshold compared to <10 % of patients without any CKD. (52)

ICD placement in hemodialysis patients is associated with higher rate of immediate (bleeding) and long-term complications (including infection and central venous stenosis/occlusion). This has to be balanced against the survival benefit ICD can potentially offer to dialysis patients. Life expectancy for the hemodialysis patient also needs to be considered when making any intervention decisions. The 2008 guidelines consider primary prevention ICD therapy to be contraindicated in patients who do not have "a reasonable expectation of survival with an acceptable functional status for at least 1 year". In a decision model analysis that weighed the potential risks and benefits, implantation of defibrillator for primary prevention was favored only for dialysis patients who were younger than 65 years of age. (53)

The treatment guidelines at this time are not very clear and based on either observational studies with conflicting conclusions or on randomized studies for non-dialysis patients. The Implantable Cardioverter Defibrillator in Dialysis patients (ICD2) study will be the first randomized prospective trial which will likely define the benefits of ICD in the prevention of Sudden Cardiac Death in Dialysis patients (54). Until we have results from this study or other randomized prospective study, an individualized treatment decision has to be made for each dialysis patient.

4.1.3.4 External cardioverter defibrillators

There are mixed conclusions among available studies about the benefits of having on-site defibrillators in the dialysis units. Majority of sudden cardiac deaths do not occur during delivery of dialysis. For those who have life-threatening arrhythmias during dialysis, defibrillators likely do prevent sudden death. These patients will likely have repeat arrhythmogenic events and unless the primary cause is identified and addressed, the mortality tends to be exceptionally high.

KDOQI guidelines recommend basic life support (cardiopulmonary resuscitation) training for dialysis unit staff and on-site capability for external cardiac defibrillation either with an automated external defibrillator (AED) or standard manual defibrillator (55).

4.2 Ischemic heart disease

4.2.1 Clinical signs and symptoms

Ischemic heart disease is very common in hemodialysis patients. Obstructive coronary artery disease can most commonly present with chest pain and exertional dyspnea similar to that in non-dialysis patients. In addition, the symptoms can be chest pain and hypotension during dialysis. A significant minority of patients can have silent myocardial ischemia and myocardial infarction. Arrhythmias and sudden cardiac death can occur secondary to myocardial ischemia during dialysis or in the interdialytic period. Anemia and left ventricular hypertrophy which are very prevalent among dialysis patients can exaggerate the ischemic effects of obstructive coronary lesion by increasing the myocardial oxygen demand.

4.2.2 Screening

Beyond a complete history and physical examination and a baseline EKG at the initiation of dialysis, the role of screening for coronary artery disease (CAD) in dialysis patients is not established. KDOQI guideline recommends a baseline echocardiogram at the initiation of dialysis and every 3 yrs after (56). The evidence behind this recommendation is rather weak.

4.2.3 Evaluation and diagnosis of ischemic heart disease

Evaluation of atherosclerotic coronary artery disease is done as part of ongoing care for dialysis patients depending on the symptoms and risk stratification. If the patients develop classical angina/ angina equivalent symptoms, recurrent hypotension, CHF unresponsive to dry weight changes or inability to achieve dry weight because of hypotension, significant LV dysfunction with EF< 40 %; evaluation for CAD is recommended (57).

The other groups of dialysis patients who need periodic evaluation for CAD are discussed below (58).

- Patients with history of coronary artery disease with complete coronary surgical revascularization (CABG) are recommended to have initial evaluation for CAD in 3 years and then annually thereafter. Patients with incomplete coronary revascularization are recommended to have this evaluation every year.
- Diabetic patients on transplant list are recommended to have evaluation for CAD annually.
- Patients on transplant list deemed high risk on Framingham risk score (>20 % per 10 yr cardiovascular event rate) are recommended to have annual evaluation for CAD.
- Patients on transplant list not considered high risk are recommended to have evaluation for CAD every three years.
- Patients on transplant list with known CAD (not revascularized or vascularized with PTCA/coronary stent) should have annual evaluation for CAD.

4.2.4 Choice of diagnostic modalities

A variety of non-invasive stress test is available. Part of the choice and usefulness of such test is dependent on the institutional expertise. Stress test however should not be a routine diagnostic test for all dialysis patients. EKG and echocardiogram can be fairly useful and informative in many stable, low risk dialysis patients who do not have a history of previous coronary artery disease. Similarly, in some patients with appropriate risk and prior history of coronary artery disease the pretest probability of a significant coronary artery disease is high enough to warrant a coronary angiogram without a need for non-invasive stress test.

Exercise EKG is not recommended because of poor exercise tolerance and a high prevalence of left ventricular hypertrophy among dialysis patients. Exercise echocardiography has similarly been found not suitable for a majority of dialysis patients (59). There have been concerns about the validity of nuclear scintigraphy on the ground that it could potentially be influenced by the abnormal metabolic milieu in renal failure.

Dobutamine stress echocardiography is a fairly reliable diagnostic test. In a study of 125 dialysis patients, all of them had coronary angiography, dobutamine stress echocardiography, and resting and exercise electrocardiography. Independent predictors of severe coronary artery disease (defined as luminal stenosis >70 percent by visual estimation in at least one epicardial artery) were a positive stress echo result (Odds Ratio of 23, 95% CI 6-88) or an abnormal resting EKG (OR 7, 95% CI 2-34). Overall, the sensitivity and specificity of dobutamine stress echocardiography was approximately 75 percent (60). The additional advantage of this test is that with the pre-test imaging we can get information on left ventricular ejection fraction, valvular disease, pulmonary artery pressure, volume status and any associated pericardial disease. The risk of arrhythmias, typically atrial fibrillation, (2-4 % versus 0.5% in non-dialysis patients) is however higher with this test (61).

Stress test using vasodilator (adenosine, dipyridamole) and imaging with nuclear scintigraphy is another widely used and perhaps equally reliable test. Though available

studies suggest that vasodilator-induced stress nuclear scintigraphy may be less sensitive than dobutamine stress test in detecting obstructive CAD in dialysis patients, it is used in many centers with equally good results. In a recent head to head study comparing dobutamine echocardiography with dipyridamole myocardial perfusion imaging in 102 dialysis patients, the latter test was found to be more specific and accurate for the diagnosis of coronary artery disease. Positive test result of myocardial perfusion imaging was predictive of fatal and non-fatal coronary events. Surprisingly, no association was observed between abnormalities on dobutamine echocardiography and patient outcome (62).
Given the lack of consistent conclusion among available studies, the choice between dobutamine echocardiography and myocardial perfusion imaging should be guided by available resource and institutional expertise.

4.2.5 Acute coronary syndrome

Like in non-dialysis patients acute coronary syndrome is diagnosed with a triad of clinical signs and symptoms, EKG changes and serum biomarkers of myocardial injury. A significant number of acute coronary events can be asymptomatic or present with atypical symptoms which may be overlooked. Dyspnea and pulmonary edema due to acute MI can be overlooked as "volume overload" in a dialysis patient; hypotension due to shock, often during dialysis may be falsely attributed to transient intradialytic hemodynamic change. This may be one of the factors for the dismally poor prognosis of acute myocardial infarction in dialysis patients. The estimated survival is only about 35 % in 2 years.

4.2.5.1 Diagnosis

Dialysis patients have a high prevalence of coronary artery disease. Outcome of an acute coronary event is time dependent and delay in diagnosis can be the biggest impediment in lowering the subsequent mortality. Index of suspicion for acute coronary event should be high among the physicians involved in the care of dialysis patients. The diagnosis as mentioned earlier is based on a triad of clinical symptoms/signs, dynamic EKG changes and elevation of cardiac biomarkers.
The EKG changes of ischemia may be difficult to interpret on a background of a pre-existing ST changes of LV hypertrophy. Similarly cardiac biomarkers may be falsely elevated (false positive) in ESRD patients. Out of the commonly used markers, Troponin I (cTnI) has been found to be a more specific marker of cardiac injury compared to both Troponin T (cTnT) and CK MB. In a prospective study of 817 consecutive patients (including 51 dialysis patients) with possible acute myocardial infarction, cTnI serum level was found to be independent of creatinine clearance while CK-MB and myoglobin correlated with creatinine clearance (63).

4.2.5.2 Treatment

After a diagnosis of acute coronary syndrome has been established, the treatment should be similar to that in non-dialysis patients. Careful attention should be paid when using certain drugs that have altered clearance in renal failure.
Patients with acute ST-segment elevation MI should receive acute reperfusion therapy preferably Percutaneous Coronary Intervention (PCI) with similar time urgency as in non-dialysis patients. When primary PCI is not available, thrombolytics should be used. The risk of significant hemorrhage with thrombolytic therapy is more than in non-dialysis patients.
Aspirin, Clopidogrel, B-Blocker and ACE Inhibitor are recommended both in both acute myocardial infarction and for the secondary prevention of future ACS. There is no

randomized controlled trial to support this recommendation in dialysis patients but these therapies have been found to be effective in retrospective observational studies in all stages of CKD (64,65). Similarly Glycoprotein 2b/3a inhibitor should be considered in dialysis patients like in non-dialysis patients. These antiplatelet agents have been shown to increase survival in high risk NSTEMI and STEMI patients undergoing PCI. These drugs act by inhibiting glycoprotein GP 2b/3a, an integrin in platelet membrane, necessary for platelet aggregation. The risk of bleeding with these drugs is higher in dialysis patients because of the underlying uremic platelet dysfunction. When used, Abciximab and Tirofiban should be considered preferred agents, since no dosing changes are required for Abciximab, and dialysis-specific dosing recommendations are available for Tirofiban. Abciximab is typically used for PCI as clearance of this drug is not affected in dialysis patients.

Hemodialysis is often deferred for patients who are admitted with an acute myocardial infarction. There is no good evidence to support this practice. The timing of dialysis should be individualized after taking into account the patients' volume / electrolyte status. With the use of thrombolytics, heparin and different platelet agents the risk of bleeding from the AV fistula/graft site may be increased. Significant hypotension should be avoided because it can put additional strain on the myocardium and also can increase the risk of stent thrombosis.

4.2.6 Chronic coronary artery disease

The medical management of stable CAD is not different than in the general population. B-Blockers are indicated to reduce afterload and myocardial oxygen demand; ACE Inhibitors to reduce afterload and for their favorable effects on ventricular remodeling; antiplatelet agents to inhibit platelet aggregation in unstable atherosclerotic plaques and statins for LDL lowering and plaque stabilizing effect. All of these drugs have been shown to have strong beneficial effects on progression of CAD and recurrence of acute myocardial infarction in multiple well-designed randomized prospective trials. But dialysis patients have traditionally been excluded from these studies, so while the conventional wisdom probably applies to dialysis patients too, some uncertainties still exist.

4.2.7 Coronary revascularization

4.2.7.1 Percutaneous Coronary Intervention (PCI) Vs Coronary Artery Bypass (CABG)

As mentioned earlier in the chapter, the mortality rate after coronary revascularization is very high (2-year 48 % mortality after bare metal stents and 43 % after coronary artery bypass surgery using internal mammary graft)(38). There have been no prospective randomized studies that have compared CABG and PCI head-to-head. Observational studies have mixed conclusions about the relative benefit of one revascularization procedure over the other. Diabetes patients who undergo CABG using internal mammary graft in general tend to do better than diabetic patients undergoing percutaneous coronary interventions (PCI).

Herzog et.al looked at the USRDS database for the long-term survival of dialysis patients undergoing coronary artery bypass comparing it to dialysis patients (n=10,941) who received drug-eluting stent (DES) in 2004-2006. The authors found DES patients had better survival at 12 months, but after 18 months CABG patients had better outcome. CABG patients receiving internal mammary grafts (68% of CAB pts, n=2356) did significantly better than those without (66). Similarly in a meta-analysis by Nevi F et al. which included 17 retrospective cohort studies from 1977 to 2002, there was no difference in mortality in patients who received CABG compared to PCI. However there was a higher mortality for CABG patients within the first 30 days compared to PCI (67). The authors pointed out that the baseline differences among the patient groups were adjusted for final analysis in only four of the studies. Given the lack of randomized prospective trial and methodological flaws with the available retrospective studies, no definite conclusion can be drawn in regards to preference of one revascularization procedure over the other.

4.2.7.2 Drug Eluting Stent (DES) Vs Bare Metal Stent (BMS)

There is again no randomized prospective trial to establish the superiority of one over the other. Many trials of Drug Eluting Stent have excluded dialysis patients. In a single center study by Ayoma et al in Japan, 88 consecutive HD patients who received sirolimus-eluting stent were compared with 78 patients who received bare-metal stent in the preceding year. There was no difference in the rate of restenosis, the primary endpoint, at 6-8 months (68). But in another single center retrospective study from Japan, there was less late in-stent stenosis and better major cardiovascular event profile with sirolimus-eluting stent. Particularly, all cause mortality and need for revascularization was lower in the DES group (69). It is difficult to draw conclusions based on small single-center non-randomized study and whether Drug eluting stent is really superior to bare-metal stent in dialysis patients is still not settled.

5. Stroke/transient ischemic attack (TIA)

Stroke is the third leading cause of death in the United States and other developed countries. Dialysis patients have a markedly elevated risk of atherosclerotic cerebrovascular disease, the substrate for stroke and transient ischemic attack. Data available for hospitalized ESRD patients show the rate of stroke to be 5-10 fold higher compared to non-ESRD patients (70). However the risk factors for stroke in dialysis patients have not been well studied and the recommendations for prevention and treatment are largely based on studies done on non-dialysis patients.

5.1 Risk factors

Hypertension, age, diabetes, malnutrition and ethnicity have been found to be associated with risk of stroke in available studies. Seigel et al. conducted a retrospective study on data collected by USRDS looking at the relationship of black ethnicity, BP and markers of malnutrition with elevated risk of stroke. Adult ESRD patients without a history of stroke or transient ischemic attack were considered for analysis. The primary outcome was hospitalization or fatal stroke. The rate of incident stroke was 33/1,000 person-years in the study sample. In a Cox proportional hazard model, after adjustment for age and other patient characteristics, three markers of malnutrition were associated with the risk of stroke—serum albumin (per 1 g/dl decrease, hazard ratio [HR] = 1.43), height-adjusted body weight (per 25% decrease, HR = 1.09), and a subjective assessment of undernourishment (HR = 1.27)—as was higher mean BP (per 10 mmHg, HR = 1.11). The association between black race varied by cardiac disease status, with blacks estimated to be at lower risk than whites among individuals with cardiac disease (HR = 0.74), but at higher risk among individuals without cardiac disease (HR = 1.24). In exploratory analysis looking at laboratory parameters and their relation to stroke risk there was no relationship between

baseline cholesterol (per 10 mg/dl increment, HR = 1.00), serum calcium, phosphorous, or parathyroid hormone and incident stroke. Patients with severe anemia with hemoglobin (<9 g/dl) were at a 22% higher risk for stroke (HR = 1.22, 95% CI = 1.00 to 1.49) (71).
While severe anemia has been considered a risk factor in observational studies, there probably is a significant risk associated with attempting to normalize hemoglobin too. In the TREAT study, the incidence of stroke was significantly higher in the treatment group receiving darbopoetin compared to the placebo group(HR 1.92; 95 % CI 1.38-2.68; P< 0.001). The median Hb concentration achieved was 12.5 gm % and 10.6 gm % in the Darbopoetin and the placebo group respectively. The primary end-point (death or non-fatal cardiovascular event) was not different between the two groups. (72)

5.2 Prevention and treatment

In general, the prevention and treatment of stroke should be along the lines of recommendations for general population. Antiplatelet agent is fairly safe and can be used for both primary and secondary prevention of stroke. The risk of stroke and need for anticoagulation with Coumadin can be assessed using the standard CHADS2 score. INR targets should be in accordance with general guidelines. The treating physician should also keep in mind the increased propensity of dialysis patients for bleeding.
The other issue is the safety and efficacy of thrombolytic therapy in acute stroke patients who present within three hours of symptom onset. In non-dialysis stroke patients thrombolytic have been shown to increase resolution of neurological deficit and improve functional outcomes. This has been validated in multiple studies. But in dialysis patients there is no prospective trial to examine the benefit and risk of thrombolytic. In the original NINDS study, the ESRD status and the renal function were not mentioned for the study population (73). While no prospective data is available for ESRD patients, guidelines from AHA do not make distinction between dialysis and non-dialysis patients for thrombolytic indication in acute stroke.

6. Peripheral vascular disease

PVD is very common in both diabetic and non-diabetic dialysis patients. Almost 15% of incident dialysis patients have a clinical diagnosis of PVD (74). The treatment and secondary prevention of PVD follow the recommendations for general population although the evidence behind this approach is weak.

6.1 Diagnosis

All dialysis patients should have a thorough examination looking for evidence of peripheral vascular disease. History of claudication, poor wound healing and weak peripheral pulse or non-healing ischemic ulcers on exam should be the basis of a diagnostic work-up. Further evaluation is done non-invasively with Ankle Brachial Index (Ankle systolic blood pressure divided by brachial systolic blood pressure), Duplex and if indicated with arteriogram. ABI is a useful screening test in most instances but can be falsely elevated due to heavy vascular calcification in dialysis patients.
Prevention begins with risk factor modification like in any other atherosclerotic disease. Smoking cessation, lipid lowering, glycemic control, HTN control and use of antiplatelet agents are important in primary prevention. The relative role of these risk factor modifications on the outcome, after PVD has already set in; is not known.

6.2 Therapy

Revascularization procedures do not have as good an outcome as in non-dialysis patients. Indications for revascularization are similar to general population, those being severe claudication, rest pain and critical leg ischemia with non-healing ulcers.

Angioplasty is preferred for amenable stenotic lesions. In a study by Kumada et al. the immediate results of angioplasty in 118 HD patients and 108 control subjects were equally good. Dialysis patients seem to have more fem-popliteal atherosclerotic lesions than iliac lesions (75). Formal surgical revascularization with bypass grafts is needed for many dialysis patients. The problems with revascularization include high peri-operative and one year mortality, delayed wound healing, loss of limb despite patent graft, prolonged hospitalization and poor rehabilitation (76). Because of all these issues, some experts recommend primary amputation, especially for patients who are non-ambulatory, bedridden and have extensive tissue necrosis and infection. Revascularization with either percutaneous or surgical intervention can be beneficial in selected dialysis patients who are ambulatory or use the affected limb for weight bearing or for transfer purpose.

7. Conclusion

Cardiovascular disease is very common in ESRD patients and is the major cause of morbidity and mortality. While we partly understand the role of traditional risk factors in the pathogenesis of cardiovascular disease, much remains to be defined as to how modification of these would translate into improved survival. Similarly more studies are needed to define the role of other non-traditional risk factors like calcium, phosphorus, anemia. Large randomized controlled trials specifically designed to answer these questions are awaited.

8. References

[1] [2] National Health and Nutrition Examination Survey (NHANES, 2003–06), National Center for Health Statistics and NHLBI.

[3] [4] [5] [6] [15] United States Renal Data System Annual Data Report 2008, Bethesda, MD: National Institute of Health, National Institute of Diabetes and Digestive and Kidney Diseases

[7] Traditional Cardiovascular Disease Risk Factors in Dialysis Patients Compared with the General Population: The CHOICE study, Longencker JC et al.(J Am Soc Nephrol 13:1918-1927, 2002)

[8] Intensive Blood Glucose Control and Vascular Outcomes in Patients with type 2 Diabetes, The ADVANCE Collaborative Group. N Engl J Med 2008; 358: 2560-72

[9] Effects of intense glucose lowering in type 2 Diabetes, The Action to Control Cardiovascular Risk in Diabetes Study Group. N Engl J Med 2008; 358:2545-2559

[10] [11] [12] Atorvastatin in Patients with Type 2 Diabetes Mellitus undergoing Hemodialysis, Wanner C, Krane V, Ritz E et. Al. N Engl J Med 2005; 353:238-248

[13] Primary prevention of cardiovascular disease with atorvastatin in type 2 diabetes in the Collaborative Atorvastatin Diabetes Study (CARDS): multicentre randomised placebo-controlled trial. Colhoun HM, Fuller JH et al. Lancet 2004; 364: 685–96

[14] Rosuvastatin and Cardiovascular Events in Patients Undergoing Hemodialysis, Fellstrom BC et al for the AURORA Study group. N Engl J Med 2009; 360:1395-1407

[16] [17] National Kidney Foundation (NKF) Kidney Disease Outcome Quality Initiative (KDOQI)Guidelines 2006
[18] Aortic Pulse Wave Velocity as a Marker of Cardiovascular Risk in Hypertensive Patients, Blancher J, Safar M et. Al. .*Hypertension.* 1999;33:1111-1117.
[19] Prognostic implications of echocardiographically determined left ventricular mass in the Framingham Heart Study. Levy D, Garrison RJ et al. *N Engl J Med.* 1990; 322: 1561–1566
[21] Blood Pressure and Mortality Risk on Peritoneal Dialysis. Udayaraj UP, Tomson CR et al. Am J of Kidney Dis 2009 53:70-78
[22] Importance of Blood Pressure Control in Hemodialysis Patient Survival. Mazzuchi N, Fernandez-Cean J et al .*Kidney International* (2000) 58, 2147–2154
[23] Home Blood Pressure Monitoring In Blood Pressure Control among Hemodialysis Patients: An Open Randomized Clinical Trial. Da Silva GV, Micon D JR et al. Nephrol Dial Transplant 24, 2009:3805-3811
[24] Cardiovascular Protection with Antihypertensive Drugs in Dialysis Patients: A Systematic Review and Meta-analysis of Randomized Control Trials. Agrawal R, Sinha AD. *Hypertension.* 2009; 53:860
[25] Effect of lowering Blood Pressure on Cardiovascular events and Mortality in Patients on Dialysis: A systematic review and Meta-analysis of Randomized Controlled Trials. Heerspink HJ, Perkovik V et al. Lancet 373:1009-1015, 2009
[26] Therapeutic options in minimizing Left Ventricular Hypertrophy. Devereux RB. American Heart Journal , Vol 139 Issue 1, Supplement 1 ; Jan 2000
[27] Pathophysiology of cardiovascular Disease in Hemodialysis patients. Meeus F, London GM et al. *Kidney International* (2000) 58, S140–S147
[28] Cardiac hypertrophy, aortic compliance, peripheral resistance, and wave reflection in end-stage renal disease. Comparative effects of ACE inhibition and calcium channel blockade. London Gm, Cuche JL et al. Circulation, Vol 90, 2786-2796, 1994
[29] Cardiovascular effects of angiotensin converting enzyme inhibition or angiotensin receptor blockade in hemodialysis: a meta-analysis. Tai DJ, Hemmelgarn BR, Alberta Kidney Disease Network.Clin J Am Soc Nephrol Clin 2010 Apr;5(4):623-30
[30] Prescription of antihypertensive agents to haemodialysis patients: time trends and associations with patient characteristics, country and survival in the DOPPS. Lopes AA, Young EW et al. Nephrol Dial Transplant 2009; 24(9):2809-16
[31] The benefit of salt restriction in the treatment of end-stage renal disease by hemodialysis. Kayikcioglu M, Ok E etal. NDT 2009; 24:956-962
[32] The mortality risk of overhydration in hemodialysis patients. Wizemann V,Marcelli D et al. NDT 2009; 24: 1574-1579
[33] Relative plasma volume monitoring during hemodialysis aids the assessment of dry weight. Sinha AD, Light RP, Agrawal R: Hypertension2010; 55: 305-311
[34] Association of elevated serum PO4, Ca _ PO4 product, and parathyroid hormone with cardiac mortality risk in chronic hemodialysispatients. Ganesh SK, Port FK et al. *J Am Soc Nephrol* 12: 2131–2138, 2001
[35] Mineral Metabolism, Mortality, and Morbidity in Maintenance Hemodialysis. Block GA, Chertow GM et al. J Am Soc Nephrol 15: 2208–2218, 2004
[36] Accelerated Atherosclerotic Calcification and Monckeberg's Sclerosis: A Continuum of Advanced Vascular Pathology in Chronic Kidney Disease. McCullough PA, Abela GS et al. Clin J Am Soc Nephrol 3: 1585–1598, 2008.

[37] Arterial Intima and Medial Calcification: Distinct entities with different pathogenesis or all the same ? Drueke TB. Clin J Am Soc Nephrol 3:1583-1584, 2008
[38] USRDS Annual Data Report 2008
[39] USRDS Annual Data Report 2006
[40] The challenge of sudden death in dialysis patients. Ritz E, Wanner C. Clin J Am Soc Nephrol 2008; 3:920-929
[41] Cause-specific mortality of dialysis patients after coronary revascularization: why don't dialysis patients have better survival after coronary intervention? Herzog CA, Gilbert DT et al. Nephrol Dial Transplant. 2008 August; 23(8): 2629–2633
[42] Immediate Coronary Angiography in survivors of out-of-hospital cardiac arrest. Spaulding CM, Carli P et. al. N Eng J Med 336:1629-1633, 1997
[43] USRDS Annual Data Report 2002
[44] Sudden Cardiac Death and Dialysis patients. Herzog CA, Passman R et. al. Semin Dial. 2008 Jul-Aug;21(4):300-7
[45] Characteristics of sudden Death in Hemodialysis Patients. Bleyer AJ, Russell G et. al. Kidney Int 69: 2268-2273, 2006
[46] Carvedilol increases two-year survival in dialysis patients with dilated cardiomyopahty. A prospective-placebo controlled trial. Cice G, Calabro R et al. J Am Coll Cardiol 41:1438-1444, 2003
[47] Prophylactic Implantation of a Defibrillator in PatientAs with Myocardial Infarction and Reduced Ejection Fraction. Moss AJ, Andrew ML et al for the Multicenter Automatic defibrillator Implantation Trial Investigators. N Engl J Med 2002; 346:877-883
[48] Prophylactic defibrillator implantation in patients with nonischemic dilated cardiomyopathy. Kadish A, Levine JH et al.Defibrillators in Non-Ischemic Cardiomyopathy Treatment Evaluation (DEFINITE) Investigators. N Engl J Med 2004; 350:2151-2158
[49] The clinical epidemiology of cardiac disease in chronic renal failure. Parfrey PS, Foley RN. *J Am Soc Nephrology* 10:1606-1615, 1999
[50] Survival of dialysis patients after cardiac arrest and the impact of implantable cardioverter defibrillators. Herzog CA, Gilbertson DT et al. *Kidney International* (2005) 68, 818–825(51)Meta-analysis of mortality in dialysis patients with an implantable cardioverter defibrillator. Sakhuja R, Bhatt DL et al. Am J Cardiol 2009; 103 : 735-741
[52] Impact of chronic kidney disease upon survival among implantable cardioverter-defibrillator recipients,Wase A, McCullough PA et al., *J Interven Card Electrophysiol* 11 (2004), pp. 199–204
[53] M.S. Amin, A.D. Fox, G. Kalahasty, R.K. Shepard, M.A. Wood and K.A. Ellenbogen, Benefit of primary prevention implantable cardioverter-defibrillators in the setting of chronic kidney disease: a decision model analysis, *J Cardiovasc Electrophysiol* 12 (2008), pp. 1-6. (47)
[54] Prevention of sudden cardiac death: rationale and design of the Implantable Cardioverter Defibrillators in Dialysis patients (ICD2) Trial--a prospective pilot study. de Bie MK, Jukema JW et al. Cur Med Res Opin 2008 Aug;24(8):2151-7
[55] [56] [57] [58] KDOQI guidelines on evaluation and management of Cardiovascular disease. *American Journal of Kidney Diseases,* Vol 45, No 4, Suppl 3 (April), 2005: p S17

[59] How to manage the renal patient withcoronary heart disease: the agony and the ecstasy of opinion based medicine. Herzog CA. JAm Soc Nephrol 14:2556-2572, 2003
[60] Dobutamine stress echocardiography and the resting but not exercise electrocardiograph predict severe coronary artery disease in renal transplant candidates. Sharma R, J.D Brecker S et al. Nephrol Dial Transplant (2005) 20: 2207–2214
[61] Dobutamine stress echocardiography for the detection of significant coronary artery disease in renal transplant candidates. Herzog CA, Dick CD et al. Am J Kidney Dis 33:1080-1090, 1999
[62] Comparison of the prognostic value of dipyridamole and dobutamine myocardial perfusion scintigraphy in Hemodialysis patients . De Vriese AS, De Geeter FW et. al. Kidney Int 76: 428-436 2009
[63] Performance of multiple cardiac biomarkers measured in the emergency department in patients with chronic kidney disease and chest pain. McCullough PA, McCord J et. al. Acad Emerg Med. 2002 Dec;9(12):1389-96.
[64] Determinants of mortality after myocardial infarction in patients with advanced renal dysfunction. Beattie JN, McCullough PA et al. Am J Kidney Dis 37:1191-1200, 2001
[65] Benefits of Aspirin and Betablockade after myocardial infarction in patients with chronic disease. McCullough PA, Manley HJ et al. Am Heart J 144:226-232, 2002
[66] Long-term Survival of Dialysis Patients in the US after Surgical versus Percutaneous Coronary Revascularization. Herzog CA, Solid C et al. Circulation 2010: 122: A12633
[67] Optimal Method of Coronary Revascularization in Patients Receiving Dialysis: Systematic Review. I F Nevis, Garg A X et al. Clin J Am Soc Nephrol 4: 369–378, 2009
[68] Sirolimus-eluting stents vs bare metal stents for coronary intervention in Japenese patients with renal failure on Hemodialysis. Aoyama T, Murohara T et. al. Circ J 72:56-60, 2008
[69] Clinical and angiographic outcomes following percutaneous coronary intervention with sirolimus-eluting stent versus bare-metal stents in Hemodialysis patients. Yachi S, Hara K et. al. Am J Kidney Dis 54: 299-306, 2009
[70] The Choices for Healthy Outcomes in Caring for ESRD (CHOICE) study. Sozio SM, Parekh RS et al. Am J Kidney Dis 54: 468-477,2009
[71] Risk Factors for Incident Stroke among Patients with End-Stage Renal Disease Seliger Sl, Stehman-Breen CO et. al. J Am Soc Nephrol 14:2623-2631, 2003
[72] A Trial of Darbepoetin Alfa in Type 2 Diabetes and Chronic Kidney Disease.Pfeffer MA, Totto R et. al for the TREAT investigators. N Engl J Med 2009; 361:2019-2032
[73] Tissue Plasminogen activator for Acute Ischemic Stroke. The National Institute of Neurological Disorders and Stroke rt-PA Stroke Study Group. N Engl J Med 1995; 333:1581-1588
[74] Factors associated with future amputation among patients undergoing Hemodialysis:results from the Dialysis Morbidity and Mortality Study Waves 3 and 4. O'Hare AM, Johansen KL et al. Am J Kidney Dis 41: 162-170, 2003
[75] Long term outcome of percutaneous transluminal angioplasty in chronic Hemodialysis patients with peripheral arterial disease. Kumada Y, Murohara T et. al. Nephrol Dial Transplant 23:3996-4001, 2008
[76] Peripheral Vascular disease-related procedures in dialysis patients: Predictors and prognosis. Plantinga LC, Jaar BG et. al. Clin J Am Soc Nephrol 4: 1637-1645, 2009

9

Cardiovascular Morbidity in Hemodialysis: The Reverse Epidemiology Phenomenon

Georgios Tsangalis
Service de Nephrologie-Hemodialyse, Centre Hospitalier "Jean Rougier", CAHORS, France

1. Introduction

The Framingham study that begun more than 60 years ago (1948) has shaped the way Western societies face cardiovascular disease (CVD). The relative impact of this study (now on its 3rd generation of participants) [1] has been so impressive that both public health authorities and the medical community have fully endorsed its results: since then, hypertension, dyslipidemia, tobacco smoking, diabetes mellitus and more recently obesity and hypertriglyceridemia are considered as the major risk factors for new cardiovascular morbidity and overall mortality.
Major advances aiming both at prevention and management have had a significant impact on survival of patients with CVD. These advances, together with the extinction of undernutrition after the 2nd World War, have led to an increase in survival and thus in the number of patients with chronic disease states (congestive heart failure, chronic kidney disease, dialysis patients, cancer etc) that survive over prolonged time periods. Numerous epidemiological studies over the last decade, have observed that in these subgroups of patients, the well established-for the general population- surrogates of cardiovascular risk and metabolic syndrome as obesity, hypercholesterolemia and hypertension are paradoxically associated with greater survival. Hence the term "reverse epidemiology paradox" was coined in medical literature.
Approximately 9% of the US adult population (about 20 million people) has chronic kidney d stage 1 (CKD-1) and 2% are receiving maintenance dialysis. It has been projected that dialysis patients will exceed 1 million by 2018. It should be emphasized that although dialysis for CKD-5 is expected to be life-prolonging, 5-year survival in the US is only about 35% for patients on dialysis [2,3]. Robust observational studies have repeatedly shown that even after adjustments for comorbidities, moderately higher levels of blood pressure, higher body mass index (BMI) and higher cholesterol levels are associated with improved survival.
This chapter will review data concerning the role of arterial hypertension, obesity, and cholesterol levels on cardiovascular morbidity and mortality in hemodialysis (HD) patients and discuss potential pathogenetic mechanisms that could possibly explain the so called "reverse epidemiology paradox".

2. Hypertension in dialysis: friend or foe?

The definition of arterial hypertension (AH) in the general population is based on observations showing a significant increase in cardiovascular morbidity and mortality over a certain level of systolic and/or diastolic blood pressure (140/90 mmHg respectively). In the general population the association of hypertension with the occurrence of new CVE is indisputable [4-6] and even patients with high normal blood pressure have an increased cumulative incidence of CVE compared to normotensive subjects.

The same definition of AH (mainly pre-dialysis blood pressure) has been used for the dialysis population as well, although data concerning the impact of pre-dialysis hypertension on the occurrence of CVE and overall mortality show significant contradiction. Elevated BP may not represent the primary risk for overall survival in patients treated with hemodialysis; several studies have failed to show that high BP is an independent mortality risk factor in this population group [7-12]. Moreover, Iseki et al [12] found a strong association between low diastolic blood pressure and risk of death in a cohort of 1243 hemodialysis patients that were followed for 5 years and Zager et al [10] noted that the relative death rate for patients with pre- or postdialysis hypotension increased to four times normal or greater than 2.5 normal, respectively.

In a different approach, Klassen et al [13] investigated whether an increased pulse pressure would be associated with increased risk of death despite the inverse relationship between conventional blood pressure measures and mortality in patients with end-stage renal disease.According to their results after a follow-up period of 1-year, multivariable Cox proportional hazards modeling showed a direct and consistent relationship between increasing pulse pressure and increasing death risk. Each incremental elevation of 10 mm Hg in postdialysis pulse pressure was associated with a 12% increase in the hazard for death (hazard ratio, 1.12; 95% confidence interval, 1.06-1.18). Postdialysis systolic blood pressure was inversely related to mortality with a 13% decreased hazard for death for each incremental elevation of 10 mm Hg (hazard ratio, 0.87; 95% confidence interval, 0.84-0.90).

Blood pressure of hemodialysis patients varies with each hemodialysis session as a result of loss of excess fluid. In a recent publication, Moriya et al [14]tried to define clearly the time point at which the blood pressure is measured. For this purpose, home BP of patients was monitored twice a day for 1 wk (morning-after waking up and evening-before sleeping). During the same week, the BP was measured in the supine position before and after each dialysis session. The BP was measured with automated devices by the same method. The authors calculated the weekly averaged blood pressure (WABP) based on these 20 mBP measurements/week. According to their results, none of the components of pre- or postdialysis blood pressure was significantly different between patients with and without cardiovascular events. Pulse weekly averaged blood pressure, age, and human atrial natriuretic peptide were significantly higher in patients who died than in survivors. Kaplan-Meier method with a log-rank test demonstrated that survival free rate from cardiovascular events and that of all-cause mortality in patients with pulse weekly averaged blood pressure ≥70 mmHg were significantly lower than those in the remaining patients

The same authors have showed that the systolic and diastolic WAB are almost completely consistent with the wake-up BP on the next day after the middle dialysis session (R^2 =0.709, P<0.0001; R^2=0.775, P<0.0001, respectively) suggesting that this measurement could be used instead of the WAB [15]. Agarwal *et al.* [16,17,18] reported the significance of self-recorded home BP three times a day during 1 week in HD patients and showed that home BP correspond to ambulatory BP and left ventricular hypertrophy in HD patients.

The above mentioned studies suggest that BP should rather be evaluated by the average of sequential monitoring during 1 wk and not by one-point measurement before or after dialysis or after waking up. Pulse pressure (PP) more accurately predicts adverse CVE than systolic+/-diastolic BP; moreover since PP is a marker of arterial stiffness (the latter being markedly increased in dialysis patients) it is logical, from a pathophysiological point of view, to use pWAB as a target index for controlling BP and a useful prognostic marker of cardiovascular events or all-cause mortality of HD patients.

An interesting approach to the reverse epidemiology paradox in HD patients (including hypertension) has been suggested by Shoji et al, based on data collected from Japanese registries. Undoubtedly, the relative risk of death from CVD in HD patients is 10−30 as compared with the general population in Europe and the US [19]. A logical approach would assume that HD patients experience 10 to 30 times more CVD events than the general population. Nevertheless, the report of the registry data in Okinawa, Japan, suggests that this is not the case; the risk of occurrence of acute myocardial infarction was 2.5 times and 4.6 times higher in male and female HD patients, respectively, than the general population [20] while the risk of stroke was 5.7 times and 8.5 times higher in male and female HD patients in their sixties, respectively, than the general population of the same age category [21]. Although these data indicate that HD patients experience more CVE, they do not suffice to fully explain the 10-30 times higher risk of death observed in these patients. An intriguing explanation suggested by Shoji et al, lies in the relative risk of death after a given CVE (fatality). In fact, death rate in 30 days after acute myocardial infarction was 22.9% for the general population and 50.8% for hemodialysis patients in Okinawa, Japan [20]. The 50% survival period after acute myocardial infarction was 7.3 years for the general population, whereas it was one month for hemodialysis patients. Also, the death rate in 30 days after stroke was 12.3% for the general population and 46.6% for hemodialysis patients in Okinawa, Japan [21].

Another possible explanation for the association of low blood pressure with higher mortality rates in HD patients is the "reverse causation" phenomenon. Reverse causation suggests that it is not hypotension or normotension, per se, that is detrimental but rather the underlying condition causing low blood pressure (congestive heart failure or continuously erroneous estimation of dry weight); in other words, the reversion of the direction of the causal pathway that is responsible for this paradoxical association.

Nevertheless, even if the association of low blood pressure and mortality is somewhat a result of poor general health, strategies that would avoid hypotension (or even low normal blood pressure) in HD patients should be implemented.

3. Obesity and cholesterol levels in HD patients

Several epidemiologic studies have shown a strong relationship between obesity and increased risk of cardiovascular disease and mortality in the general population [22-23]. Nevertheless, several studies have indicated a J or U curve effect in individuals with a low BMI [23-25]. The first study to report that overall mortality risk decreased with increasing BMI was the Diaphane Collaborative Study Group in France. Participants were young, mostly nondiabetic, French patients treated with hemodialysis during the 1970s [26]. In the 1990s, Leavy et al [27] described the predictive value for mortality over 5 years of follow-up of a number of risk factors, recorded at baseline, in a national sample of 3607 hemodialysis patients. According to their results, low BMI was independently and significantly predictive of increased mortality; moreover its independent predictive value of mortality risk persisted even 5 years later. No evidence of increasing mortality risk was found for higher values of BMI. The prospective Dialysis Outcomes and Practice Study (DOPPS) [28,29] has allowed comparison of BMI-mortality relationships in the United States and Europe and among a variety of "healthier," as compared with "sicker" hemodialysis patient subgroups, such as younger patients, never-smokers, and those with less chronic illnesses.

A BMI of 23 to 24.9 kg/m2, was associated with the highest relative mortality risk. Overall, a lower relative risk (RR) of mortality as compared with a BMI of 23 to 24.9 kg/m2, was found for overweight (BMI 25 to 29.9 kg/m2; RR 0.84; P = 0.008), for mild obesity (BMI 30 to 34.9 kg/m2; RR 0.73; P= 0.0003), and for moderate obesity (BMI 35 to 39.9 kg/m2; RR 0.76; P= 0.02). Even when patients were subdivided in different groups in respect to general health status, the results didn't change, contrary to the initial hypothesis of the investigators that reverse epidemiology may not exist in healthier or younger ESRD patients. There was a survival benefit for healthy overweight patients (BMI 25 to 29.9 kg/m2) that was even greater for the obese patients (BMI ≥30 kg/m2), and this was observed for the healthier as well as the sicker groups of hemodialysis-treated patients.

One could argue that although BMI is used as a general index to distinguish underweight, normal, overweight and obese patients, it doesn't provide information on the relative contribution of muscle and fat mass to overall body weight. This is of paramount importance since increased catabolism is common place in HD patients and this can lead to substantial decreases in muscle mass resulting in lower BMIs that could erroneously be interpreted as "normal". A recent study by Kalantar-Zadeh et al [30], investigated the relative contribution of fat versus muscle mass or their changes over time to the survival benefits of larger body size.

These investigators studied 121,762 patients receiving HD 3 times weekly from July 1, 2001, through June 30, 2006. They examined whether BMI (calculated using 3-month averaged post-HD dry weight) and 3-month averaged serum creatinine levels and their changes over time were predictive of mortality risk. They assessed muscle mass by using serum creatinine measurements since in long-term HD patients who have minimal or no residual renal function and who undergo a stable HD treatment regimen, time-averaged serum creatinine concentration is a more likely surrogate of muscle mass, and its changes over time may represent parallel changes in skeletal muscle mass[31,32]. According to their findings higher BMI (up to 45) and higher serum creatinine concentration were incrementally and independently associated with greater survival, even after extensive multivariate adjustment for available surrogates of nutritional status and inflammation. Dry weight loss or gain over time exhibited a graded association with higher rates of mortality or survival, respectively, as did changes in serum creatinine level over time. Among the 50,831 patients who survived the first 6 months and who had available data for changes in weight and creatinine level, those who lost weight but had an increased serum creatinine level had a greater survival rate than those who gained weight but had a decreased creatinine level. These associations appeared consistent across different demographic groups of patients receiving HD. These results suggest that in patients receiving long-term HD, larger body size with more muscle mass appears to be associated with a higher survival rate. A discordant muscle gain with weight loss over time may confer more survival benefit than weight gain while losing muscle. Moreover the combination of an increase in time averaged serum creatinine levels (a surrogate according to the authors of muscle mass) and total body weight is associated with higher survival rates than an isolated increase in muscle mass, suggesting that higher body fat content confers also a survival benefit in HD patients.

Several pathogenetic mechanisms have been proposed in order to explain the association of obesity with a higher survival rate in HD patients. A recent review by Kalantar-Zadeh et al has summarized these mechanisms (Table 1).

Potential pathophysiologic mechanisms concerning the Obesity paradox
Malnutrtion inflammation syndrome
Temporal delay between competitive risk factors: Increased nutrition vs malnutrition
Selection bias during progression of Chronic Kidney Disease
Sequestration of uremic toxins in fat tissue
Anti-inflammatory cytokines related to total body mass, adiponectines
TNF-α receptors
Endotoxin-lipoprotein hypothesis
Hemodynamic stability of obese patients
Neurohormonal alterations in obesity
Alteration of traditional risk factors in the uremic environment
Inverse causation
Survival bias
Advantages of obesity during human evolution

Table 1. Adapted from Kalantar-Zadeh [8,15,16].

4. Malnutrition inflammation syndrome

This hypothesis states that low BMI in HD patients is associated with increased inflammation meaning that underweight patients with ESRD would more likely become ill and would recover more slowly from illness compared with patients who have normal weight or who are obese. On the contrary, if overweight patients with an increase in adipose tissue develop a deficiency in energy or protein intake, they would be less likely to develop frank protein-energy malnutrition. This assumption, however, has not been adopted by other investigators of the obesity paradox. According to Beddhu et al, recent data suggest a cross-sectional association of high BMI or abdominal adiposity with inflammation both in persons with moderate chronic kidney disease (CKD) and in the dialysis population (33). Moreover in HD patients inflammation is associated with coronary artery calcification (34), myocardial injury as shown by elevations in serum troponin T (35), and death (36). These authors hypothesized that in HD patients, the effects of nutrition on survival are much stronger than are the effects of atherosclerotic events. Therefore, although undernourished patients have lower inflammation, they experience a higher rate of cardiovascular and noncardiovascular events than patients with normal or higher weight. On the other hand, better nutrition and adiposity, although associated with increased inflammation, oxidative stress and atherosclerotic changes is associated with better survival since it confers a survival advantage relatively to undernutrition.

5. Temporal delay between competitive risk factors: Increased nutrition vs malnutrition

It has been suggested that the obesity paradox is due to the presence of a temporal delay between competitive risk factors: a "fast killer" like the malnutrition-inflammation syndrome and a "slow killer" like obesity. It is noteworthy to bear in mind that 2/3 of dialysis patients die within the first 5 years of HD with this dramatic survival rate being worse than the 5-year survival in the majority of cancer patients. [37].

6. Selection bias during progression of Chronic Kidney Disease (CKD)

Chronic Kidney disease is associated with increased cardiovascular morbidity and mortality. In the United States almost 90% of the 20 million patients with CKD die before reaching dialysis due to cardiovascular events [38], meaning that only a small minority of these patients survive long enough to start dialysis. This observation suggests that there is a selection bias for survival, probably reflecting different genetic or metabolic profiles that determine which patients can overcome the increased risk of death in the pre-dialysis period and eventually start dialysis [39]. Arizona PIMA Indians are a typical example of this hypothesis; although they are obese and diabetic and develop CKD stage 5 rapidly, they are protected from cardiovascular disease probably because if high HDL-cholesterol levels [40]. Therefore, one can hypothesize that dialysis patients constitute a group of "survivors" that doesn't represent the totality of CKD patients and therefore the associations of high BMI and prolonged survival is erroneous in this group.

7. Sequestration of uremic toxins in fat tissue

This theory suggests that uremic toxins are sequestered in adipose tissue and therefore obese dialysis patients are "protected" more efficiently than lean dialysis patients from the deleterious effects of these toxins. A recent study has showed that a substantial reduction in body weight results in liberation in the circulation of lipophilic molecules (hexachlorobenzole, chlorated hydrocarbons) [41]. Weight loss is associated with a reduction in musculoskeletal oxidative metabolism, resulting in a decrease in anti-oxidant defensive mechanisms. [42]. The abovementioned events can possibly explain in part the in the relative risk of mortality in dialysis patients [43].

8. Anti-inflammatory cytokines related to total body mass, adiponectines and TNF-α receptors

Adipose tissue produces adiponectins and soluble receptors of TNF-α; these molecules antagonize the deleterious effects of inflammatory cytokines in the cardiovascular system resulting in an increase in cardiovascular protection. Moreover the soluble receptors of TNF-α neutralize the nocious biologic effects of this factor [44]. Leptin is mainly produced by adipocytes and metabolized in the kidney. Leptin is taken up into the central nervous system by a saturable transport system, and controls appetite. Leptin acts on peripheral tissue and increases the inflammatory response by stimulating the production of tumor necrosis factor alpha, interleukin-6 and interleukin-12. In healthy humans, serum leptin concentration is related to the size of adipose tissue mass in the body. The majority of obese subjects have inappropriately high levels of circulating plasma leptin concentrations, indicating leptin resistance. In healthy subjects increased leptin concentration constitutes a biomarker for increased cardiovascular risk. On the other hand, a recent prospective long-term study in patients with chronic kidney disease stage 5 on hemodialysis therapy showed that reduced serum leptin concentration is an independent risk factor for mortality in these patients. According to this study,a reduced serum leptin concentration is an independent risk factor for mortality in hemodialysis patients. During the follow-up period of almost 7 years the relative risk for mortality in 71 patients with chronic kidney disease stage 5 with serum leptin concentrations below the median (<2.6 lg/ l) compared with patients above the median was 1.96 (45). These data indicate that higher serum leptin concentrations might be advantageous in patients with chronic kidney disease stage 5. Other investigators showed that in patients with chronic kidney disease stage 5 leptin is not increased as a consequence of inflammation, but behaves as a negative rather than as a positive acute phase protein meaning that lower serum leptin concentrations are a marker of increased systemic inflammation.

9. Endotoxin-lipoprotein hypothesis

This hypothesis suggests that high levels of lipoproteins bind to and reduce the concentrations of circulatory endotoxines, resulting in an increased protection from their pro-inflammatory effects [46]. The same hypothesis has been suggested as an explanation to the paradox of increased survival of patients with chronic heart failure and high cholesterol levels [47].

10. Hemodynamic stability of obese patients

Obesity has been associated with higher blood pressure and therefore better endurance of ultrafiltration during HD and lower rates of hypotensive episodes [46].

11. Neurohormonal alterations in obesity

Sympathetic and renin-angiotensin system hyperactivity are associated with increased mortality both in heart failure and dialysis patients. It has been suggested that obesity diminishes the stress reponse and therefore "protects" the patient against the deleterious effects of increased acute neurohormonal activation [48].

12. Alteration of traditional risk factors in the uremic environment

Hypertension, dyslipidemia, tobacco smoking, diabetes mellitus and more recently obesity and hypertriglyceridemia are considered as the major risk factors for new cardiovascular morbidity and overall mortality in the general population. It is possible that the uremic environment and/or the water-sodium overload in HD patients can alter the function of the cardiovascular system; this scenario suggests that other non-traditional risk factors (i.e inflammation, disorders of divalent ion metabolism, secondary hyperparathyroidism, anemia, acidosis) are more important for overall survival [46].

13. Inverse causation

The association of low BMI with increased mortality may be only an epiphenomenon (in other words the result) and not the cause of the increased mortality observed in dialysis patients. This is a common source of bias in observational studies that focus only on the presence of an association without looking at the direction of causality [47].

14. Survival bias

Obesity is associated with an increase in cardiovascular morbidity and mortality in the long and not in the short term. This could be of particular importance in HD patients, since the latter don't live long enough to experience the nocious effects of obesity. It is worth noting that almost 50% of HD patients die within 5 years after starting dialysis. Therefore, HD patients "benefice" of a high BMI for as long as they live since undernutrtion is the principal "fast killer" that is responsible for the inappropriately high mortality rate observed in this population group.

15. Conclusions

Albeit the fact that the reverse epidemiology paradox may be a misnomer, its use highlights a reality frequently observed in chronic disease states that has until recently been neglected: the relative impact of "classical" risk factors for cardiovascular morbidity and mortality is if not reversed at least significantly altered. This observation is stimulating for further research that eventually could unravel the mechanisms that underlie this phenomenon and deepen our knowledge concerning the altered physiology of chronic disease states, including dialysis. Perhaps, the best explanation of the reverse epidemiology paradox relies on the constantly altered physiology observed in chronic disease; it is this "reverse" physiology that is responsible for the reverse associations between classical risk factors and CVE.

16. References

[1] Agarwal R, Andersen MJ, Bishu K, Saha C: Home blood pressure monitoring improves the diagnosis of hypertension in hemodialysis patients. *Kidney Int* 69: 900–906, 2006.
[2] Agarwal R, Brim NJ, Mahenthiran J, Andersen MJ, Saha C: Out-of-hemodialysis-unit blood pressure is a superior determinant of left ventricular hypertrophy. *Hypertension* 47:62–68, 2006.
[3] Agarwal R: Role of home blood pressure monitoring in hemodialysis patients. *Am J Kidney Dis* 33: 682–687, 1999.
[4] Axelsson J, Qureshi AR, Suliman ME, et al. Truncal fat mass as a contributor to inflammation in end-stage renal disease. Am J Clin Nutr 2004;80:1222–9.
[5] Byers T: Body weight and mortality. *N Engl J Med* 333:723–724, 1995.
[6] Dawber TR, Meadors GF, Moore Jr FE: Epidemiological approaches to heart disease: the Framingham Study. Am J Public Health Nations Health 41:279–281, 1951.
[7] DeFilippi C, Wasserman S, Rosanio S, et al. Cardiac troponin T and C-reactive protein for predicting prognosis, coronary atherosclerosis, and cardiomyopathy in patients undergoing long-term hemodialysis. JAMA 2003;290:353–9.
[8] Degoulet P, Legrain M, Reach I, *et al*: Mortality risk factors in patients treated by chronic hemodialysis: Report of the Diaphane Collaborative Study. *Nephron* 31:103–110, 1982
[9] Duranti E, Imperiali P, Sasdelli M: Is hypertension a cardiovascular risk factor in dialysis? *Kidney Int* 49(Suppl 55):S173–S174, 1996.
[10] Floege J, Ketteler M. Vascular calcification in patients with end-stage renal disease. Nephrol Dial Transplant 2004;19(suppl):V59–66.
[11] Gasowski J, Fagard RH, Staessen JA, *et al*: Pulsatile blood pressure component as predictor of mortality in hypertension: A meta-analysis of clinical trial control groups. *J Hypertens* 20:145– 60.
[12] Hidekazu Moriya, Machiko Oka, Kyoko Maesato, Tsutomu Mano, Ryota Ikee, Takayasu Ohtake, and Shuzo Kobayashi Weekly Averaged Blood Pressure Is More Important than a Single-Point Blood Pressure Measurement in the Risk CJASN March 2008 vol. 3 no. 2 416-422.

[13] Imbeault P, Tremblay A, Simoneau JA, Joanisse DR. Weight lossinduced rise in plasma poluant is associated with reduced skeletal muscle oxidative capacity. Am J Physiol Endocrinol Metab 2002;282:E574-E579.
[14] Iseki K, Fukiyama K. Clinical demographics and long-term prognosis after stroke in patients on chronic haemodialysis. The Okinawa Dialysis Study (OKIDS) Group. Nephrol Dial Transplant 2000;15:1808–13.
[15] Iseki K, Fukiyama K. Long-term prognosis and incidence of acute myocardial infarction in patients on chronic hemodialysis. The Okinawa Dialysis Study Group. Am J Kidney Dis 2000;36:820–5.
[16] Iseki K, Miyasato F, Tokuyama K, *et al*: Low diastolic blood pressure,hypoalbuminemia and risk of death in a cohort of chronic hemodialysis patients. *Kidney Int* 51:1212–1217, 1997.
[17] Jandacek RJ, Anderson N, Liu M, Zheng S, Yang Q, Tso P.Effects of yo-yo diet, caloric restriction, and olestra on tissuedistribution on hexachlorobenzene. Am J Physiol GastrointestLiver Physiol 2005;288:G292-G299.
[18] Johansen KL, Young B, Kaysen GA, Chertow GM. Association of body size with outcomes among patients beginning dialysis. Am J Clin Nutr 2004;80:324-32.
[19] Kalantar-Zadeh K, Abbott KC, Kronenberg F, Anker SD, Horwich TB, Fonarow GC. Epidemiology of dialysis patients and heart failure patient: special review article for the 25th anniversary of the seminars in Nephrology. Semin Nephrol 2006;26:118-33.
[20] Kalantar-Zadeh K, Balakrishnan VS. The kidney disease wasting: infl ammation, oxidative stress and diet-gene interaction. Hemodial Int 2006;10:315-25.
[21] Kalantar-Zadeh K, Block G, Humphreys MH, Kopple JD. Reverse epidemiology of cardiovascular risk factors in maintenance hemodialysis patients. Kidney Int 2003;62:793-808.
[22] Kalantar-Zadeh K, Kuwae N, Wu DY, Shantouf RS, Fouque D, Anker SD, et al. Association of body fat and its changes over time with quality of life and prospective mortality in hemodialysis patients. Am J Clin Nutr 2006;83:202-10.
[23] Kalantar-Zadeh K, Streja E, Kovesdy C, Oreopoulos A,Noori N, Jing J, Nissenson A, Krishnan M, Kopple J, Mehrotra R, Anke S. The Obesity Paradox and Mortality Associated With Surrogates of Body Size and Muscle Mass in Patients Receiving Hemodialysis. *Mayo Clin Proc 85(11):991-100, 2010.*
[24] Keith DS, Nichols GA, Gullion CM, Brown JB, Smith DH. Longitudinal follow-up and outcomes among a population with chronic kidney disease in a large managed care organization. Arch Intern med 2004;164:659-63.
[25] Keshaviah PR, Nolph KD, Moore HL, et al. Lean body mass estimation by creatinine kinetics. *J Am Soc Nephrol*. 1994;4:1475-1485.
[26] Klassen PS, Lowrie EG, Reddan DN, et al. Association between pulse pressure and mortality in patients undergoing maintenance hemodialysis. JAMA 2002;287:1548–55.
[27] Kushner RF: Body weight and mortality. *Nutr Rev* 51:127–136, 1993.
[28] Leavey SF, McCullough K, Hecking E, *et al*: Body mass index and mortality in "healthier" as compared with "sicker" haemodialysis patients: Results from the Dialysis Outcomes and Practice Patterns Study (DOPPS). *Nephrol Dial Transplant* 16:2386–2394, 2001.
[29] Leavey SF, Strawderman RL, Jones CA, *et al*: Simple nutritional indicators as independent predictors of mortality in hemodialysis patients. *Am J Kidney Dis* 31:997–1006, 1998.

[30] Lew EA, Garfinkel L: Variations in mortality by weight among 750,000 men and women. *J Chronic Dis* 32:563 565, 1979.
[31] Lowrie EG, Huang WH, Lew NL, Liu Y: The relative contribution of measured variables to death risk among hemodialysis patients, in *Death on Hemodialysis*, edited by Friedman EA, Boston, Kluwer Academic, 1994, pp 121–141
[32] Macleod J, Davey Smith G. Psychological factors and public health: a suitable case for treatment? J Epidemiol Community Health 2003;57:565-70.
[33] Manson JE, Willett WC, Stampfer MJ, *et al*: Body weight and mortality among women. *N Engl J Med* 333:677–685, 1995.
[34] McClellan WM, Chertow GM. Beyond Framingham: Cardiovascular risk profi ling in ESRD. J Am Soc Nephrol 2005;16:1539-41.
[35] Mohamed-Ali V, Goodrick S, Bulmer K, Holly JM, Yudkin JS, Coppack SW. Production of soluble tumor necrosis factor receptors by human subcutaneous adipose tissue in vivo. Am J Physiol 1999;277:E971-E975.
[36] Moriya H, Ohtake T, Kobayashi S: Aortic stiffness, left ventricularhypertrophy and weekly averaged blood pressure (WAB) in patients on haemodialysis. *Nephrol Dial Transplant* 22: 1198–1204, 2007.
[37] No authors listed] (2005) Excerpts from the United States Renal Data System 2004 Annual Data Report. *Am J Kidney Dis* 45 (Suppl 1): S1–S280
[38] No authors listed] (2006) Excerpts from the United States Renal Data System 2005 Annual Data Report: atlas of end-stage renal disease in the United States. *Am J Kidney Dis* 47 (Suppl 1): S1–S286
[39] Rauchhaus M, Coats AJ, Anker SD. The endotoxin-lipoprotein hypothesis. Lancet 2000;356:930-3.
[40] Salem MM: Hypertension in the haemodialysis population: Any relationship to 2-years survival? *Nephrol Dial Transplant* 14:125–128, 1999.
[41] Salem MM: Hypertension in the hemodialysis population? High time for answers. *Am J Kidney Dis* 33:592–594, 1999 68.
[42] Schrier RW, Abraham WT. Hormones and hemodynamics in heart failure. N Engl J Med 1999;341:577-85.
[43] Schutte JE, Longhurst JC, Gaffney FA, Bastian BC, Blomqvist CG. Total plasma creatinine: an accurate measure of total striated muscle mass. *J Appl Physiol.* 1981;51:762-766.
[44] Shoji T, Tsubakihara Y, Nakai S. Néphrologie & Thérapeutique (2008) 4, 223—227.
[45] Van den Hoogen PCW, Feskens EJM, Nagelkerke NJD, *et al*: The seven countries study research group. The relation between hematocrit, blood pressure andmortality due to coronary heart disease among men in different parts of the world. *N Engl J Med* 342:1–8, 2000.
[46] Vasan RS, Larson MG, Leip EP, *et al*: Impact of high-normal blood pressure on the risk of cardiovascular disease. *N Engl J* 38:1251–1263, 2001.
[47] Yeun JY, Levine RA, Mantadilok V, Kaysen GA. C-reactive protein predicts all-cause and cardiovascular mortality in hemodialysis patients. Am J Kidney Dis 2000;35:469 -76.
[48] Young EW, Goodkin DA, Mapes DL, *et al*: The Dialysis Outcomes and Practice Patterns Study (DOPPS): An international hemodialysis study. *Kidney Int* 57 (Suppl 1):S74–S81, 2000.
[49] Zager PG, Nikolic J, Brown RH, *et al*: "U" curve of blood pressure and mortality in hemodialysis patients. *Kidney Int* 54:561–569, 1998.

10

Metabolic Complications of Chronic Kidney Failure and Hemodialysis

Roman Cibulka and Jaroslav Racek
Charles University in Prague, Faculty of Medicine in Pilsen, Czech Republic

1. Introduction

Chronic kidney disease is a very real and growing problem, as indicated by demographic trends. The total number of treated patients has markedly increased during the last 30 years, and chronic kidney disease currently affects approximately 19 million adult Americans, with an incidence that is still increasing (Snyder & Pendergraph, 2005). This trend is caused by a growing percentage of elderly people in the population as well as by technical progress and broader availability of dialysis therapy. An increasing number of diabetic patients is a further important factor.

Chronic kidney disease is characterized by progressive deterioration of kidney function, which develops eventually into a terminal stage of chronic kidney failure. Chronic kidney failure has traditionally been categorized as mild, moderate, or severe. Other poorly defined terms like uremia and end-stage renal disease have commonly been applied. During the last few years, an international consensus has emerged categorizing chronic kidney failure into 5 stages according to the glomerular filtration rate (GFR) and presence of signs of kidney damage: stage 1: GFR > 90 ml/min and signs of kidney damage; stage 2: GFR = 60–89 ml/min and signs of kidney damage; stage 3: GFR = 30–59 ml/min; stage 4: GFR = 15–29 ml/min; and stage 5: GFR < 15 ml/min (Levey et al., 2005). RIFLE (from Risk, Injury, Failure, Loss, End Stage) is a modern classification of acute renal failure and it is noteworthy here (Van Biesen et al., 2006).

Stage 5 of chronic kidney failure represents the total inability of kidneys to maintain homeostasis, and this metabolic state is without treatment incompatible with life. Thus, at this stage, it is necessary to use methods that substitute for kidney function to ensure patient survival; these methods include hemodialysis, peritoneal dialysis, and other extracorporeal purifying procedures, or kidney transplantation.

Chronic kidney failure is associated with many kinds of metabolic changes caused by the kidney disease itself and also attributable to dialysis treatment. Phenomena such as accumulation or deficit of various substances and dysregulation of metabolic pathways participate and combine in the pathogenesis of these changes. In the process of accumulation, decreased urinary excretion plays a crucial role and leads to retention of metabolites in the organism (e.g., creatinine, urea, electrolytes, water, substances with middle molecular weight such as beta-2 microglobulin and other). The increased formation of metabolites through catabolic processes and alternative metabolic pathways also wields an influence. Regular dialysis treatment partly decreases this accumulation but cannot avert the overall deficit. The deficit of some important substances in chronic kidney failure can be caused by deficient intake in diet, impaired intestinal absorption, or increased losses during dialysis sessions. Disturbed synthesis of some crucial metabolic regulators (e.g., erythropoietin or active vitamin D) in kidneys also plays an important role (Cibulka & Racek, 2007).

All of the abovementioned factors lead to many serious complications for patients with chronic kidney disease during the course of predialysis and dialysis. All markedly affect prognosis and the quality of life of these patients.

Metabolic complications of chronic kidney failure and hemodialysis include basically changes in acid-base balance and changes in metabolism of proteins, carbohydrates and lipids. Furthermore, we describe disorders typical for chronic kidney disease such as renal anemia, bone mineral disease, atherosclerosis and cardiovascular disease, oxidative stress, dialysis-related amyloidosis, hyperhomocysteinemia and endothelial dysfunction.

2. Acid–base balance

Acid-base disorder is commonly observed in the course of chronic kidney failure.

Metabolic acidosis is noted in a majority of patients when GFR decreases to less than 25% of normal. The degree of acidosis approximately correlates with the severity of chronic kidney failure and usually is more severe at a lower GFR. Metabolic acidosis can be of the high-anion-gap type, although anion gap can be normal or only moderately increased even with stages 4 or 5 of chronic kidney failure (Kraut & Kurtz, 2005). In mild chronic renal insufficiency, metabolic acidosis is the result of a reduced ability to reabsorb bicarbonate, to excrete ammonia, and to eliminate titratable acid excretion (hyperchloremic, normal anion gap acidosis). In more severe renal insufficiency, organic and other conjugate anions of acids (nonvolatile acids) cannot be sufficiently excreted, and elevated anion gap acidosis appears (Kovacic et al., 2003).

Metabolic acidosis resulting from advanced chronic kidney failure is called uremic acidosis. The level of GFR at which uremic acidosis develops varies depending on a multiplicity of factors. Endogenous acid production is an important factor, which in turn depends on the diet. Ingestion of vegetables and fruits results in net production of alkali, and therefore increased ingestion of these foods will tend to delay the appearance of metabolic acidosis in chronic renal failure. Diuretic therapy and hypokalemia, which tend to stimulate ammonia production, may delay the development of acidosis. The etiology of the renal disease also plays a role. In predominantly tubulointerstitial renal diseases, acidosis tends to develop earlier in the course of renal insufficiency than in predominantly glomerular diseases. In general, symptomatic metabolic acidosis is rare when the GFR is greater than 25–20 ml/min (Oh et al., 2004).

Several adverse consequences have been associated with uremic acidosis, e.g. muscle wasting, bone disease, abnormalities in growth hormone and thyroid hormone secretion, impaired insulin sensitivity, and exacerbation of beta-2 microglobulin accumulation (Kraut & Kurtz, 2005). Other complications include negative nitrogen balance, anorexia, fatigue, impaired function of the cardiovascular system, hyperkalemia, and altered gluconeogenesis and triglyceride metabolism (Kovacic et al., 2003).

Therapy of uremic acidosis should aim to obtain a serum bicarbonate level as close to normal as possible (i.e., 22–26 mmol/l). The best way to initiate therapy is with oral sodium bicarbonate (1 tablet three times a day) and to increase the dosage as necessary. The usual tablet of 650 mg of sodium bicarbonate contains 7.5 mmol of alkali (HCO_3^- ions). Occasionally patients treated with sodium bicarbonate complain of gastric discomfort. In this case, they may use Shohl's solution (a mixture of sodium citrate and citric acid). In dialysis patients, the treatment of acidosis relies on the gain of alkali from the dialysate either as bicarbonate in hemodialysis or as lactate in peritoneal dialysis (Oh et al., 2004).

3. Protein metabolism

Patients with chronic kidney disease in predialysis stages have to keep a low-protein diet to protect kidneys against hyperfiltration and following progression of chronic kidney disease. On the other hand, a too-strict low-protein diet can have a negative effect on nitrogen balance. A safe low-protein diet should contain 0.6 g of protein/kg/day, minimally. Disorders in protein metabolism in hemodialysis patients are usually caused by combined (protein and energy) malnutrition that can be termed uremic malnutrition. It is present in approximately 20%–50% of patients on dialysis and is characterized by insidious loss of somatic protein stores (reflected in lean body mass and serum creatinine) and visceral protein concentrations (reflected in serum albumin and prealbumin concentrations) (Ikizler, 2004). Urinary losses of protein and losses of amino acids during a dialysis session may play a role as well. Metabolic acidosis is a further important factor that markedly contributes to negative nitrogen and total body protein balance in patients with chronic kidney failure (Kovacic et al., 2003).

It has been demonstrated that the presence of uremic malnutrition increases mortality and morbidity in chronic dialysis patients (Ikizler et al., 1999). It is very often combined with a chronic inflammation state in the syndrome known as malnutrition-inflammation complex syndrome (Kalantar-Zadeh et al., 2003). Chronic inflammation accelerates the catabolism and deepens the negative nitrogen balance. The malnutrition-inflammation score (MIS) is a number from 0 to 30 by which an outcome of a dialysis patient can be estimated. Its calculation includes seven components of subjective global assessment, body mass index, and serum albumin and transferrin concentrations. Higher value of MIS indicates worse outcome of a patient (Rambod et al., 2009).

4. Carbohydrate metabolism

Disorders of carbohydrate metabolism are very frequent in patients with chronic kidney failure. On the one hand, diabetes mellitus is the most common cause of kidney failure. Diabetics represent about 35% of all dialyzed patients. In these cases, the causality seems to be relatively clear.

On the other hand, a majority of dialyzed patients are not diabetics. But also non-diabetics patients with chronic kidney disease have often disorders of carbohydrate metabolism. Impaired glucose tolerance occurs together with the loss of kidney function (Alvestrand, 1997). Insulin resistance is primarily detectable when GFR is below 50 ml/min. Reduced insulin-mediated non-oxidative glucose disposal is the most evident defect of glucose metabolism, but impairments of glucose oxidation, the defective suppression of endogenous glucose production, and abnormal insulin secretion also contribute to uremic glucose intolerance (Rigalleau & Gin, 2005). Accumulating nitrogenous uremic toxins seem to be the dominant cause of a specific defect in insulin action, and identification of these toxins is progressing, particularly in the field of carbamoylated amino acids. The consequences of chronic kidney failure, such as exercise intolerance, anemia, metabolic acidosis, secondary hyperparathyroidism, or insufficient activation of vitamin D, also indirectly play a role (Rasic-Milutinovic et al., 2000).

It has been reported that insulin resistance may be related to arterial hypertension (Ferrannini et al., 1987) and may contribute to high cardiovascular morbidity and mortality in patients with chronic kidney failure (Shinohara et al., 2002). The underlying mechanism can be an impaired synthesis of nitric oxide (NO) in endothelium of patients with chronic kidney disease. It was proved that appropriately functioning endothelial NO synthase is important for the control not only of arterial pressure but also of glucose and lipid homeostasis (Duplain et al., 2001).

Disturbance in synthesis of adipocytokines may contribute to the insulin resistance and related metabolic disorders in patients with chronic kidney failure. Patients with metabolic syndrome have lower levels of adiponectin and, on the contrary, higher levels of leptin than patients without metabolic syndrome (Vostry et al., 2008).

5. Lipid metabolism

Lipid metabolism appears to be substantially influenced by the severity of renal dysfunction.

Patients with chronic kidney disease have elevated levels of triglycerides mainly because of enhanced production of triglyceride-rich lipoproteins such as very-low-density lipoproteins (VLDL) in the liver (Attman et al., 1993). Further reasons are decreased activities of hepatic lipase and peripheral lipoprotein lipase. These abnormalities in turn may be due to an inhibitory effect of hyperparathyroidism, calcium accumulation in islet cells resulting in impaired insulin action, elevated level of apolipoprotein C-III which acts as a direct lipase inhibitor, or a putative circulating inhibitor detected in uremic plasma (Shurraw & Tonelli, 2006). Hyperinsulinemia is, however, probably the main factor increasing synthesis of triglycerides and directly decreases activity of lipoprotein lipase.

Insufficient mitochondrial beta-oxidation, due to a deficit of L-carnitine, is an important factor for the development of disorder in lipid metabolism in hemodialysis patients. L-carnitine is an essential substance for transport of long chain fatty acids across the inner mitochondrial membrane into mitochondrial matrix where beta-oxidation proceeds (Cibulka et al., 2005).

Following changes in lipid metabolism are also found in many patients with chronic kidney failure. The most prominent are increased serum triglyceride levels mentioned above and low levels of high-density lipoprotein (HDL) cholesterol. Low-density lipoprotein (LDL) cholesterol levels are often normal, but the cholesterol may originate from the atherogenic small and dense LDL subclass. The apolipoprotein B-containing lipoprotein particles may undergo modifications (peptide modification of the enzymatic and advanced glycation end-product, oxidation, or glycation). Modifications contribute to impaired LDL receptor-mediated clearance from plasma and promote prolonged circulation. HDL particles are structurally altered during states of inflammation (Cibulka & Racek, 2007).

The contribution of this complex atherogenic form of dyslipidemia to cardiovascular disease in patients with chronic renal disease is not absolutely clear. Some studies reported negative results regarding the predictive power of serum lipids for the development of cardiovascular disease in these patients (Wanner & Krane, 2002). Recent findings have suggested that the development of malnutrition-inflammation complex syndrome is responsible for this phenomenon. Because malnutrition-inflammation complex syndrome leads to a low body mass index, hypocholesterolemia, hypohomocysteinemia, and other manifestations, a reverse epidemiology of traditional cardiovascular risk factors occurs in patients with chronic kidney failure (Kalantar-Zadeh et al., 2003). It means that for example hypercholesterolemia, obesity or hyperhomocysteinemia appear to be protective and paradoxically associated with a better outcome.

It is well known that HDL cholesterol level is inversely correlated with the risk of atherosclerosis. In addition to its role in reverse cholesterol transport, HDL has the ability to protect LDL particles against oxidation. The underlying mechanism by which HDL inhibits LDL oxidation is partly enzymatic. There is increasing evidence that paraoxonase 1 could be involved in this process (Mackness et al., 1993). It was proved that serum paraoxonase 1 activity is reduced in patients with chronic kidney failure. The possible causes can include reduced HDL level, altered HDL subfraction distribution, reduced paraoxonase 1 concentration and its different phenotype distribution. Another possible explanation could be that paraoxonase 1 activity is inhibited in the uremic environment. Generally, reduced serum paraononase 1 activity could also contribute to the accelerated development of atherosclerosis in patients with chronic kidney failure (Dirican et al., 2004).

Lipoprotein (a) has been identified as an independent risk factor for atherosclerotic cardiovascular disease. It was found to be consistently elevated in a considerable proportion of patients with chronic kidney disease. Plasma concentration of lipoprotein (a) is highly heritable and mainly determined by a size polymorphism of apolipoprotein (a). It has been demonstrated that the low-molecular-weight apolipoprotein (a) phenotype independently predicted coronary artery disease occurrence (Kronenberg et al., 1999). It has been suggested that the apolipoprotein (a) size and the lipoprotein (a) plasma concentration may play a synergistic role in advanced atherosclerosis.

Patients treated with peritoneal dialysis have a similar but more severe dyslipidemia compared to hemodialysis patients due to stimulation of hepatic lipoprotein synthesis by glucose absorption from dialysate, increased insulin levels, and selective protein loss in dialysate analogous to the nephrotic syndrome (Shurraw & Tonelli, 2006).

6. Renal anemia

Renal anemia, which is often associated with fatigue and cognitive and sexual dysfunction, has a significant impact on the quality of life of patients with chronic kidney failure. Anemia has been identified as an important etiologic factor in the development of left ventricular hypertrophy, an independent risk factor for heart failure and a predictor of mortality in hemodialysis patients (Cibulka & Racek, 2007).

The major cause of renal anemia in patients with chronic kidney disease is an inadequate production of the glycoprotein hormone erythropoietin because of a reduction in functional kidney parenchyma (Santoro, 2002). Furthermore, free radicals elicited from leucocytes by their contact with the dialysis membrane cause hemolysis with consecutive anemia in patients on extracorporeal renal replacement therapy (Eiselt et al., 1999). There are a number of other metabolic derangements associated with uremia that can affect the production and survival of red blood cells (e.g., uremic toxins, parathormone, protein malnutrition) (Cibulka & Racek, 2007).

The introduction of recombinant human erythropoietin has revolutionized the treatment of anemia in patients with chronic kidney failure. The majority of patients respond very well, however, about 10% of patients show some resistance to this therapy. The most common causes of that are considered iron deficiency (Santoro, 2002) and the development of malnutrition-inflammation complex syndrome (Kalantar-Zadeh et al., 2003). The erythropoietin hyporesponsiveness can further worsen symptoms that decrease the quality of life, such as an intolerance of physical work, deterioration of cognitive functions, anorexia, insomnia, or depression.

These problems are partly related to the deficit of L-carnitine mentioned above. In hemodialysis patients, a complex of complications related to the deficit of this important substance is marked as dialysis-related carnitine disorder. This disorder is a functional metabolic deficiency which can have a negative impact on erythrocyte production and survival. Laboratory studies examining the influence of L-carnitine on red blood cell function and clinical trials in hemodialysis patients support the use of L-carnitine in the setting of erythropoietin hyporesponsiveness (Golper et al., 2003).

The supplementation with iron in patients with chronic kidney disease might obviate or delay the need for treatment with erythropoietin. Oral iron is inferior to intravenous iron in patients on hemodialysis, in part because elevated serum levels of hepcidin prevent intestinal absorption of iron. Increased levels of hepcidin, a peptide hormone produced by the liver, also impair the normal recycling of iron through the reticuloendothelial system (Besarab & Coyne, 2010).

7. Bone mineral disease

Bone mineral disease or renal osteodystrophy are terms which are used to describe the skeletal abnormalities of many patients with chronic kidney disease.

Bone mineral disease is basically a multifactorial disorder of bone remodeling. It encompasses a heterogeneous group of disorders from states of high bone turnover to states of low bone turnover. High-turnover bone disease or osteitis fibrosa represents the manifestations of secondary hyperparathyroidism on bone. Low bone turnover syndromes are represented by the increasingly prevalent adynamic bone disease or less commonly, by osteomalacia. These disorders may occur in combination or alternately, each may predominate in any given patient (Gonzalez & Martin, 2001).

The most important factor which is responsible for the development of secondary hyperparathyroidism is a deficit of active vitamin D (calcitriol). Diseased kidneys cannot sufficiently hydroxylate 25-hydroxycholecalciferol, which is a precursor of calcitriol (1,25-dihydroxycholecalciferol). The deficit of calcitriol causes an inadequate absorption of calcium in the small intestine, with resulting hypocalcemia. Retention of inorganic phosphate may deteriorate this situation because phosphates impair the activity of 1-alpha-hydroxylase even more. Long-lasting hypocalcemia and coincidental hyperphosphatemia lead to the stimulation of parathyroid glands with subsequent secondary hyperparathyroidism which causes decalcification of bones (Cibulka et al., 2007). Chronic metabolic acidosis intensifies this harmful process (Kraut and Kurtz, 2005). All of these factors are closely interrelated, and while one or more of them may predominate in a particular patient during the course of chronic kidney failure, much overlap occurs (Gonzalez and Martin, 2001).

Moreover, hyperphosphatemia has been recognized as an important risk factor for cardiovascular disease mortality in patients with chronic kidney failure. It is a direct cause of vascular calcification, the cardio-bone connection (Lund et al., 2006).

The treatment of vitamin D deficiency when present in patients with chronic kidney disease is warranted since such therapy may reduce or prevent secondary hyperparathyroidism in the early stages. In patients with chronic kidney disease and GFR of 20 to 60 ml/min, nutritional vitamin D deficiency and insufficiency can both be prevented by supplementation with vitamin D_2 (ergocalciferol) or vitamin D_3 (cholecalciferol). The recommended daily allowance in individuals over 60 years is 800 IU, and for younger adults 400 IU. In patients in stage 5 of chronic kidney failure and in those on dialysis, the value of supplementation is less certain; although in dialysis-dependent patients, high doses of ergocalciferol or 25-hydroxycholecalciferol can raise the serum levels of calcitriol (National Kidney Foundation, 2004). Calcitriol himself and 1-alpha-hydroxylated derivate of calcitriol (alphacalcidiol) are also commonly used for supplementation in clinical practice.

In hemodialysis patients, the administration of L-carnitine may also have some positive effects on bone metabolism. It probably increases production of osteoprotegerin which is one of the most important regulators of osteoclastogenesis. Osteoprotegerin is a tumor necrosis factor-related cytokine which is produced by osteoblasts. It suppresses bone resorption and increases the density, area and strength of bone (Cibulka et al., 2007).

8. Atherosclerosis and cardiovascular disease

Cardiovascular disease is the leading cause of death in patients with chronic kidney failure. For every registry reporting national dialysis data in Europe, the U.S., Japan, and elsewhere, about 50% of deaths are attributed to cardiovascular disease. In comparison with the general population, dialysis patients have a greater than 20-fold increased risk of a cardiovascular death (Levey & Eknoyan, 1999). A majority of these deaths are related to atherosclerosis with subsequent myocardial infarction, cerebrovascular accidents (strokes), and ischemic events of the limbs. Additionally, patients with chronic kidney disease exhibit evidence of early and exaggerated vascular and cardiac remodeling (arteriosclerosis and left ventricular hypertrophy). The risk of cardiovascular disease and associated mortality increases in proportion to the decrease of GFR. It is significantly higher if GFR has fallen below approximately 75 ml/min. The evidence suggests that the damage is already far progressed when patients reach end-stage renal disease; thus, effective intervention must be started much earlier (Diaz-Buxo & Woods, 2006). Patients with albuminuria and normal GFR also are at increased risk (Go et al., 2004).

Evaluation of traditional risk factors, including lipid levels, blood pressure, smoking, and sedentary lifestyle, is essential (Snyder & Pendergraph, 2005).

The KDOQI (Kidney Disease Outcomes Quality Initiative) recommended a blood pressure goal of 130/80 mmHg in patients with normal urinary albumin concentrations, and a blood pressure goal of 125/75 mmHg in patients with excretion of more than 1 g of protein/24 hours (National Kidney Foundation, 2002).

The KDOQI guidelines on managing dyslipidemias in patients with chronic kidney disease recommended an LDL cholesterol goal of less than 100 mg/dl (2.60 mmol/l) (National Kidney Foundation, 2006). We use statins at moderate doses for reduction of LDL cholesterol levels.

However, as mentioned above, some patients with chronic kidney disease with the lowest cholesterol levels are the most likely to die of cardiovascular disease because low levels of cholesterol are associated with nontraditional cardiac risk factors of malnutrition and inflammation (Liu et al., 2004). Additional cardiac risk factors specific to chronic kidney failure may also play an important role in the development of atherosclerosis. Among these factors we include for example volume overload, hyperparathyroidism, uremia, anemia, endothelial dysfunction, and, especially in hemodialysis patients, oxidative stress (Cibulka & Racek, 2007).

Statins probably influence, except the LDL cholesterol levels, still other cardiovascular risk factors, namely the chronic inflammation state. It is manifested as a decrease of C-reactive protein level. Large observational studies demonstrate that statin treatment is associated with a significant reduction of mortality in dialysis patients (Shurraw & Tonelli, 2006).

9. Oxidative stress

Oxidative stress is a state in which the production of reactive oxygen species exceeds the capacity of the antioxidant defense system in cells and tissues. Reactive oxygen species are free radicals, highly reactive substances with an unpaired electron in the outer orbital, and other related reactive compounds (such as hydrogen peroxide and hypochlorous acid) that can attack lipids, proteins, and nucleic acids and alter the structure and function of these macromolecules (Klaunig et al., 1998). Specifically, LDL particles are damaged by excessive oxidation and consequently are not recognized by cell LDL receptors. They are subsequently accumulated in the blood in higher amounts and penetrate the vascular walls. This mechanism is probably the basis of atherosclerotic lesions.

Oxidative stress threatens hemodialysis patients with serious clinical complications (e.g., accelerated atherosclerosis, amyloidosis, hemolysis, and the development of the state of chronic inflammation). Free radicals originate from leucocytes, which are activated during the contact with the dialysis membrane, and also from erythrocyte iron released as a consequence of hemolysis (Eiselt et al., 1999). Intravenous administration of iron can also contribute to oxidative stress, increasing free radical production by the so-called Fenton reaction. Co-administration of ascorbic acid with the goal of mobilizing iron stores further stimulates free radical formation, possibly by reduction of Fe(III) ions to more dangerous Fe(II) compounds (Eiselt et al., 2006).

10. Dialysis-related amyloidosis

Dialysis-related amyloidosis is a frequent complication of chronic kidney failure and long-term renal replacement therapy. Beta-2 microglobulin is a major constituent of amyloid fibrils. Amyloid deposition mainly involves bone and joint structures, presenting as carpal tunnel syndrome, destructive arthropathy, and subchondral bone erosions and cysts. The molecular pathogenesis of this complication remains unknown. Recent studies, however, have suggested a pathogenic role of a new modification of beta-2 microglobulin in amyloid fibrils. Increased carbonyl compounds derived from autoxidation of both carbohydrates and lipids modify proteins in uremia, leading to augmentation of advanced glycation end-products and advanced lipoxidation end-product production. Thus, uremia might be a state of carbonyl overload with potentially damaging proteins (carbonyl stress) (Miyata et al., 1999).

Dialysis-related amyloidosis is one of the most harmful osteoarticular complications with regard to the maintenance of daily activities and quality of life in patients undergoing long-term dialysis therapy (Yamamoto et al., 2009).

11. Hyperhomocysteinemia and endothelial dysfunction

Hyperhomocysteinemia is present in the majority of patients with chronic kidney failure. They have a plasma concentration of homocysteine elevated 3 to 4 times above normal (Suliman et al., 2001). The causes are still not clear, but the possibilities include defective renal or extrarenal metabolism as a result of uremic toxicity (Perna et al., 2004).

In the general population, hyperhomocysteinemia is considered to be an independent risk factor for the development of cardiovascular disease. As mentioned above, reverse epidemiology of traditional cardiovascular risk factors occurs in patients with chronic kidney failure, so that increased homocysteine levels appear to be paradoxically associated with a better clinical outcome. The development of malnutrition-inflammation complex syndrome is responsible for this phenomenon. Plasma homocysteine concentration is higher in patients with normal nutritional status than in malnourished patients. Plasma homocysteine was inversely correlated with subjective global nutritional assessment and positively correlated with serum albumin and protein intake. Thus, serum albumin concentration is a strong determinant of plasma homocysteine concentration in patients with chronic kidney failure.

On the other hand, the toxicity of homocysteine results from the structural modification of proteins and deoxyribonucleic acid (DNA). Disruption of DNA methylation has been demonstrated to occur as a result of hyperhomocysteinemia and is associated with vascular damage (Perna et al., 2005). Homocysteine could be a principal candidate for endothelial dysfunction in patients with chronic kidney failure. Hyperhomocysteinemia may impair endothelial function by the generation of oxygen species and decreased NO bioavailability. NO is produced by endothelial NO synthase and it has many positive vascular effects. It mediates normal endothelial and vessel wall functions including antithrombosis, endothelial permselectivity, and vasomotor tone. In addition, NO suppresses cellular proliferation (e.g., of vascular smooth muscle cells) and has a quenching effect on inflammation. The function of the endothelial NO synthase is impaired in patients with chronic kidney disease (Kone, 1997). However, the precise mechanisms underlying the link between hyperhomocysteinemia and impaired endothelial function in chronic kidney failure is not quite clear. Some authors propose that accumulation of asymmetric dimethylarginine (ADMA), an endogenous inhibitor of NO synthase, could be the missing connecting link. Homocysteine is produced during ADMA synthesis and can alter ADMA catabolism mainly by inhibiting dimethylarginine dimethylaminohydrolase (Dayal & Lentz, 2005). ADMA levels are elevated in patients with chronic kidney disease, and ADMA should be considered to be a futher uremic toxin. In some studies, an increased level of ADMA has been identified as an independent predictor of mortality in patients with chronic kidney disease (Ravani et al., 2005; Cibulka et al., 2007).

In any case, influence the endothelial function in chronic kidney failure may offer a novel strategy to reduce risk for cardiovascular disease.

12. Conclusion

In conclusion, it is necessary to emphasize the importance of searching actively for chronic kidney disease. Unfortunately, it is often overlooked in its earliest, most treatable stages. Guidelines from the National Kidney Foundation's KDOQI recommend estimating GFR and screening for albuminuria in patients with risk factors for chronic kidney disease, including diabetes, hypertension, systemic illnesses, age greater than 60 years, and family history of chronic kidney disease. When chronic kidney disease is detected, an attempt should be made to identify and treat the underlying conditions as well as the secondary abnormalities. These goals include slowing disease progression, detecting and treating complications, and managing cardiovascular risk factors. Suitable treatment also includes attention to the influence of elevated blood pressure, malnutrition, anemia, hyperparathyroidism, insulin resistance, disorders of lipid metabolism, and acid–base balance. At the same time, it is necessary to continue research projects focused on other areas that may uncover new aspects of cardiometabolic risk and its influence in patients with chronic kidney disease. These areas include the development of malnutrition-inflammation complex syndrome, management of oxidative stress, and endothelium protection. Clearly, progress in management of cardiovascular disease in patients with chronic kidney disease will require collaboration with experts in the research and treatment of vascular disease.

13. Acknowledgement

This work was supported by the research project MSM 0021620819.

14. References

Alvestrand, A. (1997). Carbohydrate and insulin metabolism in renal failure. Kidney Int, 62, S48-S52.

Attman, P.O., Samuelsson, O. & Alaupovic, P. (1993). Lipoprotein metabolism and renal failure. Am J Kidney Dis, 21, 573-592.

Besarab, A. & Coyne, D.W. (2010). Iron supplementation to treat anemia in patients with chronic kidney disease. Nat Rev Nephrol, 6, 699-710.

Cibulka, R., Racek, J. & Vesela, E. (2005). The importance of L-carnitine in patients with chronic renal failure treated with hemodialysis. Vnitr Lek, 51, 1108-1113.

Cibulka, R. & Racek J. (2007). Metabolic disorders in patients with chronic kidney failure. Physiol Res, 56, 697-705.

Cibulka, R., Racek, J., Pikner, R., Rajdl, D., Trefil, L., Vesela, E., Studenovska, M. & Siroka, R. (2007). Effect of L-carnitine supplementation on secondary hyperparathyroidism and bone metabolism in hemodialyzed patients. Calcif Tissue Int, 81, 99-106.

Cibulka, R., Rajdl, D., Siroka, R., Eiselt, J., Malanova, L., Trefil, L. & Racek, J. (2007). Asymmetric dimethylarginine (ADMA) as a novel prognostic factor for survival in hemodialysis patients. Klin Biochem Metab, 15 (3), 160-163.

Dayal, S. & Lentz, S.R. (2005). ADMA and hyperhomocysteinemia. Vasc med,10 (Suppl 1), S27-S33.

Diaz-Buxo, J.A. & Woods, H.F. (2006). Protecting the endothelium: A new focus for management of chronic kidney disease. Hemodial Int, 10, 42-48.

Dirican, M., Akca, R., Sarandol, E. & Dilek, K. (2004). Serum paraoxonase activity in uremic predialysis and hemodialysis patients. J Nephrol, 17, 813-818.

Duplain, H., Burcelin, R., Sartori, C., Cook, S., Egli, M., Lepori, M., Vollenweider, P., Pedrazzini, T., Nicod, P., Thorens, B. & Scherrer, U. (2001). Insulin resistance, hyperlipidemia and hypertension in mice lacking endothelial nitric oxide synthase. Circulation, 104, 342-345.

Eiselt, J., Racek, J. & Opatrny, K.Jr. (1999). Free radicals and extracorporeal renal replacement therapy. Vnitr Lek, 45, 319-324.

Eiselt, J., Racek, J., Opatrny, K.Jr., Trefil, L. & Stehlik, P. (2006). The effect of intravenous iron on oxidative stress in hemodialysis patients at various levels of vitamin C. Blood Purif, 24, 531-537.

Ferrannini, E., Buzzigoli, G., Bonadonna, R., Giorico, M.A., Oleggini, M., Graziadeli, L., Pedrinelli, R., Brandi, L. & Brevilasqua, S. (1987). Insulin resistance in essential hypertension. N Engl J Med, 317, 350-357.

Go, A.S., Chertow, G.M., Fan, D., McCulloch, C.E. & Hsu, C.Y. (2004). Chronic kidney disease and the risk of death, cardiovascular events, and hospitalization. N Engl J Med, 351, 1296-1305.
Golper, T.A., Goral, S., Becker, B.N. & Langman, C.B. (2003). L-carnitine treatment of anemia. Am J Kidney Dis, 41 (4 Suppl 4), S27-S34.
Gonzales, E.A. & Martin, K.J. (2001). Renal osteodystrophy. Rev Endocr Metab Disord, 2, 187-193.
Ikizler, T.A., Windgard, R.L., Harvell, J., Shyr, Y. & Hakim, R.M. (1999). Association of morbidity with markers of nutrition and inflammation in chronic hemodialysis patients: a prospective study. Kidney Int, 55, 1945-1951.
Ikizler, T.A. (2004). Protein and energy: recommended intake and nutrient supplementation in chronic dialysis patients. Semin Dial, 17, 471-478.
Kalantar-Zadeh, K., Ikizler, T.A., Block, G., Avram, M.M. & Kopple, J.D. (2003). Malnutrition-inflammation complex syndrome in dialysis patients: causes and consequences. Am J Kidney Dis, 42, 864-881.
Klaunig, J.E., Xu, Y., Isenberg, J.S., Bachowski, S., Kolaja, K.L., Jiang, J., Stevenson, D.E. & Walborg, E.F.Jr. (1998). The role of oxidative stress in chemical carcinogenesis. Environ Health Perspect, 1, 289-295.
Kone, B.C. (1997). Nitric oxide in renal health and disease. Am J Kidney Dis, 30, 311-333.
Kovacic, V., Roguljic, L. & Kovacic, V. (2003). Metabolic acidosis of chronically hemodialyzed patients. Am J Nephrol, 23, 158-164.
Kraut, J.A. & Kurtz, I. (2005). Metabolic acidosis of CKD: diagnosis, clinical characteristics, and treatment. Am J Kidney Dis, 45, 978-993.
Kronenberg, F., Neyer, U., Lhotta, K., Trenkwalder, E., Auinger, M., Pribasnik, A., Meisl, T., Konig, P. & Dieplinger, H. (1999). The low molecular weight apo(a) phenotype is an independent predictor for coronary artery disease in hemodialysis patients: a prospective follow-up. J Am Soc Nephrol, 10, 1027-1036.
Levey, A.S. & Ecknoyan, G. (1999). Cardiovascular disease in chronic renal disease. Nephrol Dial Transplant, 14, 828-833.
Levey, A.S., Eckardt, K.U., Tsukamoto, Y., Levin, A., Coresh, J., Rossert, J., Zeeuw, D., Hostetter, T.H., Lameire, N. & Eknoyan, G. (2005). Definition and classification of chronic kidney disease: a position statement from Kidney Disease: Improving Global Outcomes (KDIGO). Kidney Int, 67, 2089-2100.
Liu, Y., Coresh, J., Eustace, J.A., Longenecker, J.C., Jaar, B., Fink, N.E., Tracy, R.P., Powe, N.R. & Klag, M.J. (2004). Association between cholesterol level and mortality in dialysis patients: role of inflammation and malnutrition. JAMA, 291, 451-459.
Lund, R.J., Davies, M.R., Suresh, M. & Hruska, K.A. (2006). New discoveries in the pathogenesis of renal osteodystrophy. J Bone Miner Metab, 24, 169-171.
Mackness, M.I., Arrol, S., Abbott, C.A. & Durrington, P.N. (1993). Protection of low-density lipoprotein against oxidative modification by high density lipoprotein associated paraoxonase. Atherosclerosis, 104, 129-135.
Miyata, T., Inagi, R. & Kurokawa, K. (1999). Diagnosis, pathogenesis, and treatment of dialysis-related amyloidosis. Miner Electrolyte Metab, 25, 114-117.
National Kidney Foundation: K/DOQI, clinical practice guidelines for bone metabolism and disease in chronic kidney disease, guideline 7. Accessed online at: http://www.kidney.org/professionals/kdoqi/guidelines _bone/Guide7.htm.
National Kidney Foundation: K/DOQI, clinical practice guidelines for chronic kidney disease: evaluation, classification and stratification. Am J Kidney Dis, 39 (2 Suppl 1), S1-S266, 2002. Accessed online at:

http://www.kidney.org/professionals/kdoqi/guidelines_ckd/toc.htm.
National Kidney Foundation: K/DOQI, clinical practice guidelines for managing dyslipidemias in chronic kidney disease, part 3, guideline 4. Accessed online at: http://www.kidney.org/professionals/kdoqi/guidelines_lipids/iii.htm.
Oh, M.S., Uribarri, J., Weinstein, J., Schreiber, M., Kamel K.S., Kraut, J.A., Madias, N.E. & Laski, M.E. (2004). What unique acid-base considerations exist in dialysis patients? Semin Dial, 17, 351-364.
Perna, A.F., Ingrosso, D., Satta, E., Lombardi, C., Acanfora, F. & De Santo, N.G. (2004). Homocysteine metabolism in renal failure. Curr Opin Clin Nutr Metab Care, 7, 53-57.
Perna, A.F., Capasso, R., Lombardi, C., Acanfora, F., Satta, E. & Ingrosso, D. (2005). Hyperhomocysteinemia and macromolecule modifications in uremic patients. Clin Chem Lab Med, 43, 1032-1038.
Rambod, M., Bross, R., Zitterkoph, J., Benner, D., Pithia, J., Colman, S., Kovesdy, C.P., Kopple, J.D. & Kalantar-Zadeh K. (2009). Association of malnutrition-inflammation score with quality of life and mortality in hemodialysis patients: a 5-year prospective cohort study. Am J Kidney Dis, 53, 298-309.
Rasic-Milutinovic, Z., Perunicic-Peckovic, G. & Pljesa, S. (2000). Clinical significance and pathogenic mechanism of insulin resistance in chronic renal insufficiency (part II): pathogenic factors of insulin resistance in chronic renal insufficiency. Med Pregl, 53, 159-163.
Ravani, P., Tripepi, G., Malberti, F., Testa, S., Mallamaci, F. & Zoccali, C. (2005). Asymmetrical dimethylarginine predicts progression to dialysis and death in patients with chronic kidney disease: a competing risks modeling approach. J Am Soc Nephrol,16, 2254-2256.
Rigalleau, V. & Gin, H. (2005). Carbohydrate metabolism in uraemia. Curr Opin Clin Nutr Metab Care, 8, 463-869.
Santoro, A. (2002). Anemia in renal insufficiency. Rev Clin Exp Hematol Suppl, 1, 12-20.
Shinohara, K., Shoji, T., Emoto, M., Tahara, H., Koyama, H., Ishimura, E., Miki, T., Tabata, T. & Nishizawa, Y. (2002). Insulin resistance as an independent predictor of cardiovascular mortality in patients with end-stage renal disease. J Am Soc Nephrol, 13, 1894-1900.
Shurraw, S. & Tonelli, M. (2006). Statins for treatment of dyslipidemia in chronic kidney disease. Perit Dial Int, 26, 523-539.
Snyder, S. & Pendergraph, B. (2005). Detection and evaluation of chronic kidney disease. Am Fam Physician, 72, 1723-1732.
Suliman, M.E., Lindholm, B., Barany, P. & Bergstrom, J. (2001). Hyperhomocysteinemia in chronic renal failure patients: relation to nutritional status and cardiovascular disease. Clin Chem Lab Med, 39, 734-738.
Van Biesen, W., Vanholder, R. & Lameire, N. (2006). Defining acute renal failure: RIFLE and beyond. Clin J Am Soc Nephrol, 1, 1314-1319.
Vostry, M., Rajdl, D., Eiselt, J., Malanova, L., Pikner, R., Trefil, L. & Racek J. (2008). Adipocytokines and other survival predictors in hemodialysis patients with metabolic syndrome. Klin Biochem Metab, 16 (37), 239-243.
Wanner, C. & Krane, V. (2002). Uremia-specific alterations in lipid metabolism. Blood Purif, 20, 451-453.
Yamamoto, S., Kazama, J.J., Narita, I., Naiki, H. & Gejyo, F. (2009). Recent progress in understanding dialysis-related amyloidosis. Bone, 45 (Suppl 1), S39-S42.

11

The Endothelium and Hemodialysis

Hernán Trimarchi
Hospital Británico de Buenos Aires, Argentina

1. Introduction

The endothelium is a functional barrier composed of a single layer of endothelial cells between the vessel wall and circulating blood. The human vascular bed has a combined surface area of 1000 m^2 and contains 10^{13} endothelial cells. The endothelium is the largest endocrine organ, with also important paracrine and autocrine functions (Perry & Pearson, 1989). Endothelial cells play important roles in haemostasis, vasoactivity, cellular proliferation, immunological reactions and inflammatory events. Therefore, endothelial dysfunction can lead to vasoconstriction, local ischemic phenomena and hypertension, thrombus formation and plaque growth and rupture, vascular proliferation and remodeling, and immunologic inflammation processes. Risk factors for endothelial dysfunction include old age, hypertension, diabetes mellitus, hypercholesterolemia, tobacco, menopause, male gender and obesity (Müller & Griesmacher, 2000; Raitakari & Celermajer, 2000).

Cardiovascular disease is the leading cause of mortality in dialysis patients. In large cross-sectional studies of dialysis patients, traditional cardiovascular risk factors such as hypertension and hypercholesterolemia have been found to have low predictive power, while markers of inflammation and malnutrition are highly correlated with cardiovascular mortality. However, the pathophysiology of the disease process that links uremia, inflammation, and malnutrition with increased cardiovascular complications is not well understood. In uremia, endothelial dysfunction derives from a systemic altered milieu that is partially aggravated by the dialysis treatment itself. From water quality to the type of membrane employed, many artificial factors intervene that trigger inflammatory processes culminating with endothelial damage, smooth muscle cell hyperplasia, fibrosis and vascular calcification.

The underlying vascular disease consists mainly of two types, arteriosclerosis and atherosclerosis. Arteriosclerosis is mainly characterized by premature arterial aging with loss of elastic fibers and increased stiffness. Atherosclerosis is characterized by intima-media thickening, plaque formation and luminal narrowing. Both processes may interact simultaneously, possibly via diverse mechanisms, as endothelial dysfunction, shear stress, and elastic fiber fragmentation (Fishbein & Fishbein, 2009; Guérin et al., 2008; London & Drüeke, 1997).

Endothelial dysfunction is a well-documented early phenomenon in atherosclerosis that precedes structural changes and clinical manifestations, particularly in dialysis patients (Frick & Weidinger, 2007). Decreased endothelial function is thought to primarily reflect a decreased bioavailability of nitric oxide, a critical endothelium-derived vasoactive factor with vasodilatory and anti-atherosclerotic properties (Tatematsu et al., 2007). Although endothelial dysfunction is common as renal function declines, the exact causes are not known. The effects of various uremic toxins on endothelial dysfunction and cardiovascular outcome are being studied. There is also growing evidence that asymmetric dimethylarginine, an endogenous inhibitor of nitic oxide-synthase, is involved in mediating endothelial damage and dysfunction (Kielstein & Zoccali, 2005), is primarily cleared by the kidney, is elevated in chronic kidney disease and is associated with poor prognosis in dialysis patients (Stenvinkel et al., 2008).

Increased oxidative stress is an outstanding culprit in the process of increased atherogenesis and cardiovascular morbidity and mortality found in the dialysis population. Vascular and endothelial complications accelerate as renal function is progressively decreased in the pre-dialysis population, which is potentiated in chronic kidney disease Stage 5. Increasing number of biomarkers are constantly emerging as potential culprits in this process of accelerated atherogenesis and thrombosis in haemodialyzed subjects (Himmelfarb et al., 2002).

Oxidative stress, endothelial dysfunction, inflammation, protein-energy wasting, sympathetic activation, haemostatic disturbances, endocrine disturbances, uremic retained toxins, vascular calcification and ossification, infections, anemia and its therapy, and certain haemodialysis components are amongst the main uremia-related biochemical risk factors in patients on dialysis (Stenvinkel et al., 2008). Increased levels of oxidative stress markers are present in the plasma of chronic kidney patients, which indicates that uremia is a pro-oxidant state (Himmelfarb et al., 2002). Oxidative stress seems to occur early in kidney disease evolution because oxidative markers have been documented at least as early as stage 3 (Oberg et al., 2004). Moreover, dialysis treatment seems ineffective in the correction of oxidative stress and may sometimes trigger oxidant processes, although recent data may show the opposite (Pupim et al., 2004; McGregor et al., 2003).

There exists an activated inflammatory response in 30-50% of patients with end-stage renal disease (Zimmermann et al., 1999), even before dialysis is started: C-Reactive protein levels, one of the non-specific but highly sensitive markers usually employed to assess inflammation, may also be raised by persistent infections; comorbidities as chronic heart failure or chronic angina; accumulation of oxidative stress by-products; and pro-inflammatory cytokines retained in uremia (Stenvinkel, 2001a). Chronic inflammation, mediated by pro-inflammatory cytokines and acute-phase reactants, may contribute to accelerated atherosclerosis (Stenvinkel, 2001a). Normal endothelial function is crucial for cardiovascular homeostasis. Endothelial dysfunction results in lipid accumulation at the vessel wall, smooth muscle proliferation, and vasospasm and is associated with inflammation in advanced chronic kidney disease patients (Stenvinkel, 2001b). Finally, endothelial dysfunction and inflammation is associated with oxidative stress, leading to atherosclerosis and tissue hypoxia (Handelman et al., 2001).

Vascular calcification and ossification, present in 30% to 70% of chronic kidney patients, is virtually always associated with dialysis due to both arterial intima and media disturbances, plaque formation, hypertension and atherogenesis (Sigrist et al., 2006; Schwarz et al., 2000), and is related to arterial dysfunction because it alters nitric oxide-dependent vasodilatation and increases pulse-wave velocity in dialysis patients (Raggi et al., 2007). Calcium, hyperphosphatemia and hyperparathyroidism are risk markers of vascular calcification, and vitamin D deficiency is associated with increased mortality and cardiovascular disease

(Block et al., 2005). An antagonist of vascular calcification, fetuin-A, is low in dilaysis patients and is associated with increased cardiovascular mortality (Ix et al., 2007).
Emerging evidence suggests that aberrant DNA methylation may play a deleterious role in atherosclerosis and endothelial dysfunction (Dong et al., 2002). DNA methylation changes occur during atherogenesis and may contribute to lesion development. The homocysteine precursor S-adenosylmethionine is a competitive inhibitor of S-adenosylmethionine methyltransferases and is increased in haemodilaysis patients. This phenomenon leads to unbalanced methylation in the setting of hyperhomocysteinemia. In vascular disease patients increased homocysteine and S-adenosylmethionine concentrations are associated with DNA hypomethylation (Castro et al., 2003; Valli et al., 2008). In this regard, the presence of inflammation may partly contribute to an association between homocysteine levels, endothelial dysfunction and cardiovascular outcome in dialysis subjects, resulting in part in aberrant DNA methylation (Stenvinkel et al., 2008; Teitell & Richardson, 2003).
Finally, endothelial cells modify their function in response to changes in the extracellular concentration of sodium and potassium, constantly present in dialysis patients. The control of local tissue perfusion that the endothelium exerts may play an important in vascular tone and the development of hypertension and atherosclerosis (Oberleithner et al., 2010).

2. The endothelium in normal conditions

The endothelium is a functional and anatomic barrier composed of a single layer of endothelial cells between the vessel wall and blood. The human vascular bed contains 10^{13} endothelial cells, constituting our largest endocrine organ (Perry & Pearson, 1989). Endothelial cells play important roles in vascular tone, haemostasis, cellular proliferation, immunological processes and inflammatory events. The normal endothelium regulates vascular smooth muscle tone; exerts anticoagulant, fibrinolytic and antithrombotic actions; is involved in lipid, lipoprotein and eicosanoid metabolism; is a selective barrier for the normal trafficking of molecules from the interstitial tissue to the blood stream and viceversa, and contributes to vascular growth, leukocyte adhesion, and immunological processes.

2.1 Regulation of vascular tone

The endothelium releases a wide variety of substances both vasodilators and vasoconstrictors. Relaxing factors consist primarily of nitric oxide, prostacyclin, hyperpolarizing factor, bradykinin, and adrenomedullin. Constricting factors include mainly endothelin-1, thromboxane A2, prostaglandin H2, angiotensin II and free radicals. Amongst the relaxing molecules, nitric oxide constitutes the basis of endothelium-related vasorelaxation. Nitric oxide is synthesized by nitric oxide synthase from the N-terminal of L-arginine guanidine, is an unstable molecule with a half-life of a couple of seconds. There are three forms of nitric oxide: type I or neuronal, type II or inducible, and type III or endothelial, which is specific to the endothelium. Nitric oxide synthase is stimulated by nicotinamide dinucleotide (phosphate) (NADPH) and 5,6,7,8-tetrahydrobiopterin and inhibited by powerful oxidants as superoxide anions and hydrogen peroxide (Verma & Anderson, 2002). Excess inducible nitric oxide caused by many inflammatory cytokines such as tumor necrosis factor-alpha, interleukin-1 or -6 results in an exaggerated vasodilatation, whilst interleukins-4, -8, -10 and transforming growth factor-beta decrease nitric oxide expression (Webb & Vallance, 1997). Endothelial cells release nitric oxide into the

surrounding smooth muscle cells of the vascular wall in a paracrine manner, causing vasodilatation and inhibiting their growth, and into the vascular lumen, impeding local platelet and leukocyte adhesion (Vanhoutte et al., 1997). One of the most important causes of endothelial nitric oxide release is shear stress. The physical stimulus of a faster or a pulsatile blood flow in the arterial wall leads to vasodilatation. Endogenous substances that stimulate nitric oxide release are catecholamines, vasopressin, bradykinin, histamine, serotonin, ADP and thrombin. The interaction between the normal endothelium and platelets is crucial for vascular tone stability and haemostasis.
Amongst the vasoconstrictors produced by endothelial cells, endothelin plays an important role. Endothelins are 21-aminoacid peptides classified as 1 to 3, with a half-life of approximately 2 minutes and are derived from proendothelin in a reaction catalyzed by endothelin converting enzyme. Endothelin-1 is specific to the endothelium, is released paracrinally towards the vascular wall where it exerts its powerful vasoconstrictor effect on the smooth muscle cells (Yanashigawa et al., 1988; Clozel & Fischli, 1989). The most potent regulator of endothelin-1 production and release is blood flow. An increase in blood flow results in vasodilatation due to the activation of shear stress receptors in the endothelial cells, which increases nitric oxide synthesis and release and reduces endothelin-1 production (Webb & Vallance, 1997). Other endothelin-1 stimulants include hypoxia, angiotensin-II, insulin, thrombin, low-density lipoproteins, vasopressin, transforming growth factor-beta and plasminogen activator inhibitor-1 (Webb & Vallance, 1997). The vasoconstrictor and proliferative action of endothelin-1 on vascular smooth muscle cells is mediated by A receptors, mainly in large vessels. When B receptors are activated, they also mediate vasoconstriction in small arteries and in the low-pressure venous bed. Endothelial B receptors, however, participate in other effects: clearance of circulating endothelin-1, inhibition of endothelin-1 synthesis, and paradoxically can also stimulate endothelial nitric oxide synthase activity, leading to vasodilatation and antiproliferative effects. (Webb & Vallance, 1997).

2.2 Regulation of haemostasis

The endothelial layer affects platelet function, plasma coagulation, and fibrinolysis. The physiologic role of the endothelium is to provide an antithrombotic surface; when endothelial damage occurs, the endothelium is converted into a prothrombotic layer (Cines et al., 1998). Factors with procoagulant effects on endothelial cells include reactive oxygen species, oxidized lipids, shear stress and slow blood flow, inflammation, age and certain hormones (Müller & Griesmacher, 2000). Moreover, the endothelium itself produces, according to the circumstances, both anticoagulant and procoagulant factors. The former action is mediated mainly by nitric oxide, prostacyclin, tissue plasminogen activator, thrombomodulin and antithrombin III, while the latter is starred by platelet activating factor, tissue factor, endothelin, thrombin, plasminogen activator inhibitor-1 and factor VIII. Coagulation itself results not only in thrombosis, but also stimulates inflammation and cellular growth. In fact, thrombin is involved in coagulation, anticoagulation, pro-inflammatory and anti-inflammatory processes, cell adhesion and proliferation. Indeed, there is a strong association between inflammation and coagulation at the cellular level (Esmon, 1999). The physiology of haemostasis, inflammation and thrombosis, involves adhesion of leukocytes and platelets suspended in flowing blood to the vessel wall. Recent findings underscore the importance of blood flow and of exposed vessel wall structures in these processes. Platelet-dependent haemostasis at injured vessel walls is more extensive at higher shear. However, leukocyte adhesion to endothelium increase at slow shear (Kuijper et al., 1996; Mackay & Imhof, 1993). Multiple receptor-ligand interactions are usually needed for attachment. Endothelial secreted selectins are first released, which interact with platelets for their adhesion and for platelet and endothelial synthesis of integrins. This process results in the recruitment of leukocytes through the action of intracellular adhesion molecules, vascular cell adhesion molecules and platelet endothelial cell adhesion molecules (Mulvihill et al., 2002). The next step is the migration of leukocytes to the subintimal space and later to the medial layer, where they interact with smooth muscle cells, fibroblasts and macrophages. This platelet-bridged action for leukocyte entrance into the vascular wall is independent of blood flow speed and shear (Mackay & Imhof, 1993). Finally, endothelial cells affect fibrinolysis synthesizing fibrinolyic factors and fibrinolysis inhibiting factors: Urokinase, tissue plasminogen activator, and plasminogen activator inhibitor. Briefly, tissue plasminogen activator is released from endothelial cells and cleaves plasminogen to form plasmin, a potent fibrinolytic substance in a fine physiological balance with plasminogen activator inhibitor-1, a protein also released from endothelial cells that antagonizes tissue plasminogen activator. The levels of both molecules are increased as a result of excess stimulation of endothelial cells by thrombin or as a result of endothelial dysfunction (Huber, 2001; Kuijper et al., 1996).

3. The endothelium and chronic kidney disease

Patients with end-stage renal disease are at high risk of developing cardiovascular disease and decreasing their life survival. Renal insufficiency may be part and/or cause of a systemic subclinical atherothrombotic process (Stam et al., 2003). As mentioned before, arteriosclerosis can contribute to atherosclerosis and vice versa, possibly through endothelial dysfunction, biomechanical and blood flow stress to endothelial cells, and elastic fragmentation (Guérin et al., 2008). Both processes can ultimately lead to vascular calcification and ossification, clinically assessed as an increase in arterial stiffness and hypertension (McEniery et al., 2009). Accelerated atherogenesis at any stage of chronic kidney disease may be due to the interplay of traditional and nontraditional risk factors, such as asymmetric dimethylarginine, homocysteine, advanced glycation end products, endothelial lipidosis, oxidative stress processes and inflammatory molecules (Goligorsky, 2007). Therefore, it is correct to consider endothelial dysfunction as a heterogenous syndrome, which can be focused either as a local or a systemic condition, as in chronic kidney disease; with subclinical or clinical manifestations; being reversible or irreversible according to its severity; and with many related etiologic mechanisms, as already mentioned (Goligorsky, 2007). In chronic kidney disease, endothelial dysfunction is characterized by increased plasma concentrations of endothelium-derived molecules, an imbalance between circulating endothelial cell and bone-marrow endothelial progenitor cells, or reduced endothelium-dependent vasodilatation (van Guldener et al., 1997; Rabelink et al., 2010). As renal function deteriorates, an atherogenic milieu generates due to the accumulation of uremic toxins with direct impact on the endothelium and the vessel wall, contributing to oxidative stress and enhancing a subclinical inflammatory state. In chronic kidney disease, these initial steps in endothelial dysfunction may perpetuate if not identified at the early subclinical stages, leading to atherogenesis (Ross, 1999). Decreased endothelial function is thought to primarily reflect a decreased bioavailability of nitric oxide, a molecule with vasodilatory and antiatherosclerotic properties (Tatematsu et al., 2007). Asymmetric dimethylarginine, an endogenous inhibitor of nitric oxide synthase, is involved in atherogenesis, is primarily cleared by the kidney and is elevated in kidney disease (Kielstein & Zoccali, 2005). Dimethylarginine is considered as an independent predictor of endothelial dysfunction and poor outcome in dialysis patients (Zoccali et al., 2001).

Albuminuria is another predictor of increased cardiovascular risk (de Zeeuw, 2007). Albuminuria is also associated with other cardiovascular risk factors, such as abnormalities in fibrinolysis (Annavekar & Pfeffer, 2004), inflammation (Festa et al., 2000), and dyslipidemia (Tonelli & Pfeffer, 2007). Although the nature of the links between albuminuria and vascular disease may partly be due to endothelial dysfunction, persistent low-grade inflammation also plays a role. Indeed, inflammation is associated with both endothelial dysfunction (Stenvinkel, 2001b) and albuminuria (Festa et al., 2000). Noteworthy, albeit frequently present, proteinuria seldom is considered as a cause of inflammation, protein-energy wasting and endothelial dysfunction in hemodialysis.

Albuminuria is strongly associated with increased levels of pentraxin-3, an inflammatory mediator produced by a variety of tissues and cells, mainly endothelial cells, macrophages and adipocytes, in response to proinflammatory signals (Abderrahim-Ferkoune et al., 2003; Mantovani et al., 2006). Pentraxin-3 is elevated in dialysis subjects (Boehme et al., 2007) and is being considered as a new mortality risk factor in dialysis patients (Tong et al., 2007). This suggests that it may have an additional role in the atherogenic process to common inflammatory mediators (Stenvinkel et al., 2008). Because of its extrahepatic synthesis, pentraxin-3 levels are believed to be an independent indicator of disease activity directly produced at sites of inflammation and linked to endothelial dysfunction.

Detached circulating endothelial cells may serve as potential markers of endothelial damage in kidney disease (Koc et al., 2005). These circulating endothelial cells include endothelial progenitor cells, which are bone marrow–derived, and inflammatory endothelial cells, which are thought to be detached from the vessel walls and enter the circulation as a result of vascular injury. Normally, in response to ischemic insult and cytokine stimulation, endothelial progenitor cells are mobilized from the bone marrow to act as repair cells in response to the endothelial injury. In kidney disease there exists an impaired migratory activity and/or decreased numbers (Herbrig et al., 2004) of these cells, which may have a role in neovascularization of ischemic tissue and the progression of atherosclerosis and cardiovascular disease (Hill et al., 2003). Low levels of circulating endothelial progenitor cells predicted the occurrence of cardiovascular events and death. An imbalance between the expression of circulating endothelial cells (reflecting inflammatory endothelial damage) and endothelial progenitor cells (reflecting endothelial repair capacity) seems to exist in chronic kidney disease (Stenvinkel et al., 2008). This imbalance may contribute to the pathogenesis and progression of the atherosclerosis.

In agreement with Stenvinkel et al., until the results of new studies regarding this issue become available, endothelial dysfunction should be considered a cardiovascular marker and not an etiological factor in kidney patients, intimately related to oxidative stress and inflammation (Stenvinkel et al., 2008).

3.1 The endothelium and oxidative stress

Under normal conditions, reactive oxygen species (which include various compounds such as superoxide anions, hydrogen peroxide, and hydroxyl radical) are produced in mammalian cells during energy production in mitochondria by reducing oxygen during aerobic respiration (Pieczenik & Neustadt, 2007). In addition, a variety of enzymatic and nonenzymatic sources of reactive oxygen species exist in vascular vessels as well as different tissues, among which can be included nicotinamide dinucleotide (phosphate) (NAD(P)H oxidase enzyme complex, xanthine oxidase, lipoxygenases, and cyclooxygenases (Portaluppi et al., 2004). An uncoupling of nitric oxide synthase, owing to the reduction of its cofactor, BH4, can also contribute to oxygen metabolites (Andrew & Mayer, 1999). Reactive oxygen species levels are maintained at a normal range by scavenging through various antioxidant enzyme activities such as superoxide dismutase, catalase, glutathione peroxidase, and other components such as reduced glutathione, transition metal ions, and ascorbic acid. (Blokhina et al., 2003). Reactive oxygen species are part of the organism's unspecified initial defense system. However, excessive reactive oxygen species levels can produce cellular damage by interacting with biomolecules; this imbalance, which the cellular components cannot bear long, is called oxidative stress.

As mentioned, oxidative stress takes place when the production of oxidants exceeds local antioxidant capacity, resulting in the oxidation of proteins, lipids, carbohydrates, and DNA. Briefly, oxidative stress biomarkers can be classified as derived from lipids (malondialdehyde, lipid hydroperoxides, oxidized low-density lipoprotein, advanced lipoxidation end products), arachidonic acid derivatives (F2 isoprostanes), carbohydrates (reactive aldehydes, advanced glycosylation end products), amino acids (cysteine/cystine, homocysteine/homocystine), proteins (carbonyl formation, advanced oxidation protein products) and DNA (8 hydroxy 2′ deoxyguanine) (Himmelfarb et al., 2002). Oxidative stress can occur via four different chemical pathways: Oxygen reactive species can lead to the production of advanced glycosilation end-products (carbonyl stress); to the inhibition of nitric oxide synthase (nitrosative stress); to the production of hydrogen peroxide and chlorine hydroxide (chlorinated stress); and to the generation of hydroxide species with the intervention of iron molecules (classical oxidative stress). Definitively, chlorinated stress is the most important pathway implicated in renal failure (Massy et al., 2003; Himmelfarb et al., 2001).

Uremia is a prooxidant state. Lipid peroxidation, oxidative modification of proteins and carbohydrates and certain uremic toxins themselves have been implicated in endothelial dysfunction in chronic renal disease (Himmelfarb et al., 2002; Linden et al., 2008; Oberg et al., 2004; Trimarchi et al., 2003). Moreover, numerous defects in antioxidant systems lead to a decrease in the depuration of reactive oxygen species. Oxidative stress appears to start early in chronic kidney disease (Oberg et al., 2004), but total antioxidant capacity has been observed to be excelled only in end-stage renal failure, suggesting that reactive oxygen species production start overcoming their clearance at the beginning of the decline in renal function. Finally, dialysis treatment may have contradictory effects on it, depending on the quality, modality, and duration of the procedure itself (Pupim et al., 2004; Hand et al., 1998; McGregor et al., 2003).

Although priming of polymorphonuclear leukocytes is a prominent feature in chronic kidney disease (Hörl, 2002), and myeloperoxidase is involved in chlorinated stress, the exact role of inflammation as a trigger of oxidative stress remains poorly defined in renal disease. As suggested, longitudinal studies of patients with mild chronic kidney disease are needed to resolve the issue of which is the initial culprit: inflammation or oxidative stress (Stenvinkel et al., 2008).

Oxidative stress in the kidney and vascular tissues can elevate arterial pressure via several mechanisms. Reactive oxygen species react with and inactivate nitric oxide; it also perturbs its production production by depleting the nitric oxide synthase cofactor tetrahydrobiopterin; and it contributes to accumulation of asymmetrical dimethylarginines, which in turn curtails nitric oxide production. Reduced bioavailability of nitric oxide, as a resultant of endothelial dysfunction, enhances the development and maintenance of hypertension by augmenting systemic vascular resistance, by increasing adrenergic tone, volume expansion and vascular smooth muscle cell proliferation, matrix accumulation and vascular remodeling, which are inhibited by nitric oxide and and promoted by free radicals (Wilcox, 2005). Another mechanism by which oxidative stress can cause hypertension and atherogenesis in renal failure is via nonenzymatic oxidation of arachidonic acid and formation of isoprostanes, which display vasoconstrictor, proinflammatory and antinatriuretic activity (Vaziri & Rodríguez-Iturbe, 2006; Schnackenberg, 2002). Finally, oxidative stress enhances the production of angiotensin II, which leads to increased blood pressure by promoting sodium retention and renal vasoconstriction (Navar et al., 2002). Moreover, oxidative stress increases production of endothelin-1 and the cytosolic concentration of calcium, thereby increasing vascular smooth muscle tone, systemic vascular resistance, arterial pressure and accumulation of matrix proteins (Kahler et al., 2001; Touyz, 2005).

3.2 The endothelium and inflammation

In chronic kidney disease, a state of persistent low-grade inflammation is commonly observed. Chronic inflammation is characterized by the persistent effect of a causative stimulus, which leads to destruction of cells and tissues and has deleterious effects to the body. In chronic kidney disease, especially in stage 5, the systemic concentrations of both pro- and anti-inflammatory cytokines are several-fold higher as a result of both decreased renal clearance and increased production. Several factors, both dialysis-related (*e.g.*, membrane bioincompatibility) and non–dialysis-related (*e.g.*, infection, comorbidity, genetic factors, diet), may additionally contribute to a state of persistent inflammation. In addition to putative direct proatherogenic effects, persistent inflammation may serve as a catalyst and, in the uremic milieu, modulate the effects of risk factors for wasting and vascular disease (Carrero & Stenvinkel, 2009). In the uremic milieu, in which cytokines are retained as a result of loss of residual renal function and stimulated by comorbidities and the dialysis procedure itself, such interactions should be of relevance.

As mentioned before, elevated C-Reactive Protein is associated with atherogenesis and endothelial dysfunction, and inflammation enhances cardiovascular risk and mortality in haemodialysis patients (Zimmermann et al., 1999). Tumor necrosis factor-alpha is increased in this process, and may synergize oxidative stress processes that lead to lipid peroxidation and oxidized LDL (Stenvinkel et al., 1999). Inflammation also might cause endothelial dysfunction through the stimulation of intracellular adhesion molecules in patients with chronic kidney disease as soluble Vascular Adhesion Molecule-1 (sVCAM-1) and soluble Intercellular Adhesion Molecule-1 (sICAM-1) (Stam et al., 2003).

Migration of monocytes into the vessel wall contributes to the onset and progression of atherosclerosis (Kon et al., 2011). The infiltration of monocytes and T lymphocytes in the vascular wall depends on the response to chemokines, and $CD14^{2+}CD^{16+}$ monocytes are characterized by a unique pattern of chemokine receptors, represented by the chemokine receptor 5 (CCR5). In states of inflammation, CCR5 could contribute to atherogenesis through the binding of its ligands, which in turn mediate the recruitment of inflammatory cells to the endothelium (Carrero & Stenvinkel, 2009).

Chronic kidney disease is a low-grade inflammatory process with peripheral polymorphonuclear leukocyte and $CD14^{+}/CD16^{+}$ cells being key mediators in this process (Sela et al., 2005). In fact, persistent inflammation may also be a risk factor *per se* for progression of kidney disease, as inflammatory markers are predictors of kidney function deterioration. This could be a consequence of inflammatory mediators such as tumor necrosis factor-alpha or interleukin-6 being able to act as toxins participating in uremia complications. In addition, C-Reactive protein formed locally in the renal inflammatory process reduces nitric oxide production, stimulates endothelin-1 formation, and induces some of the steps involved in the atherosclerosis process, as monocyte recruitment and foam cell formation (Labarrere & Zaloga, 2004). Elevated C-Reactive protein, interleukin-6, and fibrinogen are independent predictors of cardiovascular outcomes in patients with kidney disease (Cachofeiro et al., 2008). Inflammation could promote both renal deterioration (triggering endothelial dysfunction, atherosclerosis, and glomerular injury) and cardiovascular mortality. Inflammation is a redox-sensitive mechanism, as oxidative stress is able to activate transcriptor factors such as Nuclear Factor-kappaB, which regulates inflammatory mediator gene expression (Li & Karin, 1999). This nuclear factor is maintained inactivated in the cytoplasm by binding to inhibitory proteins. Their phosphorylation, posterior ubiquitination, and proteolysis result in the release and translocation of it to the nucleus and consequent activation of specific genes. Some of these steps seem to be affected by oxidative stress as the presence of antioxidants prevents nuclear factor-kappaB activation by reactive oxygen species (Li & Karin, 1999).

The observation that both protein-energy wasting and persistent inflammation are highly prevalent in dialysis patients and are associated with a substantially increased mortality risk has focused on the endothelium as an important target (Carrero & Stenvinkel, 2009). Because protein-energy wasting, inflammation, and atherosclerosis often coexist in the uremic milieu, these risk factors are linked. One of the main detrimental effects of proinflammatory cytokine activation in patients with end-stage renal disease is muscle depletion or sarcopenia, mediated by interleukin-6, angiotensin II and Tumor Necrosis Factor –like weak inducer of apoptosis (TWEAK) (Carrero et al., 2008).

The role of persistent inflammation as a culprit of converting the endothelium into a procoagulant and proinflammatory surface that makes the vasculature more vulnerable to the effects of other circulating risk factors is to be better determined. However, the strong associations between inflammatory markers and endothelial dysfunction in patients with chronic kidney disease support this hypothesis (Carrero & Stenvinkel, 2009).

3.3 The endothelium and uremic toxins

During the development of the uremic syndrome, losses of kidney function are accompanied by deteriorating organ function attributable to the accumulation of uremic retention solutes. Compounds that exert an adverse biologic impact are called uremic toxins. At least 115 toxins accumulate in uremia and may play an important role in the pathogenesis of the uremic sindrome (Vanholder et al., 2008). Peptides in the 10- to 30-kD range, for example, are some of the so-called "middle molecules." These peptides can be glycosylated, oxidized, or carbamylated, thereby altering their structure and function so that cell and organ dysfunction may not simply result from accumulation of these metabolites. Uremic toxins provoke oxidative stress, inflammation, hypertrophy, constriction, and coagulation through various mechanisms. Monocytes, in response to advanced glycosylation end products that accumulate in uremia, produce free radicals that provoke oxidative stress. Monocytes, in response to leptin accumulation in uremia, cause clotting. Macrophages in response to homocysteine provokes oxidative stress. Finally, leukocytes are activated by the uremic toxin p-cresol sulfate. Platelets now are recognized to accumulate uremic toxins, and the interaction between platelets and vascular smooth muscle may lead to vascular smooth muscle growth and constriction, thereby contributing to both hypertension and atherosclerosis. The uremic toxins in platelets are collectively known as diadenosine polyphosphate. Both diadenosine pentaphosphate and diadenosine hexaphosphate are strongly protein bound and poorly removed by dialysis and produce vasoconstriction or vascular smooth muscle growth (Vanholder et al., 2010). Uremic toxins can activate the endothelium to produce the following effects: (1) vasoconstriction (via asymmetric dimethylarginine, advanced glycation end product, and homocysteine); (2) inflammation (via indoxyl sulfate and advanced glycation end products); (3) oxidative stress (via asymmetric dimethylarginine, advanced glycation end product, and homocysteine); (4) or procoagulant activity. The procoagulant effect of endothelium is noted by increased procoagulant factors (increased plasminogen activator inhibitor-1 and von Willebrand factor) and reduced anticoagulant factors (e.g., tissue plasminogen activator). It follows, then, that a diverse group of toxins act on a variety of cell types to provoke oxidative stress, inflammation, vascular smooth vessel proliferation and constriction, endothelial dysfunction, and coagulation, accounting for some of the manifestations of the uremic syndrome that include hypertension and accelerated atherosclerosis.

These low molecular weight organic compounds may either exist in free water- soluble forms or bind reversibly to serum proteins, thereby altering protein functions (Vanholder et al., 1992). In kidney disease, peptides may be found in their native form or, as a consequence of exposure to the uremic milieu, become irreversibly altered resulting in changes in structure and function. Importantly, both protein-bound solutes and peptides are particularly difficult to remove by conventional dialysis treatments, and uremic retention solutes may play a role in uremia-related complications (Vanholder et al., 2008). There have been described dual effects of uremic retention solutes on leukocyte function: Blunting upon stimulation, which has been linked to infection, and basal activation linked to microinflammation, malnutrition, and atherosclerosis. The major leukocyte subtypes affected by uremic conditions are polymorphonuclear cells, specifically neutrophils and mononuclear cells of the monocyte/macrophage type 2. It is predominantly the latter cell type that is activated by uremic retention solutes, enhancing vascular damage (Vanholder et al., 2008).

Patients on haemodialysis have alterations in endothelial properties with increases in both plasminogen activator inhibitor-1 and von Willebrand factor, whereas tissue plasminogen activator decreases, suggesting a procoagulant state at the endothelial surface (Haaber et al., 1995). Regulation of vascular tone is also impaired with decreased endothelium-dependent vasodilatation, associated with the aforementioned inhibition of endothelial nitric oxide synthase by asymmetric dimethylarginine, advanced glycation end-products and homocysteine. Chronic kidney disease also induces oxidant stress and inflammation in endothelial cells and production of reactive oxygen species in cultured endothelial cells by the protein-bound uremic toxin indoxyl sulfate.

A new insight into endothelial dysfunction is also provided by the observation of circulating endothelial microparticles. The generation of endothelial microparticles is elicited *in vitro* by the presence of indoxyl sulfate (Faure et al., 2006). A remarkable characteristic of the endothelium is its capacity for continuous regeneration and repair. This involves two mechanisms: The classically described proliferation of adjacent endothelial cells and the more recently described homing of circulating endothelial progenitor cells (Vanholder et al., 2008). These latter cells may be mobilized from bone marrow in response to cytokines or ischemia or derive from circulating leukocytes. In haemodilaysis subjects, endothelial repair mechanisms are altered, representing a possible threat to vascular integrity. Some uremic toxins such as indoxyl sulfate reduce endothelial proliferation, and serum from uremic patients decreases the ability of endothelial progenitor cells to migrate. In addition, these patients generally have a decrease in the number of circulating endothelial progenitor cells (de Groot et al., 2004).

3.4 The endothelium and haemostatic disturbances

An important intermediary in the continued activation of endothelial cells is the interaction of the endothelium with platelets . The adhesion of platelets to activated endothelial cells is mediated by a glycoprotein IIb/IIIa-dependent mechanism. The activation of glycoprotein IIb/IIIa induces the expression of factors such as P-selectin that promote activation of the endothelium (May et al., 2002). Platelets recruit bone marrow-derived progenitor cells to the activated endothelium and the injured vessel wall by providing a surface that supports interaction between platelet P-selectin and the glycoprotein IIb/IIIa integrin (Rabelink et al., 2010). A relevant platelet-derived chemokine for the interaction of leukocytes with the activated endothelium is RANTES, secreted by thrombin-stimulated platelets and immobilized on the surface of the inflamed endothelium which triggers shear stress-resistant monocyte arrest. (von Hundelshausen & Weber, 2007). After their activation, membrane vesicles (0.1–1 μm in diameter) may be released from endothelial cells. Under normal conditions, phospholipid moieties in the plasma membrane are distributed asymmetrically. During microparticle formation, membrane asymmetry is lost, resulting in microparticles becoming procoagulant. (Rabelink et al., 2010). A variety of proinflammatory agents, including tumor necrosis factor, and procoagulant factors, such as thrombin, can induce the formation of endothelial microparticles. The biological effects of endothelial microparticles are largely determined by their protein and lipid composition. They might contain tissue factor, metabolic enzymes, proteins involved in adhesion and fusion processes, cytoskeleton associated proteins, or chemokines. Endothelial microparticles themselves can therefore contribute to the further activation of endothelial cells and to the initiation of coagulation, and may transfer endothelial proteins to circulating cells. Circulating levels of endothelial microparticles have been suggested to be a marker of sustained endothelial-cell activation. These circulating microparticles are elevated in dialysis patients (Mallat et al., 2000), and could be directly related to the presence of uremic toxins (Rabelink et al., 2010). The levels of endothelial microparticles in patients with end-stage renal disease positively correlate with endothelial dysfunction, as measured by flow-mediated vasodilatation, and indices of arterial stiffening. Endothelial microparticles directly impair endothelium-dependent vasodilator mechanisms in dialysis subjects, while their low levels are associated with improved survival in this population. As mentioned before, platelets also play a central role in vascular damage by inducing haemostasis and arterial thrombosis (Vanholder et al., 2010).

As discussed previously, platelets interact with coagulation factors, in particular thrombin, and during thrombin-induced aggregation, almost the entire content of platelet granules is released. Platelets from patients with renal failure have increased intracellular concentration of the diadenosine polyphosphates which act as strong growth factors for vascular smooth muscle cells. Because enhanced smooth muscle growth is a hallmark of atherosclerosis in renal failure, the increased amount of diadenosine polyphosphates in platelets may play an important role in causing increased cardiovascular damage. Furthermore, diadenosine polyphosphates are strong vasoconstrictors with direct effects on vascular tone (Vanholder et al., 2010). Thus, platelet-endothelium interaction may play an important role in hypertension and atherosclerosis in renal failure.

3.5 The endothelium and protein-energy wasting

There has been an increase of mechanisms causing syndromes of wasting, malnutrition, inflammation, and their interrelationships in individuals with chronic kidney disease. Approximately 18–75% of patients on chronic dialysis show evidence of wasting (Stenvinkel et al., 2004). This phenomenon has been referred to as uremic malnutrition, uremic cachexia, protein–energy malnutrition, malnutrition–inflammation atherosclerosis syndrome, or malnutrition–inflammation complex syndrome (Fouque et al., 2008). Many of the measures indicating the presence of wasting and abnormalities in protein–energy nutritional status can also be induced by inflammatory processes. As mentioned in previous sections, an increase in proinflammatory cytokines may cause loss of protein stores. The loss of muscle and fat stores and the present inflammation condition are likely to increase the risk of death from cardiovascular disease by promoting endothelial damage (Avesani et al., 2006). In kidney disease, there are conditions resulting in loss of lean body mass not related to reduced nutrient intake, due to nonspecific inflammatory processes, intercurrent catabolic illnesses, nutrient losses into dialysate, academia, resistance to anabolic hormones, hyperglucagonemia, hyperparathyroidism, use of prostheses, and anemia or its treatment (Fouque et al., 2008). Amongst the number of disorders that can cause wasting in patients with kidney disease, inflammation, oxidative stress, acidemia, nutrient losses into dialysate, anemia, hyperparathyroidism, and retention of uremic toxins interplay and, as shown in previous sections, cause endothelial dysfunction, leading to atherogenesis and cardiovascular disease). Elevated cardiovascular and haemodynamic markers of disease and endothelial stress as Pro-Brain Natriuretic Peptide or Troponin T are associated with wasting and inflammation in haemodialysis subjects. The employment of vascular prostheses and catheters may play a role in this abnormal setting (Trimarchi et al., 2011).

3.6 The endothelium, anemia and erythropoiesis-stimulating agents

The association of anemia with cardiovascular outcomes is well known, but underlying mechanisms are not well understood (Jurkovitz et al., 2003). However, targeting a higher hemoglobin with higher doses of erythropoiesis-stimulating agents worsens cardiovascular outcomes in dialysis individuals (Singh et al., 2006) Possibilities include a higher prothrombotic state due to hypercoagulability or a potentially toxic effect of erythropoietic agents on the cardiovascular system.(Keithi-Reddy et al., 2008) As commented before, there exists a role for inflammation in atherosclerosis in kidney subjects. There is recent evidence that tumor necrosis factor-alpha is higher and the levels of serum albumin lower in anemic compared to non-anemic dialysis subjects. The levels of interleukins -6 and -8, display increasing trends between anemic and non-anemic patients (Keithi-Reddy et al., 2008).

These cytokines have been implicated as non-traditional cardiovascular risk factors associated with an increased risk of atherosclerosis. Interleukin-6 stimulate production of C-Reactive protein, while interleukin-8 is a potent angiogenic factor that induces migration and proliferation of endothelial cells and smooth muscle cells contributing to plaque formation in atherosclerosis. (Simonini et al, 2000). One of the hypotheses promulgated to explain increased inflammation in chronic kidney disease patients is the reduced clearance of cytokines as renal function declines. Inflammatory cytokines interfere with both proliferation and differentiation of erythroid precursors by several mechanisms, including induction of apoptosis, downregulation of erythropoietin receptors, and reduced activity and synthesis of them (Weiss & Goodnough, 2005). Besides, states of vascular congestion and chronic heart failure have been shown to have elevated levels of these inflammatory markers when the renal function declines. Of the inflammatory markers, interleukin-6 is important by virtue of its actions not only on cardiovascular system but also on worsening of anemia.

However, the notion that oxygen transport capacity might increase at hematocrit values above 34% in patients with chronic renal disease is undetermined, because it has been known that when hematocrit values rise above 40% in normal subjects, oxygen transport capacity decreases as a result of the decrease in cardiac index associated with a rise in blood viscosity (Crowell & Smith, 1967). The optimal hematocrit in dialysis patients has not been defined but may be lower than that in normal subjects because of decreased arterial and ventricular compliances and impaired cardiac index. Two controlled predialysis studies (CHOIR and CREATE), which compared traditional hematocrit targets of 34% to fully normalized targets, reported either no improvement in quality of life or that increased erythropoietin dosing resulted in increased cardiovascular adverse events or hypertension (Singh et al., 2006). The mechanisms responsible for these excess cardiovascular and mortality events are not fully elucidated, but erythropoietin-stimulating agents-induced arterial hypertension is a candidate (Krapf & Hulter, 2009). The increase in systolic and diastolic blood pressure at the target hematocrit varied but reached an average of approximately 5 to 8 mmHg in systolic and 4 to 6 mmHg in diastolic blood pressure. Erythropoietin doses of 40, 80, and 120 U/kg thrice weekly for 49 weeks were associated with hypertension in 28%, 32%, and 56% of treated subjects, respectively (Krapf & Hulter, 2009). Erythropoietin induced hypertension is independent of its effect on red blood cell mass and viscosity is supported by the demonstration in rats that coadministration of erythropoietin with either a synthetic erythropoietin binding protein or an anti-erythropoietin antibody prevented erythropoietin-induced hypertension while preserving the erythropoietic response. This suggests the interesting possibility that different epitopes on the erythropoietin protein confer independent erythropoietic and haemodynamic effects. Erythropoietin induces endothelin-1 release and produces an enhanced mitogenic response in endothelial cells (Krapf & Hulter, 2009). Production of the vasodilating prostacyclin is decreased and the vasoconstricting prostanoid thromboxaneB2 is increased. In human endothelial cells, erythropoietin decreases e nitric oxide synthase expression resulting in decreased endothelial nitric oxide production. The mechanism may include increased production of reactive oxygen species and asymmetric dimethylarginine (Scalera et al., 2005). A systemic effect to blunt endothelial nitric oxide production, combined with the increased endothelin-1 response and predominance of thromboxane over prostacyclin could explain the erythropoietin-induced vasoconstrictive effect (Krapf & Hulter, 2009). Moreover, at least a subset of haemodialyzed patients exhibit an accentuated hypersensitivity to angiotensin II and norepinephrine during erythropoietin treatment, which correlated with an increase in blood pressure (Krapf & Hulter, 2009). Thus, erythropoietin-induced hypersensitivity to angiotensin II and norepinephrine, as well as increased endothelin-1 activity, are reasonable mechanisms for erythropoietin-induced hypertension in haemodialyzed patients, in part impairing endothelial relaxation (Annuk et al., 2006).

Interestingly, anemic patients treated with erythropoietin compared to erythropoietin-naive patients revealed increased levels for interleukins-6 and -8, C-Reactive protein, and tumor necrosis factor-alpha. Although the antiapoptotic effect of erythropoietin on erythroid precursors in the bone marrow is well described, its potential effect of on cytokines is less well understood (Krantz, 1991). Long-term administration of erythropoietin has been associated with decreased levels of tumor necrosis-alpha in subjects on haemodialysis, but also to enhance inflammation and ischemia-induced neovascularization by increasing the mobilization of endothelial progenitor cells (Heeschen, et al., 2003). Furthermore, erythropoietin activates vascular smooth muscle cells, endothelium, and platelets enhancing thrombogenity and loss of vasodilatory potential. An alternative hypothesis is that induction of proinflammatory cytokines by erythropoietin occurs as a consequence of acting via erythropoetin receptors on macrophages, which upon activation secrete interleukin-6,-8, and tumor necrosis-alpha, leading to chronic inflammation, protein-energy wasting and atherogenesis. Indeed, these molecules have been associated with an increased risk of death in the dialysis population (Keithi-Reddy et al., 2008). In addition, this could be one explanation for the observation of increased risk for all-cause and cardiovascular mortality in patients targeted to higher hemoglobin levels with higher doses of erythropoiesis stimulating agents (Singh et al., 2006)

3.7 The endothelium and vascular calcification and ossification

Vascular calcification is responsible for the higher prevalence of cardiovascular disease in dialysis patients. Consequently, its early detection is truly relevant in this population. Traditionally, it has been described as a patchy-like and/or a linear calcification that corresponds to intima (atherosclerosis-related) and media calcification (related to calcium/phosphorus disturbances). However, there is a current debate about the location of calcium in the artery wall and their clinical implications, as referred before (Coll et al., 2011). Calcified plaques and intima calcification appear to be the most prevalent coronary abnormalities in advanced chronic kidney disease patients, and only a small proportion present media calcification. The pattern of linear calcification is highly associated with atherosclerosis (Coll et al., 2011). Vascular calcification has been historically classified as (*1*) intima calcification associated with atheroma plaques and (*2*) medial calcification mediated by a switch of vascular smooth muscle cells to a procalcification phenotype and associated with kidney disease and disturbances in the metabolism of calcium, phosphorus, and vitamin D (Cardús et al., 2006). However several potential flaws associated with this traditional view present: First, large arteries are "elastic" arteries functioning as blood conduits, and as such have a low content of smooth muscle cells. On the contrary, small, peripheral arteries are aimed at the regulation of blood flow in the tissue, presenting a dense layer of smooth muscle cells. Traditionally it is stated that large arteries are more prone to atherosclerosis, while small vessels are more prone to calcify. Moreover, the anatomic location of calcium in the artery wall presents a singular pattern that corresponds to the calcification of the internal elastic lamina. Conversely, medial calcification is related to the control of metabolic disturbances in terms of calcium, phosphorus, and vitamin D. However, low serum phosphorus is a protective factor for developing linear calcification, underscoring the influence of phosphorus on atherosclerosis. Therefore, vascular calcification in large arteries is more prevalent in dialysis patients than in controls, and it is predominantly a linear pattern located in the lumen-intima interphase. Age, dialysis, past medical history of cardiovascular disease, atherosclerosis, and inflammation are variables significantly influencing calcification (Coll et al., 2011).

Recently, the term ossification rather than calcification of both the arterial intima and media has been proposed for kidney subjects (Stenvinkel et al., 2008). The presence of artery ossification is associated with functional estimates of arterial dysfunction, such as nitric oxide-dependent vasodilatation in dialysis patients and pulse-wave velocity (Raggi et al., 2007). Vascular ossification should be considered as a cardiovascular risk marker and not an etiological factor of cardiovascular disease in chronic kidney disease (Stenvinkel et al, 2008). Multiple new biomarkers for early detection of arterial intima and/or media ossification have emerged. Serum levels of calcium and phosphorus have become established risk markers (Block et al., 2005). Hyperparathyroidism has also been suggested as a risk factor for and a marker of vascular ossification (Stevens et al., 2004), and Vitamin D deficiency is associated with increased early mortality. The best studied inhibitor of vascular ossification is fetuin-A, the major carrier of calcium ions in the circulation. Only in chronic kidney patients stage 5 low levels of fetuin-A are associated with adversed cardiovascular outcomes (Hermans et al., 2007). The ossification regulators matrix-Gla protein, bone morphogenic proteins, osteopontin, and osteoprotegerin, promote an early and extensive vascular ossification process, and have been shown to interfere with endothelial function by decreasing nitric oxide production and altering the normal anatomic vessel wall, rendering the endothelial surface prone to calcium deposition, prothrombotic events and a more rigid vessel wall (Hofbauer et al., 2007).

4. The endothelium and haemodialysis

Endothelial dysfunction is the initial pathophysiologic step in the progression of vascular damage that precedes and leads to clinically manifest cardiovascular diseases (Vita & Keany, 2002). Endothelial dysfunction is highly prevalent in patients with advanced chronic kidney disease (Endermann & Schiffrin, 2004) and is linked to the elevated cardiovascular risk of this patient population (Tonelli & Pfeffer, 2007). The cause of endothelial dysfunction is complex and involves dysregulation of multiple pathways (Yilmaz et al., 2009).

4.1 Haemodialysis components and endothelial damage

Haemodialysis therapy may induce activation of complement and polymorphonuclear leukocytes, monocytes, or lymphocytes, depending on the dialyzer membrane used. The clinical situation is further complicated by the accumulation of uremic retention solutes and toxins, often inadequately removed during the dialysis schedule. Haemodialysis patients display evidence of elevated interleukin-1 and tumor necrosis factor-alpha release, which is followed by the stimulated secretion of interleukin-6, responsible for acute-phase protein synthesis. High levels of the circulating proinflammatory cytokines interleukins-1, -6, -13 and tumor necrosis factor-alpha are associated with mortality in hemodialysis patients (Hörl, 2002). Essential functions of polymorphonuclear leukocytes—that is, phagocytosis, oxygen species production, upregulation of specific cell surface receptor proteins, or apoptosis—are disturbed in uremia. Clinical signs and symptoms of end-stage renal disease patients are at least in part related to the accumulation of middle molecules such as beta 2-microglobulin, parathyroid hormone, advanced glycation end products, advanced lipoxidation end products, advanced oxidation protein products (formed as a result of oxidative stress, carbonyl stress, or both), granulocyte inhibitory proteins, or leptin. Currently available membrane materials do not provide long-lasting, effective reduction of middle molecules in patients who require maintenance haemodialysis (Hörl, 2002).

During haemodialysis, contact of blood with the dialyzer and dialysate also activates the kallikrein-kinin system and also induces the above mentioned inflammatory response. (Marney et al, 2009). These cytokines stimulate plasminogen activator inhibitor-1, the major physiologic inhibitor of fibrinolysis. Activation of the kallikrein-kinin could have favorable or deleterious effects on inflammation and the risk of cardiovascular events through endothelial damage. First, bradykinin causes vasodilation and stimulates the release of tissue-plasminogen activator from the endothelium, and infused bradykinin inhibits platelet aggregation. Conversely, bradykinin stimulates the inflammatory response and may have implications in atherothrombotic events in hemodialysis. Endogenous bradykinin contributes to hypotension, increased inflammation, increased oxidative stress, and increased fibrinolysis in response to haemodialysis (Marney et al., 2009).

Enhanced production of proinflammatory cytokines by dialysate pyrogens, by complement activation, or both, as well as inhibition of anti-inflammatory cytokine secretion, may contribute to the cell-mediated immunosuppression seen in dialysis patients. The presence of low and high molecular weight inhibitors of neutrophils in the plasma of uremic patients may explain, at least in part, why infections are a common cause of hospitalization and the second most common cause of death in these patients. Other middle molecules accumulate, and proteins are modified by oxidative stress, carbonyl stress, or both, contributing to the uremic syndrome.

4.2 Haemodialysis and endothelial function improval

Dialysis patients frequently present with endothelial dysfunction and a higher risk of developing atherosclerosis. Factors that impair endothelial function include lipid abnormalities, hyperhomocysteinemia, and the accumulation of inhibitors of nitric oxide synthesis (Trimarchi et al., 2002). Endothelial dysfunction can be detected long before atherosclerosis arises (Vanhoutte, 1988), and on ocassions can be improved by appropriate haemodialysis delivery (McGregor et al., 2003). Haemodialysis itself can reduce plasma endothelin-1 levels and increase the vasodilator endothelium-derived adrenomedullin (McGregor et al., 2003), which vasodilatory action is in part nitric oxide dependent (Majid et al., 1996). Asymmetric dimethyl-arginine, the nitric oxide antagonist that is elevated in uremia, can be cleared by dialysis (McGregor et al., 2003).

One of the most serious haemodynamic complications of uremia is hypotension. Symptomatic hypotension occurs in approximately 25% of haemodialysis sessions, and can restrict the amount of fluid to be removed. Many mechanisms have been proposed: Abnormalities of the response of resistance and capacitance vessels to hypovolemia and disbalanced reflex increases in peripheral vascular resistance to hypovolemia have been implicated (Hand et al., 1998). The endothelium adequate response is also altered by the uremic toxins that accumulate and by the abnormal cellular and chemical reactions between platelets, leukocytes and the endothelial cell itself. When appropriately performed and delivered, haemodialysis sessions may improve endothelial function by improving the internal milieu and by removing the toxins and inflammatory mediators that can interfere with the normal endothelium-derived vasomodulator activity (Hand et al., 1998, McGregor et al., 2003), albeit some studies have failed to support this finding (Pupim et al., 2004). Finally, as endothelial cells are highly sensitive to extracellular sodium and potassium, the chemical derangement that rules in renal failure alters the endothelial-mediated regulation of local blood flows. This effect may also has pathophysiological relevance in the development of hypertension and atherosclerosis in haemodialysis subjects (Oberleithner et al., 2010).

5. Conclusions

The endothelium is a vital organ that dynamically interacts with the whole economy, managing vital activities through the mediators it synthesizes and releases in an endocrine and paracrine fashion. It plays a main role in vascular tone and metabolic pathways. In haemodialysis, endothelial dysfunction can be caused by several factors or worsen them: Oxidative stress, inflammation, haemostatic derangements, protein-energy wasting, vascular calcification, anemia, molecular alterations and the dialytic procedure itself. They are strongly interrelated and play a major role in the initiation and progression of vascular complications, leading to the high mortality rate cardiovascular disease presents in dialysis.

6. References

Abderrahim-Ferkoune, A.; Bezy, O.; Chiellini, C.; Maffei, M., Grimaldi, P.; Bonino, F.; Moustaid-Moussa, N., Pasqualini, F.; Mantovani, A.; Ailhaud, G. & Amri E. (2003). Characterization of the Long Pentraxin PTX3 as a TNF-alpha-induced Secreted Protein of Adipose Cells. *The Journal of Lipid Research*, Vol. 44, No.5, (May 2003), pp 994-1000, ISSN 0022-2275

Anavekar, NS. & Pfeffer, MA. (2004). Cardiovascular Risk in Chronic Kidney Disease. *Kidney International*, Vol. 92, Suppl.92, (November 2004), pp 11- 15, ISSN 0085-2538

Andrew, PJ. & Mayer, B. Enzymatic Function of Nitric Oxide Synthases. (1999). *Cardiovascular Research*, Vol.43, No.3, (August 1999), pp 521-531, ISSN 0008-6363

Annuk M, Linde T, Lind L, Fellstrom B: Erythropoietin Impairs Endothelial Vasodilatory Function in Patients with Renal Anemia and in Healthy Subjects. (2006). *Nephron Clinical Practice,* Vol.102, No.1, (January 2006), pp 30–34, ISSN 1660-2110

Avesani, CM.; Carrero, JJ.; Axelsson, J.; Qureshi, AR.; Lindholm, B. & Stenvinkel, P. (2006). Inflammation and Wasting in Chronic Kidney Disease: Partners in Crime. *Kidney International*, Vol.70, Suppl., (2006), pp 8–13, ISSN 0085-2538

Block, GA.; Spiegel, DM.; Ehrlich, J; Mehta, R.; Lindbergh, J.; Dreisbach, A. & Raggi P. (2005) Effects of Servelamer and Calcium on Coronary Artery Calcification in Patients New to Hemodialysis. *Kidney International,* Vol.68, No.4, (October 2005), pp 1815-1824, ISSN 0085-2538

Blokhina, O.; Virolainen, E. & Fagerstedt, KV. (2003). Antioxidants, Oxidative Damage and Oxygen Deprivation Stress: a Review. *Annals of Botany*, Vol.91, No.2, (January 2003), pp 179-194, ISSN 0305-7364

Boehme, M.; Kaehne, F.; Kuehne, A; Bernhardt, W.; Schroder, M.; Pommer, W.; Fischer, C.; Becker, H.; Muller, C. & Schindler, R. (2007). Pentraxin 3 is Elevated in Haemodialysis Patients and is Associated with Cardiovascular Disease. *Nephrology Dialysis and Transplantation*, Vol.22, No.8, (August 2007), pp 2224-2229, ISSN 0931-0509

Cachofeiro, V.; Goicochea, M.; García de Vinuesa, S.; Oubiña, P.; Lahera, V. & Luño, J. (2008). Oxidative Stress and Inflammation, a Link between Chronic Kidney Disease and Cardiovascular Disease. Kidney International, Vol. 74, Suppl111, (December 2008), pp 4–9, ISSN 0085-2538

Cardús, A.; Parisi, E.; Gallego, C.; Aldea, M.; Fernández, E. & Valdivielso, JM. (2006). 1,25-Dihydroxyvitamin D3 Stimulates Vascular Smooth Muscle Cell Proliferation through a VEGF-mediated Pathway. *Kidney International,* Vol. 69:, No.8, (April 2006), pp 1377–1384, ISSN 0085-2538

Carrero, JJ.; Chmielewski, M,; Axelsson, J.; Snaedal, S.; Heimbürger, O.; Bárány, P.; Suliman, ME.; Lindholm, B.; Stenvinkel, P. & Qureshi, AR. Muscle Atrophy, Inflammation and Clinical Outcome in Incident and Prevalent Dialysis Patients. *Clinical Nutrition,* Vol.27, No.4, (August 2008), pp 557-564, ISSN 0954-3007

Carrero, JJ. & Stenvinkel, P. (2009). Persistent Inflammation as a Catalyst for Other Risk Factors in Chronic Kidney Disease: A Hypothesis Proposal. *Clinical Journal of the American Society of Nephrology,* Vol.4, Suppl.1, (December 2009), pp 49-55, ISSN 1555-9041

Castro, R; Rivera, I; Struys, EA.; Jansen, EEW,; Ravasco, P:; Camilo, ME:; Blom, KJ., Jakobs, C. & De Almeida, IT. (2003). Increased Homocysteine and S-adenosylhomocysteine Concentrations and DNA Hypomethylation in Vascular Disease. *Clinical Chemistry,* Vol. 49, No.8, (August 2003), pp 1292-1296, ISSN 1434-6621

Cines, DB.; Pollak, ES.; Buck, CA.; Loskalzo, J.; Zimmermann, GA.; Mc Ever, RP.; Pober, JS.; Wick, TM.; Konkle, BA.; Schwartz BS, Barnathan, ES.; Mc Krae, KR.; Hug, BA.; Schmidt, AM. & Stern DM. (1998). Endothelial Cells in Physiology and in Pathophysiology of Vascular Disorders. *Blood,* Vol.91, No.10, (May 1998), pp 3527-3561, ISSN 0006-4971

Clozel, M & Fischli, W. (1989). Human Cultured Endothelial Cells Do Secrete Endothelin-1. *Journal of Cardiovascular Pharmacology,* Vol.13, Suppl. 5, (January 1989), pp 193-196, ISSN 0160-2446

Coll, B.; Betriu, A.; Martínez-Alonso, M.; Amoedo, ML.; Arcidiacono, MV.; Borras, M.; Valdivielso, JM. & Fernández, E. (2011). Large Artery Calcification on Dialysis Patients Is Located in the Intima and Related to Atherosclerosis. *Clinical Journal of the American Society of Nephrology,* Vol.6, No.2, (February 2011), pp 303–310, ISSN 1555- 9041

Crowell, JW. & Smith, EE. (1967). Determinant of the Optimal Hematocrit. *Journal of Applied Physiology,* Vol.22, No.3 (March 1967), pp 501–504, ISSN 8750-7587

de Groot, K.; Bahlmann, FH.; Sowa, J.; Koenig, J.; Menne, J.; Haller, H. & Fliser, D. (2004). Uremia Causes Endothelial Progenitor Cell Deficiency. *Kidney International,* Vol.66, No.2, (August 2004), pp 641-646, ISSN 0085-2538

de Zeeuw, D. (2007). Albuminuria: A Target for Treatment of Type 2 Diabetic Nephropathy. *Seminars in Nephrology,* Vol. 27, No.2, (March 2007), pp 70-74, ISSN 0270-9295

Dong, C.; Yoon, W. & Goldschmidt-Clermont, PJ. (2002). DNA Methylation and Atherosclerosis. *Journal of Nutrition*, Vol.132, No.8 Suppl., (August 2002), pp 2406-2409, ISSN 0022-3166

Endemann, DH. & Schiffrin, EL. (2004). Endothelial Dysfunction. *Journal of the American Society of Nephrology*, Vol.15, No.8 (August 2004), pp 1983–1992, ISSN 1046-6673

Esmon, CT.; CT.; Fukudome, K.; Mather, T, Bode, W.; Regan, LM.; Stearns-Kurosawa, DJ. & Kurosawa, S. (1999). Inflammation, Sepsis, and Coagulation. *Haematologica*, Vol.84, No.3, (March 1999), pp 254-259, ISSN 0390-6078

Faure, V.; Dou, L.; Sabatier, F.; Cerini, C.; Sampol, J.; Berland, Y.; Brunet, P. & Dignat-George, F. (2006). Elevation of Circulating Endothelial Microparticles in Patients with Chronic Renal Failure. *Journal of Thrombosis and Haemostasis*, Vol.4, No.3, (March 2006), pp 566-573, ISSN 1538-7836

Festa, A.; D'Agostino, R.; Howard, G.; Mykkanen, L.; Tracy, RP. & Haffner, SM. (2000). Inflammation and Microalbuminuria in Non-Diabetic and Type 2 Diabetic Subjects: The Insulin Resistance Atherosclerosis Study. *Kidney International*, Vol. 58, No.4, (October 2000), pp 1703-1710, ISSN 0085-2538

Fishbein, G.A. & Fishbein, M.C. (2009). Arteriosclerosis: Rethinking the Current Classification. *Archives of Patholgy and Laboratory Medicine*, Vol.133, No.8: (August 2009), pp 1309-1316, ISSN 0003-9985

Frick, M. & Weidinger F. (2007). Endothelial Function: A Surrogate Endpoint in Cardiovascular Studies?. *Current Pharmaceutical Design*, Vol.13, No.17 (June 2007), pp 1741-1750, ISSN 1381-6128

Fouque, D.; Kalantar-Zadeh, K.; Kopple, J.; Cano, N.; Chauveau, P.; Cuppari, L.; Franch, H.; Guarnieri, G.; Ikizler, TA.; Kaysen, G.; Lindholm, B.; Massy, Z.; Mitch, W.; Pineda, E.; Stenvinkel, P.; Trevinho-Becerra, A. & Wanner,C. (2008). A Proposed Nomenclature and Diagnostic Criteria for Protein–Energy Wasting in Acute and Chronic Kidney Disease. *Kidney International*, Vol.73, No.4, (February 2008), pp 391-398, ISSN 0085-2538

Goligorsky, MS. (2007). Frontiers in Nephrology: Viewing the Kidney through the Heart-Endothelial Dysfunction in Chronic Kidney Disease. *Journal of the American Society of Nephrology*, Vol.18, No.11, (November 2007), pp 2833-2835, ISSN 1046-6673

Guérin, A.P.; Pannier, B.; Métvier, F.; Marchais, S.J. & London, G.M. (2008). Assessment and Significance of Arterial Stiffness in Patients with Chronic Kidney Disease. *Current Opinion in Nephrology & Hypertension*, Vol.17, No.6, (November 2008), pp 635-641, ISSN 1062-4821

Haaber, AB.; Eidemak, I.; Jensen, T.; Feldt-Rasmussen, B. & Strandgaard, S. (1995). Vascular Endothelial Cell Function and Cardiovascular Risk Factors in Patients with Chronic Renal Failure. *Journal of the American Society of Nephrology*, Vol.5, No.8, (February 1995), pp 1581-1584, ISSN 1046-6673

Hand, MF.; Haynes, WG. & Webb DJ. (1998). Hemdoialysis and L-arginine, but not D-arginine, Correct Renal Failure-Associated Endothelial Dysfunction. *Kidney International*, Vol.53, No.4, (April 1998), pp 1068-1077, ISSN 0085-2538

Handelman, GJ.; Walter, MF.; Adhikarla, R.; Gross, J.; Dallal, DE.; Levin, NW.; Blumberg, JV. (2001). Elevated Plasma F2-Isoprostanes in Patients on Long-Term Hemodilaysis. *Kidney International*, Vol.59, No.5, (May 2001), pp 1960-1966, ISSN 0085-2538

Heeschen, C.; Aicher, A.; Lehmann, R.; Fichtlscherer, S.; Vasa, M.; Urbich, C.; Mildner-Rihm, C; Martin, H.; Zeiher, AM. & Dimmeler, S. (2003). Erythropoietin is a Potent Physiologic Stimulus for Endothelial Progenitor Cell Mobilization. *Blood,* Vol.102, No.4, (August 2003), pp 1340–1346, ISSN 0006-4971

Herbrig, K.; Pistrosch, F.; Oelschlaegel, U.; Wichmann, G.; Wagner, A.; Foerster, S.; Richter, S.; Gross, P. & Passaurer, J. (2004). Increased Total Number but Impaired Migratory Activity and Adhesion of Endothelial Progenitor Cells in Patients on Long-Term Hemodialysis. *American Journal of Kidney Diseases,* Vol. 44, No.5, (November 2004), pp 890-894, ISSN 0272-6386

Hermans, MM.; Brandenburg, V.; Ketteler, M.; Kooman, JP.; van der Sande, FM.; Boeschoten, EW.; Leunissen, KM.; Krediet, RT. & Dekker, FW. (2007). Association of Serum Fetuin-A Levels with Mortality in Dialysis Patients. *Kidney International,* Vol.72, Vol.2, (July 2007), pp 202–207, ISSN 0085-2538

Hill, JM.; Zalos, G.; Halcox, JPJ.; Schenke, WH.; Waclawiw. MA; Quyyumi, AA. & Finkel, T. (2003). Circulating Endothelial Progenitor Cells, Vascular Function, and Cardiovascular Risk. *New England Journal of Medicine,* Vol. 348, No.7, (February 2003), pp 593-600, ISSN 0028-4793

Himmelfarb, J.; Stenvinkel P.; Alp Ikizler, T.; & Hakim, RH. (2002). The Elephant in Uremia: Oxidant Stress as a Unifying Concept of Cardiovascular Disease in Uremia. *Kidney International,* Vol.62, No.5 (November 2002), pp 1524-1538, ISSN 0085-2538

Himmelfarb, J.; McMenamin, E.; Loseto, G. & Heinecke, JW. (2001). Myeloperoxidase-Catalyzed 3-Chlorotyrosine Formation in Dialysis Patients. *Free Radical Biology & Medicine,* Vol. 31, No.10, (November 2001), pp 1163-1169, ISSN 0891-5849

Hofbauer, LC.; Brueck, CC.; Shanahan, CM.; Schoppet, M. & Dobnig, H (2007). Vascular Calcification and Osteoporosis: From Clinical Observation Towards Molecular Understanding. *Osteoporosis International,* Vol.18, No.3, (March 2007), pp 251–259, ISSN 0937-941X

Hörl WH. (2002). Hemodialysis Membranes: Interleukins, Biocompatibility, and Middle Molecules. *Journal of the American Society of Nephrology,* Vol. 13, Suppl.1, (January 2002), pp 62-71, ISSN 1046-6673

Huber, K. (2001). Plasminogen Activator Inhibitor Type-1 (part one): Basic Mechanisms, Regulation and Role for Thromboembolic Disease. *Journal of Thrombosis and Thrombolysis,* Vol.11, No.3, (May 2001), pp 183-193, ISSN 0929-5305

Ix, JH.; Shiplak, MG.; Sarnak, MJ.; Beck GJ.; Greene, T.; Wang, X; Kusek, JW, Collins, AJ; Levey, AS. & Menon, V. (2007). Fetuin-A Is Not Associated with Mortality in Chronic Kidney Disease. *Kidney International,* Vol.72, No.11, (December 2007), pp 1394-1307, ISSN 0085-2538

Jurkovitz, CT.; Abramson, JL.; Vaccarino, LV.; Weintraub, WS. & McClellan, WM. (2003). Association of High Serum Creatinine and Anemia Increases the Risk of Coronary Events: Results from the Prospective Community-Based Atherosclerosis Risk in Communities (ARIC) study. *Journal of the American Society of Nephrology,* Vol.14, No.11, (November 2003), pp 2919–2925, ISSN 1046-6673

Kahler, J.; Ewert, A.; Weckmüller, J.; Stobbe, S.; Mittmann, C.; Köster, R.; Paul, M.; Meinertz, T. & Münzel, T. (2001). Oxidative Stress Increases Endothelin-1 Synthesis in Human Coronary Artery Smooth Muscle Cells. *Journal of Cardiovascular Pharmacology,* Vol.38, No.1, (July 2001), pp 49-57, ISSN 1074-2484

Keithi-Reddy, SR.; Addabbo, F.; Patel, TV.; Mittal, BV.; Goligorsky, MS. & Singh, AK. (2008). Association of Anemia and Erythropoiesis Stimulating Agents with Inflammatory Biomarkers in Chronic Kidney Disease. *Kidney International*, Vol.74, No.6, (September 2008), pp 782–790, ISSN 0085-2538

Kielstein, J. & Zoccali, C. (2005). Asymmetric Dimethylarginine: A Cardiovascular Risk Factor and a Uremic Toxin Coming of Age?. *American Journal of Kidney Diseases*, Vol.46, No.2, (August 2005), pp 186-202, ISSN 0272-6386

Koc, M.; Richards, HB.; Bihorac, A.; Ross, EA.; Schold, JD. & Segal, MS. (2005). Circulating Endothelial Cells Are Associated with Future Vascular Events in Hemodialysis Patients. *Kidney International*, Vol.67, No.3, (March 2005), pp 1079-1083, ISSN 0085-2538

Kon, V.; MacRae, F.; Fazio, L & Fazio, S. (2011). Atherosclerosis in Chronic Kidney Disease: the Role of Macropahges. *Nature Reviews Nephrology*, Vol.7, No.1, (January 2011), pp 45-54, ISSN 1759-5061

Krapf, R. & Hulter, HN. (2009). Arterial Hypertension Induced by Erythropoietin and Erythropoiesis-Stimulating Agents (ESA). *Clinical Journal of the American Society of Nephrology*, Vol. 4, No.2, (February 2009), pp 470–480, ISSN 1046-6673

Kuijper, PHM.; Gallardo-Torres, HI; van der Linden, JAM.; Lammers JWJ.; Sixma, JJ.; Koenderman, L. & Zwaginga, JJ. (1996). Platelet-Dependent Primary Haemostasis Promotes Selectin- and Integrin-Mediated Neutrophil Adhesion to Damaged Endothelium under Flow Conditions. *Blood*, Vol.87, No.8, (April 1996), pp 3271-3281, ISSN 0006-4971

Krantz, SB. (1991). Erythropoietin. *Blood*, Vol.77, No.3, (February 1991), pp 419–434, ISSN 0006-4971

Labarrere, CA. & Zaloga, GP. (2004). C-Reactive Protein: from Innocent Bystander to Pivotal Mediator of Atherosclerosis. *American Journal of Medicine*, Vol.117, No.7, (October 1999), pp 499-507, ISSN 0002-9343

Li, N. & Karin, M. (1999). Is NF-KB the Sensor of Oxidative Stress?. *The Journal of the Federation of American Societies for Experimental Biology*, Vol.13, No.10, (July 1999), pp 1137-1143, ISSN 0892-6638

Linden, E.; Cai, W.; He, JC.; Xue, C; Li, Z; Winston, J; Vlassara, H. & Uribarri, J. (2008). Endothelial Dysfunction in Patients with Chronic Kidney Disease Results from Advanced Glycation End Products (AGE)-Mediated Inhibition of Endothelial Nitric Oxide Synthase Through RAGE Activation. *Clinical Journal of the American Society of Nephrology*, Vol. 3, No.3, (May 2008), pp 691-698, ISSN 1555- 9041

London, G.M. & Drüeke, T.B. (1997). Atherosclerosis and Arteriosclerosis in Chronic Kidney Failure. *Kidney International*, Vol.51, No.6 (June 1997), pp 1678-1695, ISSN 0085-2538

Majid, DS.; Kadowitz, PJ.; Coy, DH. & Navar, LG. (1996). Renal Responses to Intra-Arterial Administration of Adrenomedullin in Dogs. *American Journal of Physiology*, Vol.270, No.1, (January 1996), ppF200–F205, ISSN 0363-6119

Mallat, Z.; Benamer, H.; Hugel, B.; Benessiano, J.; Steg, PG.; Freyssinet, JM. & Tedgui, A. (2000.) Elevated Levels of Shed Membrane Microparticles with Procoagulant Potential in the Peripheral Circulating Blood of Patients with Acute Coronary Syndromes. *Circulation*, Vol.101, No.8, (February 2000), pp 841-843, ISSN 0009-7322

Marney, AM.;Ma, J.; Luther,JM.; Ikizler, TA. & Brown, NJ. (2009). Endogenous Bradykinin Contributes to Increased Plasminogen Activator Inhibitor 1 Antigen following

Hemodialysis. *Journal of the American Society of Nephrology*, Vol. 20, No.10, (October 2009), pp 2246–2252, ISSN 1046-6673

Massy, ZA.; Borderie, D.; Nguyen-Khoa, T.; Drüeke, TB.; Ekindjian, OG. & Lacour, B. (2003). Increased Plasma S-Nitrosothiol Levels in Chronic Haemodialysis Patients. *Nephrology Dialysis and Transplantation*, Vol.18, No.1, (January 2003), pp 153-157, ISSN 0931-0509

May, AE.; Kälsch, T.; Massberg, S.; Herouy, Y.; Schmidt, R. & Gawaz, M. (2002). Engagement of Glycoprotein IIb/IIIa (alpha(IIb)beta3) on Platelets Upregulates CD40L and Triggers CD40L-Dependent Matrix Degradation by Endothelial Cells. *Circulation*, Vol.106, No.16, (October 2002), pp 2111-2117, ISSN 0009-7322

Meltivier, F. (2007). Mineral Metabolism and Arterial Functions in End-Stage Renal Disease: Potential Role of 25-hydroxyvitamin D Deficiency. *Journal of the American Society of Nephrology*, Vol.18, No.2, (February 2007), pp 613-620, ISSN 1046-6673

Mackay, CR. & Imhof, BA. (1993). Cell Adhesion in the Immune System. *Immunology Today*, Vol.14, No.3, (March 1993), pp 99-102, ISSN 0167- 5699

McEniery, CM.; McDonnell, BJ.; So, A.; Aitken, S.; Bolton, CE.; Munnery, M.; Hickson, SS; Yasmin, S; Maki-Petaja, KM.; Cockcroft, JR.; Dixon, AK. &, Wilkinson, IB. (2009). Aortic Calcification is Associated with Aortic Stiffness and Isolated Systolic Hypertension in Healthy Individuals. *Hypertension*, Vol.53, No.3, (March 2009), pp 524-531, ISSN 1933-1711

McGregor,D.; Buttimore, A; Lynn, K.; Yandle, T. & Nicholls, M. (2003). Effects of Long and Short Hemodialysis on Endothelial Function: A Short-Term Study. *Kidney International*, Vol.63, No.2 (February 2003), pp 709-715, ISSN 0085-2538

Müller, MM. & Griesmacher, A. (2000). Markers of Endothelial Dysfunction. *Clinical Chemistry and Laboratory Medicine*, Vol.38, No.2, (February 2000), pp 77-85, ISSN 1434-6621

Mulvihill, NT; Foley, JB.; Crean, P. & Walsh, M. (2002). Prediction of Cardiovascular Risk Using Soluble Cell Adhesion Molecules. *European Heart Journal*, Vol.23, No.20, (October 2002), pp 1569-1574, ISSN 1522-9645

Navar, LG.; Harrison-Bernard, LM.; Nishiyama, A. & Kobori, H. (2002). Regulation of Intrarenal Angiotensin II in Hypertension. *Hypertension*, Vol.39, No.2, (February 2002), pp 316-322, ISSN 1062-4821

Oberg, B.; McMenamin, E.; Lucas, F.; McMonagle, E.; Morrow, J.; Iklizer, T & Himmelfarb, J. (2004). Increased Prevalence of Oxidant Stress and Inflammation in Patients with Moderate to Severe Chronic Kidney Disease. *Kidney International*, Vol. 65, No.3 (March 2004), pp 1009-1016, ISSN 0085-2538

Oberleithner, H.; Kusche-Vihrog, K. & Schillers H. (2010). Endothelial Cells as Vascular Salt Sensors. *Kidney International*, Vol.77, No.6, (March 2010), pp 490-494, ISSN 0085-2538

Perry, RG. & Pearson, JD. (1989). Endothelium- the Axis of Vascular health and disease. *Journal of the Royal College of Physicians*, Vol.23, No.2, (April 1989), pp 92-101, ISSN 1478-2715

Pieczenik, SR. & Neustadt, J. (2007). Mitochondrial Dysfunction and Molecular Pathways of Disease. *Experimental and Molecular Pathology*, Vol.83, No.1, (August 2007), pp 84-92, ISSN 0531-5522

Portaluppi, F; Boari, B. & Manfredini, R. (2004). Oxidative Stress in Essential Hypertension. *Current Pharmaceutical Design*, Vol.10, No.14, (May 2004), pp 1695-1698, ISSN 1381-6128

Pupim, L.; Himmelfarb, J.; McMonagle, E.; Shyr, Y. & Ikizler, T. (2004). Influence of Initiation of Maintenance Hemodialysis on Biomarkers of Inflammation and Oxidative Stress. *Kidney International*, Vol.65, No.6, (June 2004), pp 2371-2379, ISSN 0085-2538

Rabelink, TJ.; de Boer, HC. & van Zonneveld, J. (2010). Endothelial Activation and Circulating Markers of Endotelial Activation in Kidney Disease. *Nature Reviews Nephrology*, Vol.6, No.6, (June 2010), pp 404-414, ISSN 1759-5061

Raggi, P.; Bellasi, A.; Ferramosca, M.; Islam, T.; Muntner, P.; & Block, GA: (2007). Association of Pulse Wave Velocity with Vascular and Valvular Calcification in Hemodialysis Patients. *Kidney International*, Vol.71, No.2, (April 2007), pp 802-807, ISSN 0085-2538

Raitakari, OT. & Celermajer, DS. (2000). Testing for Endothelial Dysfunction. *Annals of Medicine*, Vol.32, No.5, (July 2000), pp 293-304, ISSN 0003-4819

Ross, R. (1999). Atherosclerosis: an Inflammatory Disease. *New England Journal of Medicine*, Vol. 340, No.2, (January 1999), pp 115-126, ISSN 0028-4793

Scalera, F.; Kielstein, JT.; Martens-Lobenhoffer, J.; Postel, SC.; Tager, M. & Bode-Boger, SM. (2005). Erythropoietin Increases Asymmetric Dimethylarginine in Endothelial Cells: Role of Dimethylarginine Dimethylaminohydrolase. *Journal of the American Society of Nephrology*, Vol.16, No.4; (April 2005), pp 892–898, ISSN 1046-6673

Schnackenberg, CG. (2002). Physiological and Pathophysiological Roles of Oxygen Radicals in the Renal Vasculature. *American Journal of Physiology-Regulatory, Integrative and Comparative Physiology*, Vol.282, No.2, (February 2002), pp R335-R342, ISSN 0363-6119

Schwarz, U.; Buzello, M.; Ritz, E.; Stein, G.; Raabe, G.; Wiest, G.; Mall, G. & Amann, K. (2000). Morphology of Coronary Atherosclerotic Lesions in Patients with End-Stage Renal Failure. *Nephrology Dialysis and Transplantation*, Vol.15, No.2, (February 2000), pp 218-223, ISSN 0931-0509

Sela, S.; Shurtz-Swirski, R.; Cohen-Mazor, M.; Mazor, R.; Chezar. J.; Shapiro, G.; Hassan, K.; Shkolnik, G; Geron, R. & Kristal, B. (2005). Primed Peripheral Polymorphonuclear Leukocyte: a Culprit Underlying Chronic Low-Grade Inflammation and Systemic Oxidative Stress in Chronic Kidney Disease. *Journal of the American Society of Nephrology*, Vol.16, No.8, (August 2005), pp 2431-2438, ISSN 1046-6673

Sigrist, M.; Bungay, P.; Taal, MW. & McIntyre, CW. (2006). Vascular Calcification and Cardiovascular Function in Chronic Kidney Disease. *Nephrology, Dialysis and Transplantation*, Vol. 21, No.3, (March 2006), pp 707-714, ISSN 0931-0509

Simonini, A.; Moscucci, M.; Muller, DW.; Bates, ER.; Pagani, FD.; Burdick, MD. & Strieter RM. (2000). IL-8 is an Angiogenic Factor in Human Coronary Atherectomy Tissue. *Circulation*, Vol.101, No.13, (April 2000), pp 1519–1526, ISSN 0009-7322

Singh, AK.; Szczech, L.; Tang, KL.; Barnhart, H.; Sapp, S.; Wolfson, M. & Reddan, D. CHOIR Investigators. (2006). Correction of Anemia with Epoetin Alfa in Chronic Kidney Disease. *New England Journal of Medicine*, Vol.355, No.20, (November 2006), pp 2085–2098, ISSN 0028-4793

Stam, F.; van Guldener, C.; Schalkwijk, CG.; ter Wee, PM.; Donker, Ab JM. & Stehouwer, DA. (2003). Impaired Renal Function is Associated with Markers of Endothelial Dysfunction and Increased Inflammatory Activity. *Nephrology Dialysis and Transplantation*, Vol.18, No.5, (May 2003), pp 892-898, ISSN 0931-0509

Stenvinkel, P.; Heimbürger, O.; Paultre, F; Ciczfalusy, U.; Wang, T.; Berlglund, L. & Jogerstrand, T. (1999). Strong Association Between Malnutrition, Inflammation, and Atherosclerosis in Chronic Renal Failure. *Kidney International*, Vol.55, No.5, (May 1999), pp 1899-1911, ISSN 0085-2538

Stenvinkel, P. (2001a). Malnutrition and Chronic Inflammation as Risk Factors for Cardiovascular Disease in Chronic Renal Failure. *Blood Purification*, Vol.19, No.2, (February 2001), pp 143-151, ISSN 0253-5068

Stenvinkel, P. (2001b). Endothelial Dysfunction and Inflammation—Is There a Link?. *Nephrololgy, Dialysis and Transplantation*, Vol.16, No.10, (October 2001), pp 1968-1971, ISSN 0931-0509

Stenvinkel, P.; Heimbürger, O. & Lindholm, B. (2004). Wasting, but not Malnutrition, Predicts Cardiovascular Mortality in End-Stage Renal Disease. *Nephrology Dialysis and Transplantation*, Vol.19, No.9, (September 2004); pp 2181–2183, ISSN 0931-0509

Stenvinkel, P.; Carrero, JJ.; Axelsson, J.; Lindholm, B.; Heimbürger, O. & Massy Z. (2008). Emerging Biomarkers for Evaluating Cardiovascular Risk in the Chronic Disease Patient: How do New Pieces Fit into the Uremic Puzzle?. *Clinical Journal of the American Society of Nephrology*, Vol.3; No.2, (March 2008), pp 505-521, ISSN 1555-9041

Stevens, LA.; Djurdjev, O.; Cardew, S.; Cameron, EC. & Levin, A. (2004). Calcium, Phosphate, and Parathyroid Hormone Levels in Combination and as a Function of Dialysis Duration Predict Mortality: Evidence for the Complexity of the Association Between Mineral Metabolism and Outcomes. *Journal of the American Society of Nephrology*, Vol.15, No.3 (March 2004), pp 770–779, ISSN 1046-6673

Tatematsu, S.; Wakino,S.; Kanda, T.; Homma,K.; Yokoshioka, K.; Hasegawa, K.; Sugano, N.; Kimoto, M.; Saruta,T. & Hayashi,K. (2007). Role of Nitric Oxide-Producing and -Degrading Pathways in Coronary Endothelial Dysfunction in Chronic Kidney Disease. *Journal of the American Society of Nephrology*, Vol.18, No.3, (March 2007), pp 741-749, ISSN 1046-6673

Teitell, M. & Richardson, B. (2003). DNA Methylation in the Immune System. *Clinical Immunology*, Vol.109, No.1 (October 2003), pp 2-5, ISSN 0091-6749

Tonelli, M & Pfeffer, MA. (2007). Kidney Disease and Cardiovascular Risk. *Annual Review of Medicine*, Vol. 58, No.2, (February 2007), pp 123-139, ISSN 0066-4219

Tong, M.; Carrero, JJ.; Qureshi, AR; Anderstam, B.; Heimbürger, O.; Barany, P; Axelsson, J; Alvestrand, A.; Stenvinkel, P; Lindholm, B. & Suliman, ME. (2007). Plasma Pentraxin 3 in Chronic Kidney Disease Patients: Associations with Renal Function, Protein-Energy Wasting, Cardiovascular Disease and Mortality. *Clinical Journal of the American Society of Nephrology*, Vol.2, No.5, (September 2007), pp 889-897, ISSN 1555- 9041

Touyz, RM. (2005). Reactive Oxygen Species as Mediators of Calcium Signaling by Angiotensin II: Implications in Vascular Physiology and Pathophysiology. *Antioxidant & Redox Signaling*, Vol. 7, No.9-10, (September-October 2005), pp 1302-1314, ISSN 1523-0864

Trimarchi, H; Schiel, A; Freixas, E. & Díaz M. (2002). Randomized Trial of Methylcobalamin and Folate Effects on Homocysteine in Hemodialysis Patients. *Nephron*, Vol.91, No. 1, (May 2002), pp 58-63, ISSN 0028-2766

Trimarchi, H.; Mongitore, MR.; Baglioni, P.; Forrester, M.; Freixas, EA.; Schropp, M.; Pereyra, H.; Alonso, M. N-Acetylcysteine Reduces Malondialdehyde Levels in Chronic Hemodialysis Patients--a Pilot Study. (2003). *Clinical Nephrology*, Vol.59, No.6, (June 2003), pp 441-446, ISSN 0301-0430

Trimarchi, H.; Muryan, A.; Campolo-Girard, V.; Dicugno, M.; Barucca, N.; Lombi, F.; Pomeranz, V.; Forrester, M.; Alonso, M.; Iriarte, R.; Díaz, ML. & Lindholm, B. (2011). Elevated Pro-Brain Natriuretic Peptide, Troponin T and Malnutrition Inflammatory Score in Chronic Hemodialysis Patients with Overt Cardiovascular Disease. *Nephron Clinical Practice*, Vol.117; No.3, (March 2011), pp 198-205, ISSN 0028-2766

Valli, A.; Carrero, JJ.; Qureshi, AR.; Garibotto, G.; Barany, P; Axelsson, J; Lindholm, B.; Stenvinkel, P.; Anderstam, B & Suliman ME. (2008). Elevated Serum Levels of S-Adenosylhomocysteine, but not Homocysteine, Are Associated with Cardiovascular Disease in Stage 5 Chronic Kidney Disease Patients. *Clinica Chimica Acta*, Vol. 395, No.1-2, (September 2008), pp 106-110, ISSN 0009-8981

Van Guldener, C.; Lambert, J.; Janssen, MJFM.; Donker, AJM. & Stehouwer, CDA. (1997). Endothelium-Dependent Vasodilatation and Distensibility of Large Arteries in Chronic Haemodialysis Patients. *Nephrology Dialysis and Transplantation*, Vol.12, Suppl.2, (1997), pp 14-18, ISSN 0931- 0509

Vanholder, R.; Hoefliger, N.; De Smet, R. & Ringoir, S. (1992) Extraction of Protein Bound Ligands from Azotemic Sera: Comparison of 12 Deproteinization Methods. *Kidney International*, Vol.41, No.4, (June 1992), pp 1707-1712, ISSN 0085-2538

Vanholder, R.; Baurmeister, U.; Brunet, P.; Cohen, G.; Glorieux, G. & Jankowski, J. for the European Uremic Toxin Work Group. (2008). A Bench to Bedside View of Uremic Toxins. *Journal of the American Society of Nephrology*, Vol. 19, No.8, (August 2008), pp 863-870, ISSN 1046-6673

Vanhoutte, PM. The Endothelium-Modulator of Vascular Smooth-Muscle Tone. (1988). *New England Journal of Medicine*, Vol.319, No.8, (August 1988), pp 512-513, ISSN 0028-4793

Vaziri, ND & Rodríguez-Iturbe, B. (2006). Mechanisms of Disease: Oxidative Stress and Inflammation in the Pathogenesis of Hypertension. *Nature Clinical Practice Nephrology*, Vol.2, No.10, (October 2006), pp 582-593, ISSN 1745- 8323

Verma, S. & Anderson TJ. (2002). Fundamentals of Endothelial Function for the Clinical Cardiologist. *Circulation*, Vol.105, No.5, (February 2002), pp 546-549, ISSN 0009-7322

Vita, JA. & Keaney, JF. (2002). Endothelial Function: A Barometer for Cardiovascular Risk? *Circulation*, Vol.106, No.6 (August 2002), pp 640–642, ISSN 0009-7322

von Hundelshausen, P. & Weber, C. (2007). Platelets as Immune Cells: Bridging Inflammation and Cardiovascular Disease. *Circulation Research*, Vol.100, No.1, (January 2007), pp 27-40, ISSN 0009-7300

Webb, D. & Vallance, P. (Eds. P. Vallance & S. Moncada) (1997). *Endothelial Function and Hypertension*, Springer Verlag, ISBN 9783642158711 Heidelberg

Weiss, G. & Goodnough, LT. (2005). Anemia of Chronic Disease. *New England Journal of Medicine,* Vol.352, No.10, (March 2005), pp 1011–1023, ISSN 0028-4793

Wilcox, CS. (2005). Oxidative Stress and Nitric Oxide Deficiency in the Kidney: a Critical Link to Hypertension? *American Journal of Physiology-Regulatory, Integrative and Comparative Physiology,* Vol.289, No.4, (October 2005), pp 913-935, ISSN 0363-6119

Yanagisawa, M.; Kurihara, H.; Kimura, S.; Tomobe, Y, Kobayashi, M.; Mitsui, Y; Yazaki, Y; Goto, K. & Mazaki T. (1988). A Novel Potent Vasoconstrictor Peptide Produced by Vascular Endotelial Cells. *Nature,* Vol. 332, No.6163, (March 1988), pp 411-415, ISSN 0028-0836

Yilmaz, MI.; Carrero, JJ.; Ortiz, A.; Martín-Ventura, JL.; Sonmez, A.; Saglam, M.; Yaman, H.; Yenicesu, M.; Egido, J. & Blanco-Colio, LM. (2009). Soluble TWEAK Plasma Levels as a Novel Biomarker of Endothelial Function in Patients with Chronic Kidney Disease. *Clinical Journal of the American Society of Nephrology,* Vol.4, No.2, (February 2009), pp 1716–1723, ISSN 1555- 9041

Zimmermann , J.; Herrlinger, S.; Pruy, A.; Metzger, T. & Wanner, C. (1999). Inflammation Enhances Cardiovascular Risk and Mortality in Hemodialysis patients. *Kidney International,* Vol.55, No.2, (February 1999), pp 648-658, ISSN 0085-2538

Zoccali, C.; Bode-Boger, SM.; Mallamaci, F.; Bendetto, FA.; Trippei, G.; Malatino, L.; Cataliotti, A.; Bellanuova, I.; Fermo, I.; Frölich, JC & Boger RH. (2001). Plasma Concentrations of Assymetrical Dimethylarginine and Mortality in Patients with End-Stage Renal Disease: A Prospective Study. *Lancet,* Vol.358, No.9299, (December 2001), pp 2113-2113, ISSN 0140-6736